Medical Sociology in Africa

Jimoh Amzat • Oliver Razum

Medical Sociology in Africa

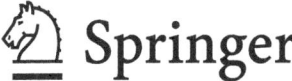

Jimoh Amzat
Department of Sociology
Usmanu Danfodiyo University
Sokoto
Nigeria

Oliver Razum
AG3 Epidemiology & Intern Public Health
Faculty of Health Sciences
University of Bielefeld
Bielefeld
Germany

ISBN 978-3-319-03985-5   ISBN 978-3-319-03986-2 (eBook)
DOI 10.1007/978-3-319-03986-2
Springer Cham Heidelberg New York Dordrecht London

Library of Congress Control Number: 2014930888

© Springer International Publishing Switzerland 2014

This work is subject to copyright. All rights are reserved by the Publisher, whether the whole or part of the material is concerned, specifically the rights of translation, reprinting, reuse of illustrations, recitation, broadcasting, reproduction on microfilms or in any other physical way, and transmission or information storage and retrieval, electronic adaptation, computer software, or by similar or dissimilar methodology now known or hereafter developed. Exempted from this legal reservation are brief excerpts in connection with reviews or scholarly analysis or material supplied specifically for the purpose of being entered and executed on a computer system, for exclusive use by the purchaser of the work. Duplication of this publication or parts thereof is permitted only under the provisions of the Copyright Law of the Publisher's location, in its current version, and permission for use must always be obtained from Springer. Permissions for use may be obtained through RightsLink at the Copyright Clearance Center. Violations are liable to prosecution under the respective Copyright Law.

The use of general descriptive names, registered names, trademarks, service marks, etc. in this publication does not imply, even in the absence of a specific statement, that such names are exempt from the relevant protective laws and regulations and therefore free for general use.

While the advice and information in this book are believed to be true and accurate at the date of publication, neither the authors nor the editors nor the publisher can accept any legal responsibility for any errors or omissions that may be made. The publisher makes no warranty, express or implied, with respect to the material contained herein.

Printed on acid-free paper

Springer is part of Springer Science+Business Media (www.springer.com)

Preface

The overall objective of this book is to provide theoretical and pragmatic discussions on medical sociology (sometimes referred to as health sociology) with African illustrations. It is an attempt to examine the various themes and topics in medical sociology with the aim of providing adequate explanations in instructive styles. It is particularly important to write from a local lens but through international perspectives. Medical sociology, although a branch of sociology, has attracted transdisciplinary relevance—especially in psychology, anthropology, health economics, medicine, nursing, history of medicine, and others. This book provides a frame of reference for those interested in the issue of society, culture, and health in general. It also intends to provide a globally renowned source and reference for academics, public health practitioners, undergraduates, and graduate students who want to improve their understanding of medical sociology.

This book emerges from the context of African experiences and perspectives, drawing classical illustrations and references from Africa. This book is adequately localised in the African context but with a global outlook. The epistemological stance of African sociology is rooted in deep cultural interpretations. Such perspective is necessary because Africa faces the majority of public health problems. The book will be useful in the teaching of medical sociology at all levels. It represents a compilation of detailed ideas about the significance and relevance of medical sociology. The book presents a shift from theoretical precepts to practical mindset within a pedagogical milieu that will aid the understanding of sociocultural or sociological approach in the study and understanding of health problems, and more importantly in the topical descriptions of medical sociology. This book is organised based on thematic issues in medical sociology. In order to represent current perspectives, recent directions in the field will be presented. As outlined in the table of contents, the work will also present more research agendas for medical sociology.

Africa bears the greatest brunt of many health problems, especially malaria, HIV/AIDS, and maternal- and child-related morbidities which are part of the health targets of the Millennium Development Goals (MDGs), set to achieve considerable alleviation of disease burden. These morbidities are preventable through effective health and illness behaviours, but millions of fatalities due to the aforementioned diseases still occur in the continent every year. Millions of others are affected by temporary and permanent disabilities annually. While there has been progress over the years at the global level, there is still insufficient progress in Africa, more specifically in sub-Saharan Africa (SSA) where the disease burden adversely affects the development processes, thereby accounting for a vicious cycle of underdevelopment. The prevalence of medical problems in Africa is rooted in the interplay of social, political, cultural, and medical factors; it is also within this holistic context that disease burden can be understood and resolved. In fact, increased focus on social/community barriers to care could prove effective in reducing the disease burden in Africa. The idea of the interplay of this myriad of factors is not new, but the factors continue to explain disease burden and persist over the years.

In order to account for a holistic perspective, the social and cultural dimensions of human health must be adequately considered. This book presents medical sociology as the study of the social patterning of health and illness (see Chap. 1) by situating health problems as a major (social) problem confronting the human being. The first chapter also presents a brief history of medical sociology and the topical coverage of the discipline to advance the relevance of the discipline in health studies and provide adequate explanations for students. The notion of health, disease, and illness as conceptual tools is the preoccupation of Chap. 2, starting with the debate of how health should be defined. The illustrations of the social manifestation of illness and cultural beliefs of illness causation from African context show the relevance of the cultural milieu in the understanding of health (see Chap. 2). The concepts of health and illness behaviours are a central part of the discourse in medical sociology (see Chap. 3). It is vital to understand health risk behaviours, and the factors influencing such behaviours.

This book is also very strong in theoretical discourse. It presents the fundamental theories in sociology under the main broad headings. The notions of the sick role by Talcott Parsons, the explanation of suicide by Emile Durkheim, and social capital theory of health constitute the landmarks in functionalist explanation of health in sociology (see Chap. 5). Then the book presents many fundamental theoretical standpoints that could guide medical sociological thinking, including Marxist analysis/political economy of health, fundamental cause theory, feminist analysis of health, Weber's social action and bureaucratic rationality health belief model, theory of planned behaviour, Suchman's stages of illness and medical care, Andersen's model of health care utilisation, social construction of illness, labelling theory, and Goffman's theories of stigma and total institution. While some criticisms of the theories are also presented, some adaptations to African contexts were illustrated stressing the need for a holistic view.

In general, a sociology of health should provide a holistic milieu in the consideration of health discourse by accounting for a multitude of dynamics and situational indices within the social and cultural spheres responsible for the health of the population. Specifically, a sociology of health problems in Africa should provide comprehensive explanations considering the social patterning of health and the community indices and sociocultural factors influencing population health. It is a well-known fact that social determinants of health (SDH) (see Chap. 4), or what could also be referred to as fundamental causes of disease, have a global relevance.

However, the impacts of these SDH are more pronounced in the context of Africa, especially in the explanation of disease of poverty such as malaria and HIV/AIDS. The question of fundamental causes has a significant link with the political economy of health (PEH) (see Sects. 6.3, 6.4), health inequalities without neglecting health transition, and the emerging disease mix, especially as a result of lifestyle factors responsible for most chronic diseases (see Sects. 3.3.1 and 4.6). Therefore, a sociology of health problems in Africa is firmly rooted in the consideration of the social production of health (see Chap. 6), interpretive perspective or social construction of health (see Chaps 7 and 8), SDH (see Chap. 4), lifestyle factors, and risk behaviours (see Chap. 3).

The concepts of medicalisation, pharmaceuticalisation, geneticisation, demedicalisation, remedicalisation, medical enhancement, and models of client-practitioner relations are adequately examined with some current illustrations (see Chap. 9). For instance, the medicalisation of pregnancy, beauty, and death are explained as illustrations in order to expose readers to how medicalisation is penetrating all facets of life. The examination of medical pluralism in Africa (the coexistence of traditional and modern health care systems) provides another opportunity to examine the realities of health care in Africa (see Chap. 10). Subsequently, the current waves of sociology of bioethics are presented by introducing the meaning and varieties of bioethics and core areas of moral perplexities in health care to advance the sociological relevance in bioethical discourse (see Chap. 11). Lastly, the hope of presenting more African illustrations informs the chapter on the sociology of health problems in Africa (see Chap. 12).

Therefore, we hope that students, instructors, and researchers interested in medical sociology (or social dimensions of health) and with interest in Africa will find this book an informative and academic resource.

Acknowledgments

This is to acknowledge the Alexander von Humboldt Foundation for providing a Georg Forster Postdoctoral Fellowship to Jimoh Amzat through which this book was written and the host institution, University of Bielefeld, AG3 Epidemiology and International Public Health, for providing a supportive academic environment.

Contents

1. Sociology and Health 1
2. Health, Disease, and Illness as Conceptual Tools 21
3. Health Behaviour and Illness Behaviour 39
4. Social Determinants/Context of Health 61
5. Functionalist Perspective on Health 83
6. Social Production of Health 107
7. The Interpretive Perspective in Medical Sociology: Part I 129
8. The Interpretive Perspective in Medical Sociology: Part II 155
9. Medicalisation and Client-Practitioner Relations 185
10. Medical Pluralism: Traditional and Modern Health Care 207
11. Towards a Sociology of Bioethics 241
12. A Sociological Study of Health Problems in Africa 265

Index 285

Abbreviations

ACT	artemisinin-based combination therapy
ADHD	attention-deficit/hyperactivity disorder
AHPs	allied health professions
AIDS	acquired immunodeficiency syndrome
ANC	antenatal care
ASA	American Sociological Association
BwO	body-without-organs
CAM	complementary and alternative medicine
CE	community engagement
CHVs	community health volunteers
CHWs	community health workers
CODESRIA	Council for the Development of Social Science Research in Africa
COPD	chronic obstructive pulmonary disease
CSWs	commercial sex workers
DHS	Demographic and Health Surveys
DNA	deoxyribonucleic acid
DTCP	direct consumer purchase
ELSI	ethical, legal, and social implications
FBOs	faith-based organisation
HB	health behaviour
HBM	health belief model
HGP	Human Genome Project
HIV	human immunodeficiency virus
HMM	home management of malaria
HRG	high-risk group
ICT	information and communication technology
IPTp	intermittent preventive treatment during pregnancy
IRBs	institutional review boards
ITN	insecticide-treated net
IVF	in vitro fertilisation
LGBT	lesbians, gay, bisexual, and transgender
MCH	maternal and child health

MDGs	Millennium Development Goals
MMR	maternal mortality ratio
MP	medical pluralism
MSTs	modern social theories
NCDs	non-communicable diseases
NGOs	non-governmental organisations
OTC	over-the-counter
PEH	political economy of health
PHB	preventive health behaviour
PHC	primary health care
PLWHA	people living with HIV/AIDS
SARS	severe acute respiratory syndrome
SCR	stem cell research
SDH	social determinants of health
SES	socioeconomic status
SHC	secondary health care
SPH	social production of health
SSA	sub-Saharan Africa
STDs	sexually transmitted diseases
TB	tuberculosis
TBAs	traditional birth attendants
TBH	traditional birth home
THC	tertiary health care
TM	traditional medicine
TPB	theory of planned behaviour
U5MR	under-five mortality rate
UNICEF	United Nations Children's Fund
VVF	vesicovaginal fistula
WHO	World Health Organisation

List of Figures

Fig. 2.1	Components of health	22
Fig. 2.2	The global burden of injuries by causes	32
Fig. 3.1	Stages of illness behaviour	48
Fig. 4.1	Social determinant of health conceptual framework	62
Fig. 4.2	Poverty and health: A bi-directional model	66
Fig. 4.3	Education and better health outcomes	68
Fig. 4.4	Components of individual behaviours and lifestyle factors in health	72
Fig. 4.5	Pathways by which occupation affects health outcomes	73
Fig. 4.6	Pathways by which discrimination and social alienation affect health outcomes	76
Fig. 5.1	Forms and dimensions of social capital with operationalization	98
Fig. 5.2	Social Capital and Health	102
Fig. 6.1	Vicious cycle of socioeconomic inequality and poor health	111
Fig. 7.1	Typology of social action	134
Fig. 7.2	The health belief model	140
Fig. 7.3	The theory of planned behaviour	146
Fig. 7.4	Suchman's stages of illness and medical care	148
Fig. 7.5	Andersen's model of health services utilisation	150
Fig. 8.1	Eight phases of the course of chronic illness	160
Fig. 8.2	Labelling framework	170
Fig. 8.3	Stigma and health	171
Fig. 10.1	Factors influencing use of traditional medicine	217
Fig. 10.2	WHO health system framework	224
Fig. 10.3	Pyramid showing the levels of care	233
Fig. 11.1	Varieties of bioethics	245
Fig. 11.2	Four principles of bioethics	256
Fig. 12.1	Map of Africa showing regions and countries	266
Fig. 12.2	Components of the community engagement approach	279

List of Tables

Table 2.1	Models for defining health	24
Table 3.1	The three stages of prevention	42
Table 4.1	Gender discrimination throughout a woman's life	63
Table 4.2	Components of poor living/housing conditions	70
Table 4.3	Occupational health hazards of agricultural work in developing countries	75
Table 4.4	Six dimensions of access to health care services	78
Table 5.1	Basic views of functionalism	86
Table 5.2	The four types of suicide	93
Table 6.1	Basic views of Marxism	109
Table 6.2	Basic views of feminism	122
Table 7.1	Basic views from the interpretive perspective	130
Table 7.2	The health belief model and potential change strategies	142
Table 7.3	The theory of planned behaviour	144
Table 9.1	Key actors and influences on medicine use/pharmaceuticalisation	190
Table 9.2	Some common types of aesthetic/cosmetic surgery	197
Table 12.1	Trends in estimates of maternal mortality ratio by five-year periods	275
Table 12.2	Levels and trends in the under-five mortality rate (1990–2011)	277

Chapter 1
Sociology and Health

1.1 Introduction

Many people (including students of sociology) often wonder about the relevance of sociology to health issues. In general, it is often a challenge to discuss the nexus between social science and health. Why medical sociology? What does sociology have to do with medicine or health? These are some of the pressing questions that require explanations. The fundamental problem starts with a lack of deeper knowledge of the meaning and focus of sociology. Therefore, it is necessary to proceed by defining sociology and briefly explaining some of its foundational focus. After this, its relevance to health will be explained.

Sociology has been variously defined since Auguste Comte coined the term in 1838. Simply, sociology is the study of human society and social problems. Sociology is the scientific study of social relations, institutions, and society (Smelser 1994). In addition, sociology can be defined as the scientific study of the dynamics of society and their intricate connection to patterns of behaviour. It focuses on social structure and how the structures interact to modify human behaviour, actions, opportunities, and how the patterns of social existence engender social problems. Social institutions include kinship, economic, political, education, and religious institutions. The institutions are like pillars that hold up society because they are the constituent parts of the social system (society). These parts are interdependent and interrelated with specialised functions towards the survival of the society. This is why the human society is often referred to as a social system. Every institution fulfils some functional imperatives. The family institution supports the procreation and socialisation of new members of society while the economic institution deals with the production and exchange of goods. The economic institution employs people from the family institutions, and the family in turn needs the goods and services produced by the economic institution. The health institutions are organised to cater to the well-being and survival of human beings.

Generally, sociology employs scientific approach to study and develops generalisations about human patterns, groupings, and behaviour. In a more concise definition, the American Sociological Association (ASA) defined sociology "as the study of social life, social change, and the social causes and consequences of human behaviour".

Social life is the most central part of the focus of sociology; it implies the connection which an individual holds with others in the society. To sociologists, social life or interaction is the essence of human existence. The process of social interaction itself may put individuals at risk of some communicable disease such as tuberculosis (TB), severe acute respiratory syndrome (SARS), and measles. In terms of communicable diseases, mere contact with an infected person (in the process of social interaction) can normally put others at risk. The investigation of social "causes" and consequences is basic in sociological research. There is often a problem of biomedical reductionism, assuming "only the germ causes the disease" without an interrogation of the social conditions enabling vulnerability to diseases. For instance, commercial sex work puts an individual more at risk of human immunodeficiency virus (HIV) than many other occupation groups: that is a kind of occupational condition, which is a risk factor for HIV.

1.2 Health Problems as Social Problems

The historical focus of sociology is on social problems in human society. Social problems include health problems, crime, deviance, violence, poverty, inequality, population problems, delinquency, and institutional instability. Social forces such as modernisation and industrialisation marked the beginning of unprecedented social alteration, especially since the beginning of the eighteenth century. This social change led to a number of problems as a result of changes in the relations of production. The industrial revolution led to new forms of production systems, community relations, migration, urbanisation, and especially new forms of employer-employee relations. Industrialisation marked the overthrow of the family as an economic unit. This was a tremendous change in the social system with resultant consequences, hence emerging social problems such as unemployment, poverty, child labour, gender discrimination, crime, and health problems. This is not to argue that all these problems only emerged during the industrial revolution, but they rapidly multiplied during that period. Social problems are conceived as strains within the system, seen as the product of certain objective conditions within the society, which is inimical or detrimental to the realisation of some norms or values for members of the society (Lyman et al. 1973, p. 474). Any issue that threatens the well-being or survival of the society is regarded as a social problem. Weber (1995, p. 9) defined social problems "as a social phenomenon that is damaging to the society or its members, is perceived as such, and is socially remediable."

It is important to note that just as crime is damaging to the society or individual, so is any health problem. Apart from this fact, a social problem can be identified through the following characteristics, which include:

1. **It is an objective condition.** This implies that it can be empirically defined. A social problem exists as a condition that can be verified. Even when subjective interpretation may be required, a social problem is an *evidence-based* problem, not just mere perception of an individual but a general knowledge that is usually

definite. This represents a utilitarian view, which holds that social problems are objective things, or what Durkheim regarded as social facts (Smelser 1996). Smelser observed that the assertion is like the medical model which views social problems as a form of disease with an identifiable cause, definite symptoms, and calls for a cure.

2. **It has social aetiology or could be linked to it.** This implies that a social problem emanates from the pattern of social interaction, organisation, association, or simply is engendered by social conditions. This point should be noted as a relevant perspective in explanation of human health/diseases and not an absolute explanation. For instance, Wellcome (2002, p. 30), summarising Day Karen's research report, observed that "... Falciparum parasite [malaria] we see today arose about 3200–7000 years ago—an era that coincides with the dawn of agriculture in Africa. This was a time of massive ecological change, when humans began to live in large communities and the rainforest was being cut down for slash-and-burn agriculture... there was also a major change in the mosquito vector at that time, when it began biting humans instead of animals... " It is further observed that P. *falciparum* migrated with Africans to other parts of the world. This means that the process of migration aids the spread of malaria. This is why Smelser (1996) also observed that the increasing world traffic of people would internationalise many health problems. It is for this reason that HIV, first diagnosed in the United States in the early 1980s (Jackson 2002), is now a global problem. Moreover, some diseases are rooted in genetics or heredity, thereby multiplying through marriage patterns or human relationships. Holtz et al. (2006, p. 1665) observed that it is impossible to understand population health without considering the social origins of diseases—"the risk of exposure, host susceptibility, course of disease, and disease outcome; each is shaped by the social matrix... " Social conditions are now invoked as fundamental causes of diseases in human society because such conditions affect exposure to diseases, as well as course and outcomes of diseases (see Chap. 4 for social determinants of health, Sect. 6.4 for fundamental cause theory).

3. **It poses social damage.** A social problem often incapacitates the individuals in a society. As poverty prevents individuals from satisfying basic needs, so, too, health problems prevent individuals from functioning effectively as members of society. A health problem may reduce the functionality of an individual within the social system. Invariably, a social problem is inconsistent with the normative value of the society. Society wants its members to be healthy, and the unattainability of this desire shows a discrepancy between social value and reality. Such a discrepancy represents a social problem.

4. **It affects the collectivity.** A social problem is different from a personal problem in that the former affects a substantial number of people in the social system (see Harris 2013). Health problems are ubiquitous like other problems such as crime and poverty. There may be a geographical variation in the magnitude or frequency, but most social problems are a pandemic. It is thus a problem when a significant number of people believe that a certain condition is, in fact, a problem (Kerbo and Coleman 2007), and it constitute a problem to their social existence or wellbeing.

5. **It requires social action.** Social problems require collective action. The solution to any social problem does not reside in just any individual; it requires the majority to act in order to ameliorate the problem. It may necessitate institutional or community approaches. Health problems also require collective action. This is why there has been a lot of implementation of research and policy engagement to improve the health of the people. This is also why health issues often appear in development agendas.

The aforementioned attributes qualify health problems as social problems. This is separate from the social dimensions of health problems, which will be examined later in this book. Health problems can also come with other dimensions apart from the aforementioned attributes. It may not only be socially damaging but also biologically damaging. Often, a health problem may move from being biological pathology to social pathology or vice versa. Whichever form it takes, it constitutes a pathology that must be remedied by the society. Sociology has been relevant ever since Comte conceived it as a science that would provide *salvation* from all the social problems confronting the world. Improved relevance of sociology in human society will alleviate human suffering and provide equitable well-being. Therefore, the application of sociological methods and perspective and attention to the social dimensions of disease should provide a vital step forward in disease control.

Apart from the fact that health problems constitute a major social problem, it is important to further stress the relevance of sociology to health. First, in this case, it is human health. It is about the people, community, and society. The health of the society cannot be grasped without understanding the intricacies of the community or society itself. George Simmel conceived of human society as an intricate web of multiple relations—of people in constant interaction with one another (Coser 2004), of people who are bound with common fate, norms, values, sociospatial conditions, exposures, and opportunities. It is about the health of people who build and share similar health institutions or who live, for instance, in an African rainforest where they are exposed to mosquito bites every day. It is also about the health of the community that has access or otherwise to simple preventive measures for malaria or diarrhoea. Health is about the society where there is self-accountability to take up smoking and bear the associated health risks. As mentioned earlier, any issue concerning the social collectivity is of enormous interest to sociology. Simply, health is one such issue of interest because it concerns the people and also affects the patterns of social interaction.

Apart from focusing on the people, health is intrinsic to human functioning or existence. It confers a form of capacity on the individual to perform social functions in human society. Human value or existence is enhanced by good health. Good health is instrumental to human survival and is required to strive for the basic necessities of life. As a contributing member of the social systems, one needs good health, and lack of this threatens the pattern of social interaction with other members in the social system. Health indicators have been used to assess the level of development in a society. It is also used as a measure of chance of survival in human societies. This is why health is a social value both at the individual and collective levels.

1.3 Medical Sociology Defined

Medical sociology is simply the application of sociological perspectives and methods in the study of health issues in human societies with a skewed focus on the sociocultural milieu that accounts for human health and illness. These perspectives include sociological theories and tools, which can be applied in the analysis of human health. In this case, the individual is examined as a member of the society, who partakes in the day-to-day functioning of the social system. The pre-comprehension is that humans exist within a socio-spatial milieu, which often affects their health. Such social conditions and the nature of human interaction are instrumental to the well-being of every individual in society. It is also assumed that the nature of social interaction and networking is a part of the determinants of human health. Sociologists are interested in issues regarding human health and employ systematic procedures to examine social phenomena. They have relied on quantitative and qualitative techniques to establish universal laws governing human societies. The essence of the methods is to look at the social links that can explain sociocultural linkages to health issues. In any case, medical sociology is the application of sociological theories, knowledge, and concepts to issues of health and illness (Hafferty and Castellani 2006).

Medical sociology can also be defined as the scientific study of the social patterning of health. In this case, it is a study of how social factors (e.g., class, race, gender, religion, ethnicity, kinship network, marriage, educational status, age, place, and cultural practices) influence human health. The idea of social patterning indicates that these social factors could be the determinants of human health status (see Chap. 4). It is in this sense that some diseases may be referred to as diseases of poverty (e.g., malaria and TB) because they are much more prevalent in poor regions or among the poor. For example, a person residing in a slum is at a higher risk of being exposed to certain diseases which a person in affluent area may have lower risk of being exposed to. Medical sociology is distinct in its approach because it considers the "import that social and structural factors have on the disease and illness processes as well as on the organisation and delivery of health care" (Hafferty and Castellani 2006, p. 334). Hafferty and Castellani further observed that these factors also include culture (e.g., values, beliefs, normative expectations), organisational processes (e.g., hospital setting), politics (e.g., health care policy, health budget, political ideology), economic system (e.g., capitalism, the costs of health care), and microlevel processes such as socialisation and identity formation.

Apart from pure research, medical sociologists are also interested in implementation or applied research. This involves the implementation of interventions to improve the health of the population through community engagement and participation in policy formulation and implementation. As Kaminskas and Darulis (2007) noted, medical sociologists utilise applied sociological methods—such as needs assessment, social impact assessment, and case management options—in health care settings using evaluation research methods. This area of applied research has attracted a lot of grants and promoted collaboration with others in the medical field through a multidisciplinary approach to health management.

Cockerham (2001) further observed that medical sociology has actually established itself as a strong subfield of sociology and removed itself from being a subordinate of medicine. He provided four major reasons for the strong academic locus of the subfield. First, the extension of focus from acute to chronic diseases strengthens the relevance of sociology to medicine because of the key roles of social condition and social behaviour in the prevention, onset, and management of chronic disorders. Medical sociologists are more relevant in the analysis of social conditions of health than physicians. Second, medical sociology has focused extensively on issues relating to clinical medicine and health policy. Third, success over the years in medical sociological research has promoted the professional status of medical sociologists in the analysis of the social patterning of health. Fourth, medical sociologists have studied medical practice and policies—at times with a critical stance to expose some blind spots.

1.4 A Brief History of Medical Sociology

Medical sociology has become a substantive subfield of sociology. It can be argued that medical sociology began with the conception of sociology by August Comte (1896) through his concept of organismic analogy. This can be a deductive argument since Comte did not intend to establish medical sociology as a subfield and did not attach the importance of sociocultural issues in health. Comte, and later Herbert Spencer (1891, 1896), extensively compared human society to a biological being. Spencer observed that the universe consists of organic (living), inorganic (nonliving) and super-organic (society) entities. The idea of organismic analogy is that the human society has similar characteristics as that of the biological organism. The similarities include growth and development, differentiation of parts, specialisation of functions, interrelatedness, and interdependence of parts. The parts of the society include the social institutions, which work harmoniously for the survival of the society. The argument further relates that if one part is damaged, it will adversely affect other parts of the society. Health institution may be affected if the political institution is corrupt or not responsive to aspirations of the citizens. This is part of the reasons why strong political will is required in implementation of health programs.

The theory of Marx and Engels explains that economic infrastructure is the foundation on which other superstructures of the society rely. Inequalities in income translate to other forms of inequalities in human society, including health inequalities. This is why Marx's proposition has been widely applied in all facets of life including health inequalities, accessibility to health care and allocation and distribution of health resources and infrastructures (see Sects. 6.2 and 6.3 for further elaboration). Another major landmark is the work of Emile Durkheim (1897/1951) on suicide. This is directly related to medical sociology since it is about the issue of death. Durkheimian perspective on suicide will be explained in detail later (see Sect. 5.3.2 for further elaboration). The perspective examines the influence of social factors in self-termination of life. Durkheim identifies two major factors, which fluctuate

1.4 A Brief History of Medical Sociology

to increase or decrease propensity to suicide. These factors are social regulation and integration. This has been a major sociological perspective in the analysis of suicide because it was a theory derived from empirical investigations. The works of Max Weber on bureaucratic rationality and social action have also been substantially applied in medical sociology to explain the organisation of health care institutions and why and how people care for others (see Sects. 7.3 and 7.4 for further elaboration).

At the time these classical sociological scholars (August Comte, Emile Durkheim, Max Weber, and Karl Marx) were writing, they did not have medical sociology in mind; however, their works provided the landmark for the development of a subfield of sociology called medical sociology. The works created the foundation for the emergence of sociological perspectives and methods that can be applied in the study of social patterning of health.

In 1848 Rudolf Virchow (a German physician) laid the foundation of social medicine (Holtz et al. 2006) by advocating for the relevance and consideration of social factors in human health and disease. While this set a new agenda for medicine, it opened a wide passage for the social sciences involvement in the understanding of human health. The early 1900s marked the beginning in the study of sociological dimension of medicine, especially with the works of Charles McIntire ("The Importance of the Study of Medical Sociology," published in 1894), along with other scholarly works of that period including the book by Elizabeth Blackwell (1902) and another by James P. Warbasse (1909), both on medical sociology (Bloom 2002; Hafferty and Castellani 2006, p. 332).

In the 1950s, Talcott Parsons (1951) published a groundbreaking work with a section on the application of functionalism in medical sociology. He dedicated a substantial part of his work to the elaboration of the sick role, explaining the social trajectories of the sick within the social system and how the health institutions can support individuals to return to normal roles in the society (see Sect. 5.3.1 for further elaboration). Parsons recognised the relevance of medicine for the society and drew attention to illness as a form of social deviance and the importance of sick role as a mechanism of social control (Freidson 1962; Stacey and Homans 1978). This is the first conscious application of sociological theory in the understanding of human illness. The sick role concept facilitated the expansion of other areas of research including the patient-physician relationship, illness behaviour, medicalisation of deviance, and medical professionalism (Hafferty and Castellani 2006). The works of Freidson (1961a/1962, 1961b) and Mechanic (1966, 1968) also promoted the relevance and understanding of medical sociology.

Conrad (2007) described Eliot Freidson's works as revolutionary in medical sociology. Freidson (1961, 1970a, 1975) devoted his time to the study of professionalism and professionalisation in medicine which presents a comprehensive view of the social and professional dynamics of medicine with a particular reference to how disease and illness are constructed, power relations between the physician and patients, division of labour, ethical conducts, increasing commercialism, and bureaucratic control in medical practice. Freidson's works were landmarks in the development of medical sociology. He practically demonstrated the relevance of sociology in medicine and health studies in general by situating his studies within applied domains.

During the same period, Glaser and Strauss (1965, 1968) also examined the social process of death and dying, and Erving Goffman (1961, 1963) released a masterpiece, *Asylums*, which introduced the concept of stigma and total institution (see Sects. 8.4.2 and 8.4.3 for further elaboration). The *Asylums* focused mainly on the study of mental health patients and health care institutions. It was a remarkable breakthrough in the application of medical sociology to the study of health care institutions. The work of Goffman has been one of the most successful sociological pieces in the management of patients and health care institutions. The concern of this subsection is to trace the development of medical sociology: Chapters 5, 6, 7, and 8 will expand some of the substantive theories of medical sociology.

The development of academic journals (e.g., *Journal of Health and Social Behaviour*; *Social Science and Medicine*; *Sociology of Health and Illness* in 1979) in the discipline, especially in the 1960s, also aided the development of the discipline (Hafferty and Castellani 2006); and now there are many other dedicated and related journals including *Health and Place, Health Affairs, Women and Health, Reproductive Health Matters, Social Theory and Health, Medical Anthropology, The Lancet, Social History of Medicine*, and many others.

Furthermore, not only do medical sociologists proclaim self-relevance to medicine but medical scientists have increasingly come to the realisation that a number of significant health care issues are outside the walls of the hospitals, pharmaceutical and medical laboratories. Clausen (1963, p. 1) observed that it has become apparent that "the understanding of health and disease requires a holistic approach in which the social and cultural aspects of human behaviour are appropriately related to the biological nature of every human being and the physical environment in which he[/she] lives." Clausen further observed that the emphasis upon the holistic approach to medical science and comprehensive health care has moved medicine to seek the services of social scientists, notably in connection with public health, preventive medicine, and psychiatry. In short, there is an unprecedented *sociolisation* of medicine, a term used by Barbour (2011) to describe how sociology has come to shape the profession of medicine, and to add to it, how sociology shapes the understanding of health and illness in the society.

From the 1960s onwards, there has been increasing popularisation of medical sociology with many departments of sociology now having specialisation in medical sociology as an option, especially for graduate programs. Cockerham has observed that medical sociology comprises one of the largest and most active sociological specialties in the developed world and the subdiscipline is expanding in Asia, Africa, Latin America, and other regions. Specifically, Africa has not been left out in this development as medical sociology is now recognised as a subfield of sociology. Medical sociology is growing in strength and importance in South Africa (Gilbert 2012) like in other African countries. There is a growing realisation that social issues are relevant and significant in explaining population health in Africa and elsewhere. The study of sexual behaviour and other social aspects of HIV/AIDS seemingly demonstrate the sociological milieu in the understanding of health. The first crops of medical sociologists in Africa were trained in western societies, specifically in the United Kingdom and United States. Now, the number of those trained in Africa is increasing, coupled with a demand for medical sociologists in health intervention in Africa.

Many medical sociologists from Africa now partner with their counterparts from other continents in addressing international health. Medical sociologists also collaborate with non-governmental organisations (NGOs) to address social determinants of health in communities. Likewise, there are many social science institutes in Africa (e.g., the Council for the Development of Social Science Research in Africa [CODESRIA]), which have incorporated health discourse as a priority. The introduction of the Health Institute by CODESRIA to train and offer small grants to young social scientists interested in health issues is part of this brilliant effort.

1.5 Topical Description of Medical Sociology

Many scholars have described medical sociology in various ways: sociology of health and illness or health sociology. "Medical sociology" is more encompassing to describe the broad aspect of sociology dealing with medicine and health in general. One particular description is that of Straus (1957), who averred that medical sociology consists of sociology of medicine and sociology in medicine. Straus (1957, p. 203) observed that "[s]tudies of the profession (of medicine) and those dealing with the organization of health resources are primarily in the sociology of medicine [while] teaching activities and research in which the sociologist is collaborating with the physician in studying a disease process or factors influencing the patient's response to illness are primarily sociology in medicine." Straus made the distinction as a result of activities and affiliations of 110 medical sociologists.

Straus (1999, p. 109) further reiterated that sociology in medicine involves "activities that were associated with achieving the educational, research, or clinical goals of medicine. These were often collaborative with health professionals and occurred within health or medical institutions. They were carried out most frequently by sociologists who held appointments in health professional-schools, hospitals, or other health-care organisations." On the other hand, sociology of medicine is close to what could be described as sociology of health and illness. It involves the study of social factors in disease aetiology, incidence, prevalence, distribution, social response to health and illness, therapeutic process, and community health needs.

Initially, Straus (1957) thought it was not feasible for a sociologist to engage in the sociology in and of medicine together; however, later he (1999) observed that because of crosscutting intellectual development, it is now feasible. Therefore, the distinction "of and in" is merely the distinction of activities, not that of persons involved. Medical sociology has now grown into a full subdiscipline of sociology with more diverged activities as a result of intellectual and research domains. It is now possible to present a topical description of medical sociology without a topical differentiation between that of sociology in or of medicine. Therefore, another major concern of students of sociology or professional is a clear topical description of medical sociology. It is imperative to explain the intellectual domain of medical sociology. The first major attempt at this was by David Mechanic (1968), who highlighted a number of intellectual domains of medical sociology. Apart from the fact that there are still some new developments, a re-explanation of some of the domains in line with currents trends is necessary.

1.5.1 Social Aetiology of Disease

Medical sociology primarily focuses on the social causes of disease. Social causationism entails direct and indirect (social) exposure to diseases. While a medical doctor will simply note that a patient has HIV, a sociologist is more interested in the sexual network of the patient since HIV can be acquired through the process of sexual interaction with others in the society. This pattern of sexual relation is a social determinant. Another explanation is that the decision to engage in protective sex is entirely that of the parties involved. A medical sociologist is more interested in the "push" factors that expose individuals to any disease. Another example is the high prevalence of vesicovaginal fistula (VVF) in sub-Saharan Africa (SSA). There are many social issues that expose women to the risk of VVF, which include age at marriage, access to maternal care, maternal education, and gender inequality, which prevent many women from obtaining permission for their partners to attend health facilities. Some of these issues are sociocultural issues, which need to be addressed in order to reduce the incidence of VVF in SSA.

The notion of social aetiology is embedded in risk factors, most of which occur at the individual or societal level (see Chap. 4 on social determinants of health); however, some risks have to do with the norms and values of the societies. For instance, a culture which promotes gender inequality or male hegemony puts women at a risk of gender violence including sexual abuse and female infanticide. The assertion that lifestyle and living conditions could expose individuals to diseases is not new and has been a major focal point in preventive medicine. Particularly in the developing world, vulnerability to disease often has less to do with germs than with the so-called social causes—factors such as income, education, gender, occupation, housing, and access to health services. Social deprivation is a key predictor of distribution of diseases and life expectancy. The social causes also include poor sanitation, nutritional deficiencies, poor infrastructures (e.g., water supply), lack of safety at work, overcrowded or poorly maintained housing, environmental pollution, stress, and lack of exercise due to a sedentary lifestyle. The social causes can also be explained in terms of the lack of education on preventive measures or appropriate health behaviour.

These social causes often found in the social condition of the individuals or societies constitute the primary crux of medical sociology. The relevance of medical sociology can be assessed based on the efforts in addressing these social causes.

1.5.2 Cultural Beliefs and Social Response to Illness

Cultural beliefs and responses have direct consequences for both preventive measures and cure-seeking behaviour. Illness perception is usually conceived in terms of local definition of the illness—its perceived cause(s), vulnerability, severity, and perceived modes of transmission. This illness perception or local understanding and cultural beliefs also constitute a part of the core focus of medical sociology. There is a cultural repertoire for recognising, diagnosing, or defining the illness condition

(Alubo 2008; Erinosho 2006). Illness is a deviation from societal norms and values, usually manifested through failure of an individual to perform his/her normal roles in the society. The course of illness is determined not merely by biomedical factors but also by the way the patients define and respond to the illness.

The response to illness often reflects a society's medical beliefs about the causes of health problems, choices of treatment options, and other health-related concerns. Feyisetan et al. (1997) noted that certain disease-specific and non-disease-specific cultural beliefs may influence people's health and health-seeking behaviour. This is why it is important to consider cultural beliefs and practices of the people when designing measures and programs aimed at improving their health (Comoro et al. 2003; Feyisetan and Adeokan 1992; Jegede 2002). It is further noted that the adoption of both preventive and curative methods may also depend on people's conception of the causes of illness and on their level of conviction about the efficacy of the preventive and curative methods (Feyisetan et al. 1997).

For instance, at the beginning of the HIV crisis in Africa, the problem was about people's belief in the reality of the disease. For several years, the "HIV is real" campaign was widespread. The response then was very weak. In general, people who doubt the reality of a disease would not adopt any preventive measure. By the time the reality of AIDS (acquired immunodeficiency syndrome) was incontrovertible (at least to the general majority), the havoc had already been caused—HIV has eaten deep into all fabrics of the society and thousands of people are losing their lives daily. Additionally, there were a lot of causal misconceptions surrounding HIV/AIDS at the societal level, which also stymies adoption of both preventive and treatment options.

1.5.3 Sociology of Medical Care and Hospital

The concerns of this aspect are on the sociocultural aspects of medical care and hospital as a (social) institution. There are often options in medical care, especially traditional and modern approaches (Alubo 2008). This interaction of plural systems of health care may be complementary, competitive, or even conflicting. Choice is usually modified by the cultural belief system in the community. Another main issue is the cost of seeking medical care in relation to affordability and quality of services from medical institutions. These are interwoven issues that have constituted focal points in medical care. Another significant issue is the gender context of medical care and hospital. Analysis of gender issues in terms of care providers and receivers is vital in medical care. At times, experts analyse the importance of cultural competence in health care delivery and desirability of gender concordance (patient-practitioner) in health care.

There is also a significant focus on the hospital as a social or total institution, a small society or a home of the vulnerable population. This aspect also attempts to explain the competing interests for managing the patients in the hospital environment, and consider how these interests or influences manifest, and are resolved in the delivery of care. The experiences of patients and quality of service delivery (especially patients' satisfaction with care) are also part of the focus. This aspect also attempts to examine perceptions of and social relations within health care institutions—the patient-practitioner, practitioner-practitioner relationships, work-related difficulties and adjustments, and the role of health professionals in society.

Sociologists also tend to unravel the bureaucratic structures in medical care or hospitals and how such structures influence health care delivery systems. What is the impact of *red tapism* on service delivery? How do standardisation or organisation hierarchies pattern the service delivery system? How are the health professionals responding to the changing bureaucracy in the medical setting? How are or can health workers be motivated to achieve the goals of health organisation or policies? All of these questions constitute parts of the research focus of medical sociologists.

In addition, power relations within the hospital management are also part of sociological research. There are resultant power scuffles that often affect health care delivery systems. The constituent units in the hospital (medical doctors [including various specialists], pharmacists, nurses, administrative staff [e.g., accountants and personnel officers], laboratory professionals, and other cadre employees [down to the lowest cadre such as cleaners]) have sometimes been in conflict as a result of power relations in work contacts. Conflict often arises as a result of interrelated and interdependent tasks and, in some cases, unclear definition and demarcation of tasks, especially among related professionals (e.g., physicians and physiotherapists in the management of a fracture). These power relations have been a core part of medical sociological research.

1.5.4 Sociology of Psychiatry or Social Psychiatry

Psychiatry is a medical subdiscipline that works most closely with the social sciences, especially sociology. The thrust of social psychiatry is on the social and cultural context of mental health and illness. Social psychiatry is concerned with the cultural and social factors that engender, precipitate, intensify, or prolong maladaptive behaviour and complicate the management of mental disorders. It is also defined as a field of psychiatry based on the study of sociocultural and ecologic influences on the development and course/trajectory of mental diseases. Because of evidence-based social aspects of mental health, social psychiatry is perhaps the most visible aspect of mental health management. It also leads to the emergence of subprofessionals in psychiatry, known as social psychiatrists. Mental health has much to do with lifestyles and social conditions. In fact, most manifestations of mental disorders depict the contravention of normal standards of behaviour in the society. This implies that in most cases, a mental disorder is recognised through excessive abnormal behaviour within the social system. Hence, there was a shift in psychiatric ideology to the patient's behaviour and social relationships (Pilgrim and Rogers 1994).

Community psychiatry approach has been a major management approach in psychiatric treatment. This approach takes cognisant of the socio-spatial environment and the roles of significant others in the rehabilitation and re-integration of those with mental disorders. Positive support from such links will facilitate the rehabilitation and re-integration of the patients. Medical sociologists have been actively involved in the management of the patients and implementation of research necessary to improve patient management styles. There is also a growing body of research on the handling of patients in psychiatric hospitals, focusing on the use of physical and medical restraints and violence.

Social stigmatisation of the mentally ill is also part of the research focus in medical sociology (see Sect. 8.4.1 on labelling and mental illness). Stigmatisation prevents proper re-integration of the patients and may lead to relapse of the mental health condition following a worsening social condition of the patients. This is why medical sociologists often prioritise how to reduce social stigmatisation among all categories of patients. Most importantly, the works of Erving Goffman (1961, 1963) on total institution (see Sect. 8.4.3) and stigma (see Sect. 8.4.2) have been the major guiding theoretical underpinnings in social psychiatry and social reaction to illness/diseases. More often, community psychiatry depicts the de-institutionisation approach advocated by the *Goffmanians* in order to minimise alienating experiences and estrangement of the patients. The aforementioned issues constitute some of the areas of involvement of medical sociology in psychiatry.

1.5.5 Social Transition and Heath Care

There are dual aspects of social transition as it relates to health care—a change in both the society and health care itself. Change in the society might inform change in health care and there could also be meaningful development in health care as a result of improved technology. Medical sociologists are interested in both. They are riveted in social dynamics and responses of various facets of social organisation. Social change is constant; hence, human society is constantly undergoing numerous forms of social transition. The health care institutions have continuously been responding to changes in all sectors of the society. As a result of changes in the economic systems, for instance, some societies practise a capitalist health system, while others adopt a socialised health care system with embedded variations in how the systems are implemented. Medical sociologists are interested in how social transitions, whether political or economic, affect health care systems. They are interested in the course, causes, and consequences of such social transitions in the health care sector.

Apart from the institutional focus regarding social change, medical sociologists also study how such changes affect health and illness behaviour of the individuals. Both the individual and the institution often respond to change. In this regard, it is important to document what social change means for the health of the community. Social change may also affect vulnerability to different forms of diseases. Modern inventions create possibilities in health care systems and also raise copious sociocultural apprehensions. The advancement in information and communication technology makes telemedicine possible and improves diagnosis and treatment of patients. The Human Genome Project (HGP) continues to create more possibilities in health care systems. We are now living in a world with assisted reproductive technology, stem cell research, and nanotechnology. Many individuals now desire to enhance their bodies instead of treating disabilities. The possibility of transplantation leads to a proliferation of organ markets. These are some typical examples of issues generating new research directions in the sociological study of health and change.

1.5.6 Traditional Medicine/Complementary and Alternative Medicine

Ethno-medicine, or traditional medicine (TM), has been one of the major focal points of sociological research (see Sect. 10.2 for further elaboration). The utilisation of TM in the prevention and treatment of diseases has been intensively researched by sociologists in an attempt to understand the sociocultural context associated with the continuous patronage of TM. What informs the choice of TM? How prevalent is the use of TM? Are patients getting results from TM? What is the cultural basis of the belief in TM? Are there diseases that are only amenable to TM? How does TM differ from the biomedical norm in the definition of disease, perception of symptoms, and treatment? How can TM be recognised and incorporated into the general health care system? How is TM itself organised as a health care alternative? What is the place of TM in health care policy? Is TM complementary or alternative to modern medicine? What are the limitations of TM in health care? These are some of the questions that sociologists want to answer.

In some countries, there is constant tension between traditional and modern medicine, especially as an alternative health care system. Unfortunately, most of the practices of TM are not amenable to science and are grossly less advanced than modern medicine. But the incessant reliance in some communities on TM informs its recognition as part of health care institutions. Such recognition is also necessary as most of such societies have limited access to modern health care. In addition, TM seems to be the closest health care system to underserved communities. More importantly, there is an argument that it conforms to the belief system of the community. It is because of these aforementioned reasons that sociologists are concerned about the developments in TM.

1.5.7 Sociology of Bioethics

There is now sociology's engagement with bioethics, a field of growing interest that is defined by its concern with moral questions in biomedicine (De Vries 2003; Petersen 2011), whether it is called sociology in bioethics or sociology of bioethics (see Chap. 11 for further elaboration). The field of medical ethics or bioethics in general is multidisciplinary because the ethical dilemma in health care requires the inputs and understanding of various professionals. Some of these moral perplexities are part of societal concerns for equity, equality, and justice in health care. A majority of these issues are sociocultural issues and general ethical or moral standards of behaviour in the society. This is why sociological insights are necessary if the ethical conundrums presented by medicine are to be successfully resolved in practice. The most vital tool in medicine is the "human body." The body is a place where medical practices and interventions are exercised. The human and his/her body have a significant place in sociological impetus. Sociologists collaborate in resolving moral challenges in health care practice and research. Humphreys (2008, p. 51) observed that the sociological approach has brought out some interesting perspectives, especially unintended consequences of behaviours that bioethics (and research ethics) may not have anticipated.

While the field of sociology of biomedical ethics is still emerging, especially in SSA, a number of medical sociologists hold interest in it. In developed countries, there is a growing relevance of bioethicists in health care regulations and practices. Sociologists generally want to understand how ethical challenges can be resolved within the limits of societal conscience and how moral values and ethical behaviours are embodied and lived by social agents. How do ethical resolutions conform to the cultural milieu of the society? How are resolutions in the best interest of the individual? What are the future implications of ethical resolutions? How do medical practices incline with the norms and values of the society? How can we structure the development of new technology and its application within the moral values of the society? Sociologists have often challenged bioethics to look beyond principlism (Petersen 2011). Humphreys (2008) noted that sociology of bioethics has concentrated on social processes within bioethical debate, on role relationships, and on the norms, values, and beliefs of those engaged in the bioethical endeavour. Invariably, sociology now has keen interest in the relevance of social processes in the understanding of moral uneasiness posed by some advancement in biomedical sciences such as biobanks, stem cell research, biotechnology, nanotechnologies, genetic testing, clinical trials, transplantation, and medical enhancement.

1.5.8 *Heath Policy and Politics*

One major factor that greatly influences the health of the society, beyond the handling of a stethoscope or syringe in the hospital, is *health policy and politics*. Health politics is about who gets what health resources, why and when. Such politics involves the creation of medical schools; construction of health facilities; recruitment and deployment of health personnel; determination of health workers' benefits and their motivation, procurement, and provision of equipment; appointment of health care administrators; and initiation, formulation, and implementation of national, regional, or community health care policies. These issues are really crucial and are usually not under the control of the physicians, but rather the politicians or political leaders. This further signifies that a number of fundamental issues are beyond the confines of the hospital walls that must be properly considered in order to improve the health of the people.

Medical sociologists in particular are interested in the community or societal processes in the formulation of health policy. Most sociological questions include, among others: What are the social consequences of health care policy on the health of the community? Which policy is working, which is not, and why? How does health policy affect access to health care? What are the attitudes towards health policy? Who benefits from a particular policy and why? How can policies be modified to get better results? How are health facilities distributed and why? How adequate are health personnel and are they properly motivated to deliver national health policies? What is the influence of political will or political agenda on health care prioritisation? All of these questions are often treated using sociological perspectives and methods.

The intricacies involved in health care politics are often overwhelming and often require unparalleled attention if population health must be improved. In most SSA countries, there is paltry health political will, which accounts for poor health care facilities and, hence, high prevalence of health problems. There is often an insufficient budget and diminutive political will to implement the best practices, which explain the high rate of mortality from preventable diseases each year. The meagre foreign aid is mismanaged and good health policies often turn ineffective. There are critical issues for health policy and politics, which, if addressed, could improve population health in many countries. This is why medical sociologists consider health politics a part of the crux of the discipline.

1.5.9 Social Epidemiology

This is the study of the sociocultural factors in the distribution, incidence, and prevalence of health problems in human society. Jegede (1996) defined social epidemiology as the study of the disease process; its occurrence in population groups; those social and cultural factors that affect their incidence, prevalence, and distribution; and the host response in disease prevention and control in human population. Social epidemiology often focuses on what Krieger (1994, 2001) described as the multifactorial aetiology or web of causation—an array of social determinants of health distribution, an interplay of host, agent, and environment. There are numerous interconnected risk factors in the social system, which exposes individuals to the agents of diseases. These multifactorial links constitute the focus of social epidemiologists. It is through the understanding of the multicausality of disease that the differential distribution of diseases can be explained. One fundamental principle in social epidemiology is that humans are embodied agents (both socially and biologically). The interplay of these embodiments plays significant roles in risk exposure and susceptibility. Social epidemiology is a marriage of sociological frameworks to epidemiological studies (Krieger 2001), which represent a holistic approach.

1.5.10 Sociology of Dying and Death

Medical sociologists are also interested in patterns of mortality in human society. The major focus is on the social factors responsible for differential mortality rates in different social groups and societies in general. Issues such as income, gender, race, education, marital status, and occupation are associated with death rates. Sociologists study the interplay of these factors with risk exposures. Life expectancy in various nations is also unconnected with social conditions. There is strong relevance of sociological frameworks in the analysis of death in human society.

Apart from this, death is also a biosocial issue. It is biological because of the failure of biological organ(s) in the body, which often signifies death. Certification of death is thus a biomedical necessity. Social death could, however, occur before (biological) death. The inability to be a functioning member of the society due to total social incapacitation, and signals the expectation of (biological) death. Apart from this, death itself is a form of social transition; a new form of being that creates a vacuum, which often signifies emptiness of social roles. This implies that death has significant social repercussions for the affected individuals and the society at large. Hence, society often prepares to cater for the social blankness created by death. Bryant (2002) observed that society shapes social structure to constrain and contain the disruptive effects of death.

Furthermore, one of the primary interests is on the causes of death in human society—especially those causes that have links with sociocultural issues. Such causes are usually studied sociologically and historically. This will expose the social patterns of death: which group dies more from what ailment and why. What are the sociological explanations of the exposure of the group to a particular ailment in the society? More so, sociologists are also interested in passage rite for the dead. Different societies respond and receive death in various ways. Other issues of interest include notions of good and bad death, death and social institution, social responses to death, political economy of death, death and religion, death after life, life after death, and increasing versus decreasing life expectancy across the globe.

1.5.11 Medical Education

The bedrock of sociology of medical education is the prioritisation of health and social origin of medical education, which has profound implications for knowledge orientation and dissemination, organisational arrangements, and access to such education. It focuses on current issues affecting medical students, the profession, faculty members, and the impact of medical education on the society at large. Light (1988, p. 307) also observed that "the changing locus of medical education in the matrix of social, cultural, political, and organizational forces exhibited by the health care system calls for the attention of medical sociologists." A number of research priorities in sociology of medical education include: how social changes affect delivery and content of medical education; access to medical education among various social groups;

orientation of medical education; outcomes of medical education; and health policy and medical education. Mechanic (1990) averred that focus of this area also includes how to improve medical curricula, cultural competence in medical education, and ethical behaviour of medical professionals as well as the study of the pattern and context of professional socialisation.

References

Alubo, O. (2008). Ontological response to illness. *Jos Journal of Social Issues, 6*, 1–16.
Barbour, R. S. (2011). The biographical turn and the 'sociolization' of medicine. *Medical Sociology Online, 6*(1), 15–25.
Blackwell, E. (1902). *Essays in medical sociology*. London, England: Ernest Bell.
Bloom, S. W. (2002). *The word as scalpel: A history of medical sociology*. Oxford: Oxford University Press.
Bryant, C. D. (2002). Sociology of death and dying. In C. D. Bryant & D. L. Peck (Eds.), *21st century sociology: A reference handbook* (pp. 156–166). California: Sage Publications.
Clausen, R. (1963). Health, society, and social science. *The ANNALS of the American Academy of Political and Social Science, 346*(1),1–8.
Comoro, C., Nsimba, S. E. D., Warsame, M., & Tomson, G. (2003). Local understanding, perceptions and reported practices of mothers/guardian and health workers on childhood malaria in a Tanzanian district—implications for malaria control. *Acta Tropical, 87*, 305–313.
Comte, A. (1896). *The positive philosophy*. Vol II & III, Trans Version by Harriet Martineau. London: George Bell & Sons.
Conrad, P. (2007). Freidson's revolution in medical sociology. *Health, 11*, 141–144.
Coockerham, W. C. (2001). Medical sociology and sociological theory. In W. C. Coockerham (Ed.), *The blackwell companion of medical sociology* (pp. 3–22). Massachusetts: Blackwell Publishers Ltd.
Coser, L. A. (2004). *Masters of sociological thought: Ideas in historical and social context*. 2nd edn. New Delhi: Rawat Publication.
De Vries, R. (2003). How can we help?: From sociology 'in to sociology of' bioethics. *Journal of Law, Medicine & Ethics, 32*, 279–292.
Durkheim, E. (1897/1951). *Suicide: A study in sociology*. NY: The Free Press.
Erinosho, O. (2006). *Health sociology for universities, colleges and health related institutions*. Ibadan: Sam Bookman.
Feyisetan, B. J., Asa, S., & Ebigbola, J. A. (1997). Mothers' management of childhood diseases in Yorubaland: The influence of cultural beliefs. *Health Transition Review, 7*, 221–234, 175.
Feyisetan, B. J., & Adeokun, L. (1992). Impact of child care and disease treatment on infant mortality. In E. Van de Walle, G. Pison, & M. Sala-Diakanda (Eds.), *Mortality and society in Sub-Saharan Africa* (pp. 145–159). Oxford: Clarendon Press.
Freidson, E. (1961a/1962). The sociology of medicine. *Current Sociology, 10–11*, 123–140.
Freidson, E. (1961b). *Patients' views of medical practice*. NY: Russel Sage Foundations.
Freidson, E. (1970a). *Profession of medicine: A study of the sociology of applied knowledge*. NY: Dodd, Mead.
Freidson, E. (1970b). *Professional dominance: The social structure of medical care*. Chicago: Atherton.
Freidson, E. (1975). *Doctoring together: A study of professional social control*. New York: Elsevier.
Gilbert, L. (2012). The report on sociology of health in Africa. *Newsletter of the Research Committee on Sociology of Health, 55*, 5–6.
Glaser, B. G., & Strauss, A. L. (1965). *Awareness of dying*. Chicago: Aldine.
Glaser, B. G., & Strauss, A. L. (1968). *The time for death*. Chicago: Aldine.
Goffman, E. (1961). *Asylum: Essays on the social situation of mental patients and other inmates*. Garden City: Anchor.

References

Goffman, E. (1963). *Stigma: Notes on the management of spoiled identity*. London: Penguin Books.
Hafferty, F. W., & Castellani, B. (2006). Medical sociology. In Clifton D. Bryant & Dennis L. Peck (Eds.), *21st century sociology: A reference handbook* (pp. 331–338). Califonia: Sage Publications.
Harris, S. R. (2013). Studying the construction of social problems. In J. Best & S. R. Harris (Eds.), *Making sense of social problems: New images, new issues* (pp. 1–10). Boulder: Lynne Rienner Publishers.
Holtz, T. H., Holmes, S., Stonington, S., & Eisenberg, L. (2006). Health is still social: Contemporary examples in the age of the genome. *PLoS Medicine, 3*(10), e419. doi:10.1371/journal.pmed.0030419.
Humphreys, S. J. (2008). The sociology of bioethics: The 'is' and the 'ought'. *Research Ethics, 4*(2), 47–51.
Jackson, H. (2002). *AIDS Africa: Continent in crisis*. Harare: SAfAIDS.
Jegede, A. S. (2002). The Yoruba cultural construction of health and illness. *Nordic Journal of African Studies, 11*(3), 322–335.
Jegede, A. S. (1996). Social epidemiology. In E. A. Oke & B. E. Owumi (Eds.), *Readings in medical sociology* (pp. 52–71). Ibadan: Resource Development and Management Services.
Kaminskas, R., & Darulis, Z. (2007). Peculiarities of medical sociology: Application of social theories in analyzing health and medicine. *Medicina (Kaunas), 43*(2), 110–117.
Kerbo, H. R., & Coleman, J. W. (2006). Social problems. In C. D. Bryant & D. L. Peck (Eds.), *21st century sociology: A reference handbook* (pp. 362–369). California: Sage Publications.
Krieger, N. (1994). Epidemiology and the web of causation: Has anyone seen the spider? *Social Science & Medicine, 39*(7), 887–903.
Krieger, N. (2001). Theories of social epidemiology in the 21st century: An ecosocial perspective. *International Journal of Epidemiology, 30,* 668–677.
Light, D. W. (1988). Toward a new sociology of medical education. *Journal of Health and Social Behaviour, 29*(4), 307–322.
Lyman, S. M., Johnson, J. M., & Warren, C. A. B. (1973). Social problems and social order. In J. D. Douglas (Ed.), *Introduction to sociology: Situations and structures*. New York: The Free Press.
Mechanic, D. (1966). Response factors in illness: The study of illness behavior. *Social Psychiatry, 1*(1), 11–20.
Mechanic, D. (1968). *Medical sociology: A selective view*. NY: The Free Press.
Mechanic, D. (1990). The role of sociology in health affairs. *Health Affairs, 9*(1), 85–97.
Parsons, T. (1951). *The social system*. Glencoe: Free Press.
Petersen, A. (2011). Can and should sociology save bioethics? *Medical Sociology Online, 6*(1), 2–14.
Pilgrim, D., & Rogers, A. (1994). Something old, something new...: Sociology and the organisation of psychiatry. *Sociology, 28*(2), 521–538.
Smelser, N. (1994). *Sociology*. Cambridge: Blackwell.
Smelser, N. J. (1996). Social sciences and social problems: The next century. *International Sociology, 11*(3), 275–290.
Spencer, H. (1891). *The study of sociology*. NY: D. Appleton & Co.
Spencer, H. (1896). *The principles of sociology*. NY: D. Appleton & Co.
Stacey, M., & Homans, H. (1978). The sociology of health and illness: Its present state, future prospects and potential for health research. *Sociology, 12,* 281–307.
Straus, R. (1957). The nature and status of medical sociology. *American Sociological Review, 22*(2), 200–204.
Straus, R. (1999). Medical sociology: A personal fifty year perspective. *Journal of Health and Social Behavior, 40*(2), 103–110.
Warbasse, J. P. (1909). Medical sociology: A series of observations touching upon the sociology of health and the relations of medicine to society. New York: D. Appleton.
Weber, L. R. (1995). *The analysis of social problems*. Massachusetts: Allyn and Bacon.
Wellcome News. (2002). *Research directions in malaria*. (Suppl. 6). London.

Chapter 2
Health, Disease, and Illness as Conceptual Tools

2.1 Introduction

There has not been an absolute consensus on the definitions of health, disease, and illness, even though these concepts are central not only in medicine but also in the health social sciences (e.g., medical sociology, health psychology and medical demography). These are parts of the conceptual tools in various medical-related fields. A definition of each concept is imperative because they constitute parts of the analytical tools in medical sociology. The lack of consensus often prevents uniformity of interpretations and generates more polemics. One wonders why there has not been consensus, despite the long history of medicine. The concepts are multidimensional, complex, and often elusive. For instance, Larson (1999) observed that disagreements about the meaning of health are common because health is imbued with political, medical, social, economic, and spiritual components. It is subject to various conceptualisation and interpretations. While all the concepts have their foundations in medicine, a biomedical perspective of health or disease may not be comprehensive enough. However, a fusion of the various perspectives often presents a complex definition like the WHO's definition of health. This is why the debate on the definition of health is still ongoing. That the debate continues is not a problem as refinement of definition could lead to a better conceptualisation.

2.2 How Should Health be Defined?

The concept of health presents a form of ambiguity because it is multidimensional, complex, and sometimes elusive. Notwithstanding, various scholars, apart from the definition given by the WHO, have defined the concept. Although it is not the first definition of health, the WHO's definition will still be the starting point because it is relatively old and has been central to the debate on the meaning of health. WHO (1948) defined health as *a state of complete physical, mental, and social well-being, not merely the absence of disease and infirmity*. The definition is holistic, and it presents three major interrelated components of health (see Fig. 2.1).

Fig. 2.1 Components of health

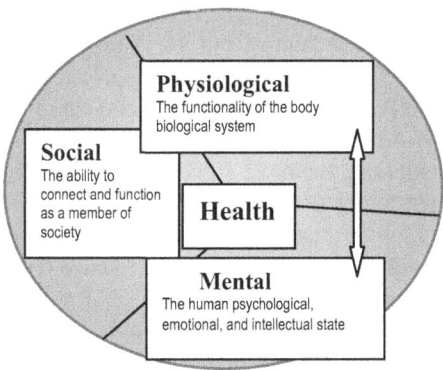

1. **The physical**: this is the physiological or biological component of the definition. It simply implies the maintenance of homoeostasis. This is often used to infer a soundness of the body. Most often, disease represents a malfunction of a part of the body system or an intrusion of harmful organisms such as a virus or parasite. This may cause a breakdown of the individual affected. This physiological aspect is the most important biomedical criterion in the determination of health. For someone to be healthy, his/her biological components must be in order. A major diagnosis procedure involves a determination of what could be wrong with any component of the body or detection of any intrusion of any anti-body by tracing the pathways of the disease from underlying causes to pathology in the human body system and examination of any emerging of symptoms. Determining this may involve a series of laboratory tests or clinical examinations. One may be certified as healthy if there is no detection of any biological hitch.
2. **The social**: this represents the behavioural aspect of human health. Being a member of society is being in the network of social interaction and being able to fulfil social roles and expectations. If an individual is not active in the social network, it represents a form of social pathology— an abnormality, which is an infraction on the norms and values of society. The social also incorporates the spiritual dimension. The spiritual aspect could be personal to the individual by connecting to the world of reality and divinity. Larson (1999) observed that since the WHO's definition of health, medicine has treated individuals as social beings whose health is affected by social behaviour and interaction.
3. **The mental**: this indicates the psychological, emotional, and mental status of the individual. Emotional apathy, fixation, and maladjusted personality constitute a part of the manifestation of illness. Huber et al. (2011) observed that the mental aspect of health signifies the possession of a "sense of coherence," which includes the subjective faculties enhancing the comprehensibility, manageability, and meaningfulness of any circumstances.

The WHO's definition has been heavily criticised since it was conceived in 1946 after the Second World War (see Callahan 1973; Bice 1976; Pannenborg 1979; Wood 1986; Simmons 1989; Saracci 1997; Jadad and O'Grady 2008; Huber et al. 2011; Godlee

2011; Awofeso 2012). For instance, Awofeso (2012) observed that the definition is inflexible and unrealistic. He claimed that the inclusion of the word "complete" in the definition makes it unlikely for anyone to be healthy for a reasonable period of time. Godlee (2011) also noted that the definition is absolute and therefore unachievable for most people in the world. The definition presents an absolute ideal situation by combining the three aspects of human life. It is often difficult, if not impossible, to gain complete contentment in all the aspects. It is observed that since health is a goal, not only of the health care system but also individual and the society at large, it is ideal for a body like WHO to present a realistic definition that can be operationalised and achievable (Godlee 2011).

In addition, Saracci (1997) also submitted that the WHO's definition of health is problematic and it should be reconsidered. Saracci observed that the definition equates health with happiness—that a disruption of happiness could be regarded as a health problem. He further argued that the WHO's definition reflects that health is boundless. More so, Huber et al. (2011, p. 2) opined that the WHO's definition is problematic because it impliedly declares people with chronic diseases and disabilities definitively ill. The definition further minimises "the role of the human capacity to cope autonomously with life's ever changing physical, emotional, and social challenges and to function with fulfilment and a feeling of wellbeing with a chronic disease or disability" (Huber et al. 2011, p. 2). Despite several decades of criticisms, the WHO has not reviewed the definition. The idea of a definition is to present a holistic view that is meaningful not only for individuals but also as a (definitive) tool in scientific investigation. The idea is not to advance an operational perfection that is unchangeable. Perhaps, there is yet a review because there has not been a more holistic and measurable alternative definition of health. The question is simple: are other definitions of "health" more operational?

2.3 A New Definition of Health?

Several other scholars have proposed other definitions of health, which can be used in light of changing global health circumstances. Some of these definitions will be critically examined; however, the essence of examining other definitions is not to defend the WHO's definition or to render such alternative definitions as immaterial. After some strictures of WHO's definition of health by Saracci (1997, p. 1410), he proposed a definition of health as "a condition of wellbeing, free of disease or infirmity, and a basic and universal human right." Impliedly, this definition also defined those who are living positively with chronic disease as unhealthy. It presents a health as a basic right, which is also problematic. In most parts of the world, health is a commodity with an insurance premium, a price-tag, or it requires a pool from the public tax. This also seems like a theoretical proposition that is not operational. It does not really account for the multidimensionality of health. Therefore, it may not be considered a holistic and viable alternative to the WHO definition.

Table 2.1 Models for defining health. (Source: Larson 1999, p. 125)

Medical model	The absence of disease or disability
World health organization (WHO) model	State of complete physical, mental, and social well-being and not merely the absence of disease or infirmity
Wellness model	Health promotion and progress toward higher functioning, energy, comfort, and integration of mind, body, and spirit
Environmental model	Adaptation to physical and social surroundings—a balance free from undue pain, discomfort, or disability

Bircher (2005, p. 1), on the other hand, defines health as "a dynamic state of well-being characterised by a physical and mental potential, which satisfies the demands of life commensurate with age, culture, and personal responsibility." While this is stylishly holistic, it is contentious due to the use of other concepts (e.g., age and culture) without unified definitions. For instance, culture is complex, dynamic, and relative. This may imply that the definition of health will also be relative and probably depend on the circumstances or societies. Additionally, does the definition refer to biological age or social construction of age? This is part of the complicatedness as the concepts used are not specific.

In an attempt to proffer a more acceptable perspective in the face of the continuous debate, Larson (1999) proposed that health should be conceived using multiple models: medical, the WHO, wellness, and environmental models. A combination of these models will be more holistic beyond the use of only the WHO model or other definitions. Table 2.1 presents the models of defining health. One major problem with model-based definition is that there could be more models than expected. The model-approach does not present a whole definition. Later, every profession will likely present a model of health beyond common understanding, and this will generate more issues. The major strength of this approach is that it emphases the multifactorial context of the concept of health.

Following the argument that there could be more models, a social model will dwell on Parsonian definition that defines health as "the state of optimum capacity of an individual for the effective performance of the roles and tasks for which he has been socialized" (Parsons 1972). This is more a sociological approach to health—a conceptualisation of health as a social element. Health in this sociological sense is more inclined towards human capacity to fulfil their obligations, participate in social activities (including work), and fulfil role expectations in the society in the face of structural limitations. This conception is connected with both physiological and mental models of health in the sense that the source of a social incapacitation could be from a biological or mental limitation. The social model does not debunk the biomedical model. The model is complementary to the medical model and signifies a perspective that is central in medical sociology.

In a recent development, Huber et al. (2011) defined health as *the ability to adapt and self-manage in the face of social, physical, and emotional challenges*. This definition was initially proposed in 2008 (see Jadad and O'Grady 2008). The definition seems to be receiving some considerations, especially because of the use of "adaptation." While the WHO's definition stresses on *a complete state*, this definition proposes *adaptive capacity*. Lancet Editorial (2009, p. 781) commented, "Health is

2.3 A New Definition of Health?

an elusive as well as a motivating idea. By replacing perfection with adaptation, we get closer to a more compassionate, comforting, and creative programme for medicine—one to which we can all contribute." The major strength of this definition is that it takes account of the shift in health challenges in the twenty-first century. Unlike the period before World War II when acute diseases were more prevalent than chronic diseases, now the latter constitutes a greater burden. Chronic diseases require behavioural adjustments in terms of self-care or management (see Sects. 2.6.2 and 8.3). This is why the idea of adaptation seems to be more current than that of "a complete state."

With a critical stance, the definition by Huber et al. is also problematic. First, adaptation does not mean the absence of diseases or infirmity. Adaptation may signify a number of limitations such food or activity restrictions or behavioural constraints. Second, it may also mean continuous treatment or dependence on medication. In the case of a chronic disease, adaptation does not nullify the self-awareness of (undesirable) state of health. The shortcomings of the definition also create opportunities for more deliberations.

Recognising the diversity, relativity and complexity of health, Blaxter (1990, 2010) presents a descriptive analysis of health. One of the major dimensions of health identified by Blaxter (1990, 2010) is the lay concept of health. This implies how different individuals define health, which explains the relativity of the concept. The lay concept of health is essentially subjective because it is based on people's own assessment and judgment of whether they are healthy or not. Blaxter (1990, p. 40) observed that the most "usual way of measuring self-perceived illness, as distinct from the presence or absence of disease, is by means of symptom lists." To the lay population, absence of symptoms means health. From this perspective, Blaxter (1990) identified the three "states" of health: freedom from illness, ability to function, and fitness. In this regards, health is also perceived as energy and vitality in terms of fitness for functions: physical, social and normative activities.

Blaxter (2010) argued that health could be defined, constructed, experienced, acted out, and it is also dynamic. Definitions of health are often for operational use like the previous definitions that have been considered. Construction of health stems from the lay perspective or individual's appraisal of state of health, which can be good or bad. Such construction also includes what a particular society qualifies as "health." For instance, labelling reactivity (people's reaction to a particular condition) might influence designation or conceptualisation of health or illness in a particular society (see sect. 8.4.1 for labeling theory). Experiential knowledge of health is phenomenological—derived from feeling of wellness or otherwise, which emanate from the presence or absence of personal discomfort and pain. In terms of "enactment" of health, the central consideration includes what people do to maintain their health. Health is also a dynamic attribute because it fluctuates across biographical, historical and contextual milieus. The state of health varies across lifespan, and is influenced by a number of factors including personal (e.g., lifestyle) and structural factors (e.g., access to health care) (see Chapter four). The conceptualisation of disease will be the focus of next section.

2.4 Disease as a Conceptual Tool

Health has been conceived in a biomedical model as the absence of disease while the holistic definition from the WHO signifies that health is not a mere absence of disease. Whichever form the definition takes, the question now is "what constitutes a disease?" One major issue is that disease is often conceived from a biomedical point of view. It can also have behavioural manifestations, especially with regard to human functionality. The definition of health is complex, so also is the definition of a disease. If the lack of health can be defined as not a mere absence of a disease or infirmity, this signifies that there are a number of germ- and non-germ-related (medical) conditions that can signify the presence of a disease. This, however, also makes the definition of a disease complex because of variations in its conceptions. Mainly, Boorse (1975, 1977) was engrossed in a practical and philosophical discussion of what health and disease may entail. He defined disease as a type of internal state which impairs health (i.e., reduces one or more functional ability below typical efficiency). One major criticism of this definition is the use of "typical efficiency," which implies the presence of a reference group in the definition of disease (Kingma 2007; Stempsey 2000) as a kind of comparative analysis. This view is often referred to as a bio-statistical theory (BST) of health and disease. Kingma (2007) argued that human species are different in functional capacity: what is normal in one group can be abnormal in another and vice versa. Therefore, Boorse's definition of health or disease is only valid depending on the reference group.

Despite this criticism, Boorse's arguments have been a significant reference point in the discussion of health and diseases. Boorse discussed seven major themes that are prominent in the discussion of what health or a disease entails. It is important here to examine the seven themes in line with the notion of disease and see how important or otherwise those themes could be in identifying a disease.

1. **Pain, suffering and discomfort**: generally what is called disease accounts for human suffering by inflicting pain and discomfort, sometimes unbearable, thereby necessitating palliative care, like terminal sedation. Whitlow is a typical condition that could impose considerable pain on the sufferer, although it requires a simple medical procedure to resolve. A reason why the argument about pain may not be sufficient is because there are a number of normal procedures that require medical attention as a result of pain and discomfort, but are not diseases, such as teething, menstruation, childbirth, and abortion.
2. **Treatment by physicians**: normally diseases require the attention of medical doctors. A disease should be treatable. However, Boorse submitted that there are some conditions that cannot be treated, and doctors also attend to a number of conditions that are not diseases. With medicalisation of life, there are medical expansions beyond treatment of disease, such as certification of fitness for a study or travel. More so, circumcision, body modification or enhancement, and family planning procedures cannot be regarded as diseases but require attention of a physician.

3. **Statistical normality**: the species' average level of performance becomes a yardstick for determining normality and abnormality. There is also a measure of statistical normality of clinical variables such as blood pressure, basal metabolism, weight, sugar level, height, pulse, and respiration. Any measure beyond the normal range is usually termed as an abnormality or a disease condition and signifies the need for medical attention. When normal blood pressure ends, there begins hypotension or hypertension. This average of normality is derived from the rate of mortality or functionality within normal and abnormal ranges. It is assumed that mortality or dysfunctionality is often higher when below or above normal ranges. This may not always be the case as clinical variables are measures of probability or propensity to a disease.
4. **Disability**: disease could also lead to many forms of disability. Poliomyelitis is a typical example of a disease that can cause physical deformity. In another case, a disease may reduce active participation of an individual in the social network, such as the inability to walk or stand. Pregnancy, for instance, could not count as a disease even though it comes with some limitations. A number of skin diseases may not count as disease since they may not present with disabling effects.
5. **Adaptation**: the ability to adapt to the environment has also been categorised as a form of healthiness while those who are not fit are presumably diseased. Lack of adaptation prevents an individual from meeting the average level of a species' functionality. The presence of eumelanin pigmentation in the skins of black Africans helps in adapting to their environment, but it does not mean those with pheomelanin pigmentation cannot survive in Africa or that Africans cannot survive elsewhere. Environmental can even inflict suffering on humans in the process of adaptations.
6. **Homeostasis**: health is a state of bodily equilibrium while disease is a state of homeostatic failure. But the process of human growth as Boorse observed is itself leading to homeostatic disequilibrium.
7. **Value**: disease is undesirable while health is desirable. Health is thus a social value in human society. However, it is also impossible to exclusively delineate disease from the point of undesirability. Conditions such as shortness and ugliness cannot be counted as diseases even though they may not be desirable.

Furthermore, *a disease can also be defined as a state in which human capacity fluctuates and represents a deviation from biomedical standard or normal human condition.* Disease often requires medical intervention. As noted earlier, not all that conditions which require medical intervention constitute disease. A disease is a pathological state which can be diagnosed through a competent medical analysis. Disease, however, does not always mean there must be a pathological agent such as a virus or bacterium. Conditions such as infertility, gunshot wound, fracture, drowning, and other forms of injuries/accidents also qualify as disease because they represent an infraction on normal human condition.

More so, Fabrega (1973) explained that diseases usually present with a *biological discontinuity*. Biological discontinuity signifies the presence of pathology in any part of the body or bodily inactivity due to an injury. Some diseases have pathological agents (e.g., onchocerciasis [worm infection], trypanosomiasis [spread by the bite of the tsetse fly], dracunculiasis [guinea worm], trachoma [bacterial infection], malaria [parasites spread through a mosquito bite]), some are mere deformities or birth defects (e.g., brain injury, autism, spinal bifida), while some are the actual breakdown of organs (e.g., renal failure, blindness) or organ functional problems (e.g., impotency, ectopic pregnancy). All these diseases have to do with biological problems and constitute apparent forms of diseases.

Furthermore, Temple et al. (2001, p. 807) proposed a definition of disease with three basic elements—"disease is *a state* that places individuals at *increased risk* of *adverse consequences*." The first element, "a state," implies a physiological or psycho-social condition which explains susceptibility to risk. Second, risk includes the possibility of impairment. Certain conditions put individuals at a risk of diseases in the future. Therefore, both preventive and therapeutic measures could be provided to avert or ameliorate adverse consequences or undesirable situations. Meanwhile, adverse consequences include morbidity, disability, or mortality. The definition adequately extends to genetic conditions in humans.

Despite these enormous arguments on the biomedical model of disease, it is important to note, as Temple et al. (2001) observed, that disease is "a fluid concept influenced by societal and cultural attitudes that change with time and in response to new scientific and medical discoveries." One major example that is often cited is the classification of obesity. In the pre-industrial era, obesity was a sign of affluence and good living, while in the modern era it is a disease with enormous research and development of medical interventions (including surgical procedures) to "cure" obesity. Apart from the medical risks of obesity, the social and modern reconstruction of beauty as a slim body figure also affects attitudes towards obesity. In addition, homosexuality was previously considered a disease but is now normalised in many societies (Nordenfeldt 1993).

2.5 The Realities of Illness

Illness and disease have been major traditional concepts in sociology and medical sciences. The important role of these concepts for human-related medical endeavours was re-emphasised by Nordenfeldt (1993). These concepts are interwoven and often require some analytical clarifications. Most often, people use the words interchangeable. As conceptual and practical tools, they are not the same. The essence of this section is to make some conceptual clarifications of these concepts and not to join the body of unending debate evident in the works of various scholars (including Boorse 1975, 1977; Hesslow 1993; Nordenfeldt 1993; Stempsey 2000; Tengland 2007). More importantly, sociologists have laid more claims on the notion of illness because it is more of a behavioural concept than a medical one. Undoubtedly, illness has a number of undeniable social, moral, and legal contexts.

In a simple illustration, disease is a form of pathology or medical problem, defect, or impairment, while illness is a manifestation of such an impairment, defect/pathology, or disability. Illness is a presentation of a medical condition in a way that limits the functional capability of an individual in the society. This is why

2.5 The Realities of Illness

Nordenfeldt (1993) observed that to be ill is to be in pain, to be anxious, or to be disabled. The notion of illness fits appropriately into the concept of sick role described by Parsons (1951). It is a situation when an individual consciously feels that he/she is unhealthy, sometimes as a result of discomfort and pain. Therefore, illness is the *live-experience of a diseased condition*. While a diseased patient might not *be real* (i.e., without a self-awareness of the condition), an ill patient is real.

It can simply be observed that *disease makes people ill*. An individual is thus ill to some degree if there is some vital goal of his/her which cannot be completely realised (Nordenfeldt 1993). Illness is a progression from the mere presence of a medical problem or condition to the presentation of disabling symptoms and signs. The underlying meaning is that *it is possible to have a disease without being ill* and vice versa—invariably it is possible to have a disease without any awareness of it. Boorse (1975) advanced some clarifications on the character of illness.

1. An illness is a reasonably serious disease with incapacitating effects that make it undesirable. It is a condition that is obviously undesirable because of its negative attributes.
2. Illness requires treatment. It is a condition, which can be described as a medical problem in terms of impairment, defect, or disability and thus requires medical attention.
3. Illness is often a valid excuse for normally criticisable behaviour. This implies that an ill person may not fulfill normative roles and expectations. Instead of criticising an individual, people will affirm that he/she is incompetent due to illness. This implies there is a diminished moral accountability for the ill.
4. Determination of illness is bound by appropriate normative judgments or a sociocultural context. This implies that illness is a relative term as it could vary by culture, place, individual, and time. The cultural notion of illness determines the kind of response and how serious some medical conditions could be termed as mild, serious, or negligible.

From the foregoing discussion, it is evident that illness is culture-bound. It is socioculturally defined. This is why Fabrega (1973) and Garro (2000) observed that illness is a universal human experience with a cultural meaning. They observed that culture is a tool, which both enables and restrains interpretive possibilities regarding an illness. This cultural interpretation of illness is inevitable and important in a number of ways.

1. The first major interpretation is the normative definition of illness, when an individual could be declared ill. In fact, the significant other may play a major role in identifying illness and referring the individual to an appropriate care sector. There are cultural frameworks for recognising a disease/illness through its signs and symptoms.
2. The second is aetiological categorisation—an attempt to determine why an individual is ill. Cultural and historical experiences affect this causal classification of illness (see Sect. 2.7). If it is an illness that is common in the community, a remedy may be available without much process of diagnosis.

3. The third is the evaluation of therapeutic options. This is often influenced by aetiological classification. Different societies have a number of causal explanations. Although natural causation is predominant in western societies, there are other etiological classifications. The same situation applies to the non-western societies. Fabrega (1973), for instance, opined that the social definition of illness forms the basis of a decision about medical treatment.
4. The last aspect is reintegration into the social system following perceived wellness. This is also very important as the society plays a large role in absorbing a previously ill individual back into the social system. This is often problematic in the case of mental illness as stigmatisation may arise which may eventually affect the illness prognosis.

2.6 Disease/Illness Categories

There are various ways in which illnesses can be categorised. For the purpose of this sociological explanation, categorisation based on acute, chronic, accident, and mental illness is adopted. This categorisation also has sociological significance in terms of the dimensions of the diseases. It is also important for medical sociologists to be aware of the nature of diseases and some basic biomedical aetiologies and modes of transmission.

2.6.1 Acute Disease/Illness

An acute illness could be mild, moderate, or severe. Acute illness is by definition a self-limiting disease, which is mostly characterised by a rapid onset of symptoms. These symptoms may be very intense and resolved in a short period of time and, in some cases, could be life-threatening. Most contagious diseases are acute in nature. The term "acute disease" is often an indication of duration of the illness compared to chronic or sub-acute illness. Some examples of acute diseases include influenza or the flu, bronchitis, tonsillitis, sore throat, appendicitis, ear aches, organ failure, and breathing difficulties. Some acute diseases come with the prefix "acute" including severe acute respiratory syndrome (SARS), acute disseminated encephalomyelitis, and acute bronchitis. Specifically, attributes of acute diseases include:

1. **Self-limiting**: acute diseases have short durations or a limited short course. It is easy to predict that the disease will only last a few days. This also means that the disease could be resolved by itself sometimes without medical intervention.
2. **Sudden or rapid onset**: more often than not, acute diseases inflict humans unaware. An individual may wake up in the morning and discover he/she has the flu. The disease is often rapidly progressive.
3. **Communicable**: most acute diseases can easily be contracted even by mere contact with a sufferer. Sometimes they lead to outbreak (e.g., a cholera outbreak) and kill many people within days of its spread.

4. **Urgent care**: acute diseases often require urgent medical attention. If prompt care is not taken, the individual may die in a matter of a few days or weeks.
5. **Rapid resolution**: most often, response to treatment is very quick. If an individual is hospitalised, it could be for a few days. It means that it can also be rapidly resolved.

2.6.2 Chronic Disease/Illness

The burden of chronic diseases is increasing in the world. Such illness has also been part of the focus of many sociological studies because of peculiar attributes and their increasing burden all over the world. The WHO set a goal to reduce the burden of chronic disease by 2 % every year, thereby saving up to 35 million lives by 2015 (WHO 2005). The goal was set following a realisation that chronic diseases are the major cause of death in almost all countries, accounting for up to 60 % of all causes of deaths: 4.9 million people die as a result of tobacco use; 2.6 million people die as a result of being overweight or obese; 4.4 million people die as a result of raised total cholesterol levels; 7.1 million people die as a result of raised blood pressure (WHO 2005). A chronic disease/illness often presents as a medical condition, which makes an individual perceptually and perpetually ill. Major chronic diseases include heart disease and stroke (cardiovascular diseases), cancer, asthma, chronic obstructive pulmonary disease (chronic respiratory diseases), diabetes, obesity, ulcers, sickle cell diseases, and hypertension. Chronic diseases have a significant impact on the population health and by 2015 will be a leading cause of death in Nigeria and many other poor countries (WHO 2005).

The characteristics of chronic diseases include:

1. **Slow onset**: this is the major attribute of chronic diseases. It may take several years to develop or to manifest any form of symptom. Smoking takes a long time to affect the smokers. Cancer may take several years to manifest even when one has the risk. Chronic diseases have a slow progression.
2. **Protracted course**: Even when a chronic disease is symptomatic, the sufferer may live with it for several years, especially with proper medical management. For this reason, chronic diseases impoverish millions of (already poor) households because such diseases often gulp a lot of expenditures: its management is usually protracted and expensive.
3. **Usually non-communicable**: chronic diseases are sometimes called non-communicable diseases (NCDs). One cannot contract a majority of the chronic diseases by mere contact with a sufferer. However, based on the other four attributes of chronic illness/diseases, HIV/AIDS is a chronic disease that can be transmitted from one person to the other (see Sect. 12.3).
4. **Chronic diseases are not self-limiting**: the medical condition often gets worse with age or time. This implies that they have a long span and are often irreversible. Even when the disease pathogens are removed, the condition may reappear.

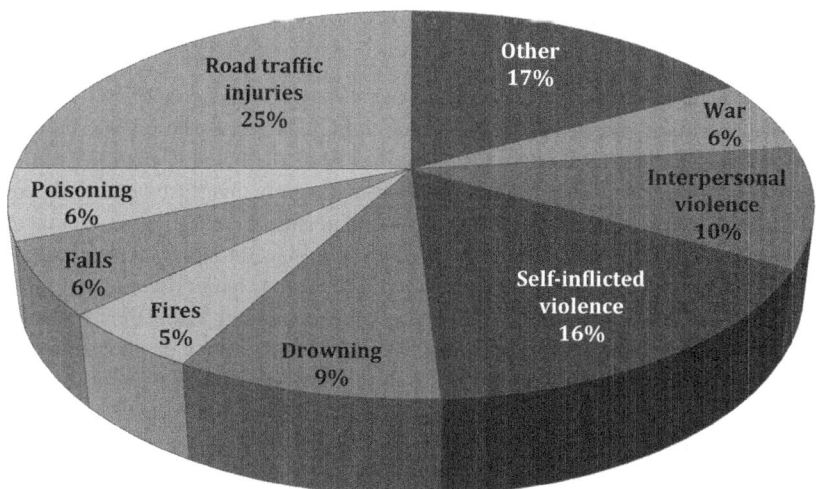

Fig. 2.2 The global burden of injuries by causes (Source: Peden et al. (2002, p. 9))

5. **Treatable but not curable**: chronic diseases are preventable, and they can also be managed, but a majority are not curable. This is why the diseases constitute a major health burden in the world today.

2.6.3 Injuries or Accidents

Injuries or accidents also constitute another form of health problem. An injury is usually sudden and may lead to a serious or permanent disability or death. Most of these medical conditions are always in the emergency unit or on a priority list in any triage system. Road accidents are the major sources of accidents especially, in the developing world. Workplace injuries also account for a substantial number of deaths each year. Most accidents are usually unintentional and random. Injuries or accidents include drowning, fire-related burns, fall-related injuries, poisoning, interpersonal violence, self-inflicted injuries, and war injuries. Approximately, more than 5 million people die and over 100 million suffer from non-fatal injuries (sometimes permanent disabilities) annually (Peden et al. 2002; WHO 2010). While the global percentage of deaths from road traffic injuries is about 25 %, the percentage in Africa is about 45 % (WHO 2010). Figure 2.2 shows the global distribution of injuries by cause. Management of injuries require rapid and responsive health care and other relevant agencies.

2.6.4 Mental Disease/Illness

Mental health simply refers to the level of psychological well-being of an individual. This often has to do with the brain vis-à-vis thought, feelings, sensation, and intuition. About 14 % of the global burden of disease has been attributed to neuropsychiatric disorders (Prince et al. 2007). Mental problems frequently manifest with behavioural changes that represent an infraction on the social norms of the society. A mental disorder is socially disastrous to the individual and could lead to total incapacitation or exemption from normal roles in the society. There are two major divisions of mental illness, which include neurosis (minor) and psychosis (major). While the former does not usually involve organic (brain) breakdown, the latter usually does. Examples of neurosis include: obsessive-compulsive disorder, anxiety disorders, post-traumatic stress disorder, phobia, dissociative disorder, minor depression, hypochondria, hysteria, and puerperal neurosis. Psychosis involves loss of contact with reality. It is generally the worst form of mental disorder. Examples of psychosis include bipolar disorder, schizophrenia, depression, substance-induced mental disorder, dementia (Alzheimer), delusional disorder, and epilepsy. A mental disorder may not necessarily lead to death, but it is disabling—it could be acute or chronic. Sartorius (2007) observed that stigma attached to mental illness is the main obstacle to the provision of care for people living with mental disorders. The stigma is a mark or label on those who are ill and their generations (see Sect. 8.4.2 for the theory of stigma).

2.7 Cultural Beliefs of Illness Causation

In all cultures, there are cultural classifications of disease aetiology or lay understanding of illness. This is usually based on the traditions and belief systems. This implies that cultural beliefs affect the perception of aetiology of diseases (Sylvia 2000). Most of these beliefs are not coherent with the biomedical beliefs and are sometimes unscientific. Irrespective of value judgment about such beliefs, the realities of such beliefs cannot be debunked, so also the realities of such causal connections. It is often the case for scientists to consider some local beliefs about causality implausible, inexplicit, and inconsiderable in scientific explanations. However, local beliefs are relevant in understanding the population health and in drawing behavioural interventions. Sometimes, such beliefs are misconceptions, which need to be addressed. Specifically, disease causation is often divided into four types: natural, supernatural, mystical, and hereditary/genetic.

2.7.1 Natural Causes

A natural cause refers to the biomedical explanation of a disease. This conforms to the germ theory of disease. The explanation is based on pathogenic causation such as microbial agents including viruses, bacteria, worms, and fungi. This also includes injuries and accidents such as broken bones and the ingestion of bad substances into the body. O'Neil (2006) observed that other forms of natural causation include :

1. Organic breakdown or deterioration (e.g., tooth decay, heart failure, senility)
2. Obstruction (e.g., kidney stones, arterial blockage due to plaque build-up)
3. Imbalance (e.g., too much or too little of specific hormones and salts in the blood)
4. Malnutrition (e.g., too much or too little food, insufficient proteins, vitamins, or minerals)

This explanation is sometimes called mechanistic or naturalistic explanation of disease causation. The diseases categorised with natural causes can be clinically or medically diagnosed. Traditional African societies hold a coherent view on the biomedical explanation of illness as it relates to natural causes, although some diseases may be explained based on multiple causalities. For instance, small pox may be explained from a natural cause, and it can also be attributed to anger of the god of small-pox (called *Sanpanna*) among the Yoruba of western Nigeria. This means that, despite the natural cause attached to a disease, there could be other explanations, and sometimes multiple therapies have to be employed.

2.7.2 Supernatural Causes

There is also a supernatural causation of illness. As Conco (1967) and Omonzejele (2008) explained, this is the spiritual construction invoked to explain the "uncommon or out-of-the-ordinary" types of sickness. It is further observed that it is made use of at a point where ordinary empirical methods of treatment and explanation have failed. This typically deals with divine attribution of illness. With the emergence of modern religions, such as Christianity and Islam, there is attribution of diseases to God. Such diseases may come as punishment for misdoings or sins. References to divine infliction of diseases/plagues can be cited from both the Bible and Quran in historical times. Especially among most religious adherents, there is a fatalistic belief that disease or health comes from God. Such infliction will usually present with medically unexplained symptoms or with medically explained symptoms that are beyond medical remedies. This is a part of the belief system and such diseases require pleasing the God through repentance, fasting, and prayers.

Disease could also come from the gods, spirits, deities, and other supernatural entities such as wizards and witches. This traditional perspective of illness describes a different source of evil (illness) caused by invisible spirits that exist within and outside human social boundaries (Foster 1976). These spirits inhabit trees, rivers, lakes, mountains, and deserted places around the habitation (Bhasin 2007, p. 6). In most African societies, there are gods or deities of the land who need to be appeased from time to time, both at the individual and community levels. Lack of appeasement from either of the levels could be detrimental. The people of the Kalahari Desert also attribute diseases and health to Hishe (god). So also the Bantu of South Africa (like many other groups in Africa) believes that supernatural entities can inflict pain or disease on individuals. Conco (1967, p. 288) specifically explained that

2.7 Cultural Beliefs of Illness Causation

> [i]n varying degrees most rural Africans believe that it [supernatural causation] explains all complexes of extra-ordinary diseases. They also believe that it is true, and this implies that they are psychologically convinced, though they cannot give conclusive empirical grounds for its truth. It is a metaphysical article of faith, and as such it cannot be verified or falsified empirically, though it always has some claim to being factual.

The belief in supernatural causality is widespread in both rural and urban communities and across groups whether educated or not. Foster (1976) and Garro (2000) noted that, among several people, there is a wide belief in the supernatural cause of illness: the Mono of Liberia and Abron of Cote d'ivoire believe that death is usually caused by external forces. Jegede (2002, 2005) observed that among the Yoruba of western Nigeria, illness can be traced to enemies (*ota*), witchcraft (*aje*), sorcery or wizard (*oso*), gods (*orisa*), and ancestors (*ebora*). The belief of the supernatural causes of illness is still highly prevalent and central in the explanation of illness in Africa (Omonzejele 2008).

In cases of supernatural causes, diseases are diagnosed through spiritual means, especially through consultation with religious clerics or traditional healers. It is believed that these categories of people have spiritual power to detect and prescribe a course of action in the treatment of illness. Such therapeutic procedures are not amenable to science or are simply beyond empirical comprehension and explanations.

2.7.3 Mystical Causes

The mystical causes are a part of what Foster (1976) described as a personalistic cause of illness. Mystical retribution is defined as acts in violation of some taboo or moral injunctions, which could lead to illness (Murdock 1978). In traditional African societies, illness can result from the violation of vital norms and values of the society. These norms are often concerned with the traditions and spirituality of the community. Specifically, many African societies believe that some individuals have "evil eyes" or possess a mystical power that can be used to inflict pain or illness on other people in the society.

Illness as a result of mystical causes also present with symptoms that cannot be explained medically or where explanation is possible, biomedical treatment is futile. Such patients are often referred to the traditional or faith-based healers for appropriate deliverance or salvation from such illness.

2.7.4 Hereditary and Genetic Causes

Hereditary diseases can be passed from one generation of same family to another. While heredity is linked with genetics, not all genetic disorders are heritable. Most hereditary or genetic diseases have natural causes, and some of them can be explained from supernatural causes. Many African societies (e.g., the Yoruba of West Africa) believe that madness can be inflicted on a family and it can continue from one generation to the other. The Yoruba call hereditary disease *aisan idile*, literarily translated as "a family disease." Treatment depends on the perception of the aetiology, whether natural or supernatural. Some biomedical hereditary/genetic diseases include autism, cancer, dwarfism, sickle cell anemia, cystic fibrosis, albinism, color blindness, myotonic dystrophy, porphyria, and some forms of mental illness (e.g., Huntington's disease). Hereditary diseases have effects on the relationship patterns in the society as many individuals may not marry from a family where a hereditary disease is perceived to exist.

One critical way of perceiving hereditary or genetic disease is through fatalism, especially among Islamic communities of Africa. This is the attribution of such a condition to the will of God claiming it has been destined that a person would have such a medical condition. The Yorubas call this *kadara* or *ayanmon* (i.e., destiny). Especially in heritable genetic disorders in children and adults, this fatalistic idea prevails. The idea can also be applied in cases of injuries and accidents. This idea serves as a coping mechanism and aids reintegration into the society. Since it is the will of God, discrimination is termed against the will of God. It helps the individual to live and surrender to destiny, fate, or an act of God. Unfortunately, the idea does not help in preventive measure. Fatalistic individuals tend to accept everything that comes their way—if it has been destined, it is beyond human preventive measure.

In conclusion, this chapter has dealt with a lot of issues regarding health, disease, and illness. It starts with the polemics on the definition of health by de-constructing some of the available definitions. In the case of health, the goal is to work towards a state of perfection. No matter how health is defined, nobody can be in a perfect state—whether "adaptation" or "a state of completeness" is used. This argument does not, however, mean that available definitions should not be reviewed.

References

Awofeso, N. (2012). Re-defining 'Health'. (Re: Üstün & Jakob 2005). http://www.who.int/bulletin/bulletin_board/83/ustun11051/en/. Accessed 5 May 2012.
Bhasin, V. (2007). Medical anthropology: A review. *Ethno Med, 1*(1), 1–20.
Bice, T. (1976). Comments on health indicators: Methodological perspectives. *International Journal of Health Services, 6,* 509–520.
Bircher, J. (2005). Towards a dynamic definition of health and disease. *Medicine, Health Care and Philosophy, 8,* 335–341.
Blaxter, M. (1990). *Health and lifestyles*. New York: Routledge.
Blaxter, M. (2010). *Health* (2nd ed.). Cambridge: Polity.
Boorse, C. (1975). On the distinction between disease and illness. *Philosophy of Public Affairs, 5,* 49–68.
Boorse, C. (1977). Health as a theoretical concept. *Philosophy of Science, 44,* 542–573.
Callahan, D. (1973). The WHO definition of 'health'. *The Hastings Center Studies, 1*(3), 77–87.
Conco, W. Z. (1967). The African Bantu traditional practice of medicine: Some preliminary observations. *Social Science & Medicine, 6,* 283–322.
Fabrega, H. Jr. (1973). Towards a model of illness behaviour. *Medical Care, 11*(6), 470–484.
Foster, G. M. (1976). Disease etiologies in non-western medical system. *American anthropologist, 78*(4), 773–782.

References

Garro, L. C. (2000). Cultural meaning, explanations of illness, and the development of comparative frameworks. *Ethnology, 39*(4), 305–334.

Godlee, F. (2011). What is health? *British Medical Journal, 343,* d4817.

Huber, M., Knottnerus, J. A., Green, L., van der Horst, H., Jadad, A. R., Kromhout, D., Leonard, B., Kate L., Loureiro, M. I., van der Meer, J. W. M., Schnabel, P., Smith, R., van Weel, C., & Smid, H. (2011). How should we define health? *British Medical Journal, 343,* d4163. doi:10.1136/bmj.d4163.

Jadad, A. R., & O'Grady, L. (2008). How should health be defined? *British Medical Journal, 10;* 337, a2900. doi: 10.1136/bmj.a2900.

Jegede, A. S. (2002). The Yoruba cultural construction of health and illness. *Nordic Journal of African Studies, 11*(3), 322–335.

Jegede, A. S. (2005). The notion of 'were' in Yoruba conception of mental illness. *Nordic Journal of African Studies, 14*(1), 117–126.

Kingma, E. (2007). What is it to be healthy? *Analysis, 67*(294), 128–133.

Lancet Editorial. (2009). What is health? The ability to adapt. *Lancet, 378*(9666) 781. doi:10.1016/S0140-6736(09)60456-6.

Larson, J. S. (1999). The conceptualization of health. *Medical Care Research and Review, 56*(2), 123–136.

Murdock, G. P., Wilson, S. F., & Frederick, V. (1978). World distribution of theories of illness. *Ethnology, 17*(4), 449–470.

Nordenfeldt, L. (1993). On the relevance and importance of the notion of disease. *Theoretical Medicine, 14,* 15–26.

Omonzejele, P. F. (2008). African concepts of health, disease, and treatment: An ethical inquiry. *Explore: The Journal of Science and Healing, 4*(2), 120–126.

O'Neil, D. (2006). Explanation of illness. http://anthro.palomar.edu/medical/med_1.htm. Accessed 10 May 2012.

Pannenborg, C. (1979). *A new international health order: An inquiry into the international relations of world health and medical care*. The Netherlands: Sijthoff and Noordhoff.

Parsons, T. (1972). Definition of health and illness in the light of American values and social structure. In E. G. Jaco (Ed.), *Patients, physicians and illness* (pp. 107–127). New York: Free.

Peden, M., McGee, K., & Sharma, G. (2002). *The injury chart book: A graphical overview of the global burden of injuries*. Geneva: WHO.

Prince, M., Patel, V., Saxena, S., Maj, M., Maselko, J., Phillips, M. R., & Rahman, A. (2007). No health without mental health. *Lancet, 370,* 859–877.

Saracci, R. (1997). The World Health Organization needs to reconsider its definition of health. *British Medical Journal, 314,* 1409–1410.

Sartorius, N. (2007). Stigma and mental health. *Lancet, 370,* 810–811.

Simmons, S. J. (1989). Health: A concept analysis. *International Journal of Nursing Studies, 36*(2), 155–161.

Stempsey, W. E. (2000). A pathological view of disease. *Theoretical Medicine, 21,* 321–330.

Sylvia, O. (2000). Disease etiology and traditional African society. *Africa, 55*(4), 583–590.

Temple, L. K. F., McLeod, R. S., Gallinger, S., & Wright, J. G. (2001). Defining disease in the genomics era. *Science, 293,* 807–808.

Tengland, P. (2007). A two-dimensional theory of health. *Theoretical Medicine and Bioethics, 28,* 257–284.

Wood, P. H. N. (1986). Health and disease and its importance for models relevant to health research. In B. Z. Nizetic, H. G. Pauli, & P. G. Svensson (Eds.), *Scientific approaches to health and health care* (pp. 57–70). Copenhagen: World Health Organization.

WHO. (1948). Preamble to the constitution of the WHO. Geneva.

WHO. (2005). *Preventing chronic diseases: A vital investment*. Geneva: WHO.

WHO. (2010). *Violence, injuries and disabilities: A biennial report 2008–2009*. Geneva: WHO.

Chapter 3
Health Behaviour and Illness Behaviour

3.1 Introduction

Having discussed the conceptions of health, disease, and illness in the previous chapter, this chapter presents another major theme in medical sociological studies: health and illness behaviours. Health and illness behaviours for various kinds of medical conditions have been widely researched in sociology. Sociologists continue to investigate how people respond to their health or illness condition. The basic concern includes the what, how, and why of health and illness behaviours. Generally, understanding human behaviour has been the bedrock of sociological studies. Sociologists want to understand, explain, control, and predict human behaviours. Understanding human behaviour involves the comprehension of the motivation behind behaviour. Why do people behaviour the way they do? What are the factors that trigger a particular behaviour in any given situation? In health-seeking behaviour, it is important to understand what people may or usually do in case of any concern about their health. For instance, what would people do to prevent cancer or any other illness conditions? Would people stop sun-bathing to prevent skin cancer or use a condom to prevent HIV? Understanding the use of appropriate preventive and treatment measures is a central focus in the study of health and illness behaviours.

3.2 Towards a Definition of Health Behaviour

Health behaviour (HB) is synonymous with preventive health behaviour (PHB). It refers to a person's way of preventing a disease, defect, injury, and disability. In what has been cited as a classic definition, Kasl and Cobb (1966, p. 246) posited that "health behaviour refers to those activities undertaken by a person believing himself [or herself] to be healthy, for the purpose of preventing disease or detecting it in an asymptomatic stage." In other words, HB is an individually approved, socially appraised, and medically recommended action voluntarily undertaken by a person who believes himself or herself to be healthy that tends to prevent the occurrence of an undesirable health condition or detect it in an asymptomatic stage (Alonzo 1993).

The critical issue in the definition is that the individual perceives himself or herself to be healthy and carries out certain modalities to avert the occurrence of ill-health. This is why HB is the same as PHB.

Closely related to HB is protective health behaviour, which is defined as "any behaviour performed by a person, regardless of his or her perceived or actual health status, in order to protect, promote, or maintain his or her health, whether or not such behaviour is objectively effective toward that end" (Harris and Guten 1979, p. 18). In this case, action is performed regardless of the health status of the individual. This implies that an individual may have perceived good health or not. Whether HB or protective health behaviour, one common ground is that it is a form of behaviour regarding personal health among individuals. Such behaviour may be objectively effective or not. This mostly happens as a result of lack of knowledge about appropriate medically recommended preventive health practices. For instance, use of appropriate malaria preventive measures is still low in many malaria endemic countries (Karanja et al. 2002, Amzat 2011). Invariably, medical sociology is immersed in showing patterns of behaviour whether effective or not in prevention and disease control. In either case, there could be intervention to intensify the effective behaviour or change the ineffective behaviour.

> Furthermore, HB includes activities engaged in and modalities used by the individual voluntarily, and in specific instances under threat of sanction, and by society to (a) prevent and (b) detect disease, defect, injury and disability, (c) promote and enhance health, and (d) protect the individual and collectivity from risk of and actual disease, defect, injury and disability (Alonzo 1993, p. 1024).

For instance, the regulations regarding a driver's licence are to protect the society from untrained drivers who may cause accidents. Health behaviour may involve simple adoption of preventive devices or advance diagnostic checks. A wide range of HB practice may include moderate eating, adequate sleep, keeping emergency phone numbers, getting enough relaxation, procurement of first aid kit at home, regular medical checkups, avoidance of unsafe environments, watching of weight, regular exercise, limit or avoidance of smoking, avoidance of overworking, limiting foods like sugar and fats, seeking health tips from professionals, and limiting or avoidance of alcoholic beverages.

The aforementioned are general health behavioural tips, although preventive health behaviour could be disease specific such as protected sex to avoid sexually transmitted diseases (STDs) including HIV, the use of insecticide treated nets (ITN) to prevent malaria, or the immunisation of children against deadly childhood diseases (e.g., measles and polio). For instance, on the prevention of malaria, Nuwaha (2002), in a study in Mabara, Uganda, claimed that avoiding mosquitoes was the most common approach to preventing malaria. Other preventive strategies mentioned include improved sanitation, clearing of bushes around homes, good nutrition, burning mosquito coils, and taking anti-malarial drugs. Findings from a study among market women in Nigeria also confirmed this as a majority of respondents claimed they utilised many measures including herbal remedies, indoor insecticides, and coils (Jegede et al. 2006).

A study also investigated aspects of adolescents' health-enhancing behaviours in four African countries (Kenya, Namibia, Uganda, and Zimbabwe). It was observed that up to 70 % of the participants engaged in many healthy practices including non-tobacco use, limiting alcohol consumption, non-drug use, washing hands before eating, were abstinent or had used a condom during their last sexual encounter, physically active for at least 60 min per day, and walk or bike to school (Peltzer 2009, p. 172). These are part of the general health practices that often enhance the health of an individual. If such preventive practices are widespread, this could improve the health status in Africa.

An empirical study (Harris and Guten 1979, p. 28) established the importance of the concept of HB. The study concluded that

1. Practically everyone performs at least some regular, routine behaviour for the purpose of protecting his or her health, and most people perform many, as well as a wide range, of these behaviours. This is still valid as everyone is immersed in protecting his/her health. Illness is generally undesirable and people implement many modalities to avert the occurrence of diseases. Right from childhood, individuals are socialised to know risky behaviours to health. Individuals grow to modify and intensify various forms of HB.
2. Activity concerning nutrition and eating habits is part of the most common health behavioural patterns. In fact, some individuals even skip food in order to control their weight and remain healthy. Other common PHB include rest and relaxation, physical activity, and other personal health practices.
3. Empirically identified dimensions of PHB include personal health practices, safety practices, preventive health care, environmental hazard avoidance, and harmful substance avoidance. Prevention is the key to good health. This is why implementation of health behaviour could save individuals from health costs, pain, or defect.
4. The study noted that PHB does not vary substantially by health condition. This implies that regardless of health condition, an individual implements various dimensions of health practices to remain healthy. It is thus important to add that certain social determinants (e.g., class, education, and age) modify such practices.

3.3 Health Behaviour and Interventions

Health behaviour has been conceived as preventive health practices. Clark and Leavell (1953) proposed three stages of prevention. They identified primary, secondary, and tertiary preventions. It is possible to prevent the occurrence of disease (primary) or to avoid extreme damage (tertiary). Table 3.1 shows the stages and activities in various stages of preventions. The primary prevention occurs before the occurrence of the disease. It involves protective and preventive activities such as health education, marriage counselling, genetic screening, a good standard of nutrition, vaccination or immunisation, personal hygiene, environmental sanitation, protection against occupational hazards, protection from accidents, taking of balanced nutrients, and avoidance of other risk behaviours.

Table 3.1 The three stages of prevention

Stage of prevention	Stage of disease	Primary objectives	Interventions
Primary	Pre-disease	Disease avoidance	Health promotion Information, education and enlightenment, preventive actions
Secondary	Latent disease	Early detention	Screening and detection, Prompt treatment and limitation of disability
Tertiary	Symptomatic disease	Minimise damage or pain	Drug compliance/adherence, recuperation or recovery process, rehabilitation and re-integration

Secondary prevention (also called health maintenance) involves perception of the possibility of ill-health and resultant activities to arrest the disease process and restore health. This involves various detection activities such as HIV testing and other forms of screening aimed at detecting what could be wrong. One of the aims of health maintenance is to avoid pathological damages and deter the communicability of infectious disease. At this stage, the individual implements action necessary to identify specific illnesses or conditions at an early stage and seeks professional help for prompt intervention to prevent or limit disability. The third stage is tertiary prevention, which aims at reducing the negative impact of established disease by restoring function and reducing disease-related complications (Sosa-Estani et al. 2012). This is the stage of recuperation (after adequate treatment). At the stage, an individual is expected to comply/adhere with a therapeutic regimen. The goal of this stage is to prevent complications, further damages, and pain from the disease. The essence of tertiary prevention is to regain health and resume functional roles. In cases of chronic diseases, this stage involves a positive living with the condition.

Health behaviour interventions often focus on individuals at high risk (or high risk groups [HRG]) and risk behaviours. The HRG includes those individuals who, as a result of their social conditions and biological attributes, are exposed to certain diseases in the society. Heinemann et al. (2012) observed that risk factors are genetic, physiological, behavioural, and socioeconomic characteristics of individuals that place them in a cohort of the population that is more likely to develop a particular health problem or disease than the rest of the population. Risk does not automatically translate to development of a disease condition. Risk is often combined with exposure for a disease to occur. For instance, Heinemann et al. further observed that risk has three major categories in cardiovascular disease. The first category includes somatic factors, which mainly include body characteristics such as blood pressure and body weight. The second includes behavioural factors such as smoking, poor nutrition, lack of physical exercise, high alcohol consumption, and drug abuse. The third are strains including exposure in the occupational, social, and private spheres. The second and the third factors are of utmost importance in this discussion—how behavioural patterns and structural factors put an individual at risk of certain disease conditions.

In addition, some diseases have defined risk groups such as kwashiorkor among children. Due to a high level of poverty, some African children are at risk of being underweight and micronutrient deficiency, which could account for the high prevalence of kwashiorkor in the region. Another leading cause of burden of disease and vulnerability in Africa includes poor social amenities such as water, sanitation, and hygiene. The high prevalence of diarrhoea is due to poor water supply. Critical deprivations and poor infrastructure are also adverse factors that affect risk exposure.

In the case of malaria in Africa, certain groups have been identified to have a high risk of contracting malaria. The most vulnerable group is children under five years old. WHO (2012) has observed that young children stand a high risk of malaria infection and are vulnerable to severe malaria disease when infected; 85 % of all malaria deaths occur in children in Africa (WHO 2012). The under-five children are yet to develop protective levels of immunity against malaria parasites. Pregnant women are also vulnerable because the immunity of women is impaired during pregnancy. Low birth weight and severe anaemia are common results of malaria in pregnancy. It has been noted that poverty breeds malaria and malaria impoverishes people and the society due to the amount of household income devoted to malaria prevention and treatment.

Mosquitoes usually breed in poorly planned neighbourhood where there is standing water. Because of the poor housing facilities, there might be poor sanitation facilities in most poor households. Most windows and doors might not be screened to prevent mosquitoes from entering the home. The poor usually have little or no access to information and education about public health. They might not have basic knowledge of ITN or available drugs. Therefore, they continue to engage in risk behaviour. Most of the available treatment and preventive measures may also not be affordable to them. Refugees (or internally displaced persons) and migrants or seasonal workers who move from malaria-free areas to malaria-endemic ones are also at greater risk because they have inadequate protective immunity. This is why travelers, especially those coming from malaria-free areas, need to take medical precautions when entering malaria-endemic areas.

3.3.1 Risk Behaviours

Risk behaviours are actions or personal dispositions that expose individuals to diseases. *Health-risk behaviour* can also be defined as any activity undertaken by people with a frequency or intensity that increases risk of disease or injury (Steptoe and Wardle 2004). Heinemann et al. (2012) observed that some risk behaviours make some individuals vulnerable to more than one disease. For example, cigarette smoking is associated with coronary artery disease, stroke, and lung cancer. In addition, risk behaviours sometimes exhibit an indirect relationship with a disease condition. A study, for instance, found that sexting among youth is correlated with early sexual initiation, which could lead to teenage pregnancy or risky sexual behaviour and may expose the individual to sexually related problems (Dake et al. 2012; Temple et al. 2012). Sexting is the act of sending sexually explicit messages or photographs, primarily between mobile phones and other chat-enabled networks or devices. Like in other continents, sexting is becoming a prominent problem among African youth who have access to forms of information technologies thereby exposing adolescents especially to sexual content and promoting sexual "experimentation."

From the foregoing discussions, it can be observed that there are five basic forms of health risk behaviours. Some of these risk behaviours have been explained among various groups in different studies (Mpofu et al. 2006; Greif et al. 2011; Lundberg et al. 2012).

3.3.1.1 Sedentary Lifestyle

Sedentary lifestyle signifies inadequate physical exercise; it is common among Africans. Some individuals engage in limited physical activities, which could account for the accumulation of fat deposits and increased propensity to being overweight or obese. Derman et al. (2008) observed that regular physical activity in the form of exercise training has the ability to prevent or delay the onset of certain illness and disease. This is because physical activity acts on the cardiovascular system and could induce "favourable changes in metabolism, body mass and body composition" (Derman et al. 2008). Most people in Africa consume a lot of carbohydrate-based solid food, and there is often no program for moderate physical activities.

3.3.1.2 Alcohol and Drug Use

A high intake of alcohol has been liked with various ill-health conditions. Many individuals still do not drink "responsibly." Apart from refined beer, there are locally brewed alcohols in many African societies. Such brews usually have a very high alcohol content. Drinking is often a daily affair. Alcohol use is increasing among women across African countries (Martinez et al. 2011). Alcohol-related morbidities include mental health disorders such as substance dependence and depression, and physical morbidities such as liver diseases and HIV infection (Hulka and Moorman 2008; Marmorstein 2009; Shuper et al. 2010). Apart from alcohol, the use of ingestible drugs is gradually becoming a social problem. Some over-the-counter drugs are frequently abused. Mostly, various forms of cough syrups are now consumed indiscriminately. The cough syrups are mainly licit drugs, but because of loose pharmaceutical regulation in most African cities, they can be bought and consumed without any medical prescription.

3.3.1.3 Smoking Behaviour and Tobacco Use

Smoking behaviour is a major cause of morbidity and mortality. Smoking of tobacco is a risk factor of many diseases (e.g., cardiovascular diseases) while dependence on tobacco is also a disease. For instance, most smokers in South Africa start smoking habits from childhood and adolescent stages (Mashita et al. 2011). Thus many of them smoke throughout their lifetime. In North Africa, smoking is very common among all categories of the population. Egypt has the highest rate of smoking in the developing Arab world—daily smokers constitute 33.5 % of the total population, of which 19.6 % is under the age of 15 (Islam and Johnson 2007). The ban of tobacco adverts in many African countries has not yielded the desired results as the trend is still increasing. Apart from smoking, tobacco is used in other forms like drinking as tea, mixed with food, or sniffed.

3.3.1.4 Sexual Behaviour

Unprotected sexual contact and multiple sexual partners have been implicated in many deadly diseases. Such diseases include chlamydia, genital warts, herpes, gonorrhea, hepatitis, syphilis, and HIV. Some of these diseases could lead to permanent functional disability or even death. The low life expectancy in Africa is partly a result of HIV, which affects all age groups. Unprotected sex and the commercialisation of sex (or transactional sex) are common risky sexual behaviours. Unprotected sex involves sex without any form of protection, such as condoms. In Madagascar, there is a high prevalence of unprotected sex (informally called one-night stands) at social venues such as parties, clubs (pubs), and hotels (Khan et al. 2008). Commercial or transactional sex implies sex in exchange for monetary gains or other forms of favours. Commercial sex workers (CSWs) are usually at high risk of STDs, especially in instances in which sex without protection can be negotiated for higher monetary costs.

Forced sex and early sexual experiences are also pervasive and a constituent part of risk accumulation. Sexual violence is on the rise: 31 % of women in Tanzania, 59 % in rural Ethiopia (WHO 2005); 13–16 % in Kenya (WHO 2005; Adudans et al. 2011), and 10 % of adolescents in South Africa have been sexually abused. A study in ten southern African states (Botswana, Lesotho, Malawi, Mozambique, Namibia, Swaziland, Zambia, Zimbabwe, Tanzania, and South Africa) revealed that 19.6 % (4,432/25,840) of female students and 21.1 % (4,080/21,613) of male students aged 11–16 years had experienced forced or coerced sex (Andersson et al. 2012). The high prevalence of forced sex is part of the reason for the high incidence of HIV/AIDS in the region. Apart from STDs and HIV, teenage pregnancy and abortions are part of the consequences of risky sexual behaviours. Annually, over 6 million abortions are carried out in Africa with less than 5 % carried out under safe conditions (Guttmacher Institute 2012). Abortion is still illegal in a majority of the African countries, hence, illegal abortions are performed with limited safety precautions, which often results in a very high number of complications or mortality.

3.3.1.5 Dietary Behaviour

The first major danger of dietary behaviour is poor nutrition. This may imply nonavailability of food at all. Famine is prevalent in many parts of Africa, such as Niger, Somalia, Ethiopia, Malawi, and Rwanda. In this case, it is a national tragedy which imposes constrain on food intake (dietary behaviour). Many people are diseased or die as a result of famine. Apart from famine, poor nutrition also involves intake of an inappropriately balanced diet. This may also be a result of poverty. More than 41 % of people in sub-Saharan Africa live on less than $ 1 per day, and 32 % is undernourished (Hunger Project 2012). Most people consume food but without adequate calories or nutrients for good health. This is why there is a high prevalence of childhood deaths or stunted growth as a result of malnutrition.

Another dimension of poor nutrition is an unbalanced diet, often manifest in terms of too high a consumption of carbohydrates and fatty foods. This accounts for increasing rates of obesity in Africa. Although in many African societies, obesity is often perceived as evidence of good living, there is a gradual awareness of the dangers of obesity. Dietary behaviour has been linked with the prevalence of diabetes in Africa. In sub-Saharan Africa, prevalence and burden of type-2 diabetes are rising quickly, owing to rising rates of obesity, physical inactivity, and urbanisation (Levitt 2008), and the rate of undiagnosed diabetes is high and sufferers who are unaware of the disease are at a very high risk of chronic complications (Mbanya et al. 2010). Another extreme end is a deliberate malnutrition to control weight. This form of behaviour could also lead to a number of eating disorders such as anorexia and bulimia nervosa. These disorders are not confined to the western world as they have also been frequently reported in Africa (Szabo and Allwoood 2004, 2006).

In conclusion, most behavioural interventions often focus on *risk takers*, or those who engage in behaviours that put them at risk of certain diseases. It is important to note that some public health interventions focus on other social circumstances or determinants of health (see Chap. 4). The focus of intervention on the health-risk behaviour is vital in disease control (Băban and Crăciun 2007). This is the bedrock of all prevention, protection, detection, and promotion activities both at individual and societal levels.

3.4 Towards a Definition of Illness Behaviour

Illness behaviour is a concept that was introduced in the late 1950s by David Mechanic to depict the "variability in reactions to symptoms and illness, and to identify the various socio-cultural, environmental and psychological factors that affect such reactions" (Mechanic 1995, p. 1208). Illness behaviour is further conceived as "the varying ways individuals respond to bodily indications, how they monitor internal states, define and interpret symptoms, make attributions, take remedial actions and utilise various sources of informal and formal care" (Mechanic 1962, 1995). Inaction is also a form of response to illness. One major difference between health and illness behaviour is that in the former, the person defines himself or herself as healthy and tries to maintain his/her health status or detect if there could be anything wrong, while in the latter, the person defines himself/herself as ill and tries to find ways of recuperating. In other words, illness behaviour is the way an individual believing himself or herself to be ill interprets and responds to signs and symptoms in order to achieve wellness.

3.4 Towards a Definition of Illness Behaviour

Invariably, there is a health problem or condition affecting the individual. Some may require prompt care, especially in the case of acute diseases. The lived experience of illness and desire to restore health are often a personal responsibility of the individual. This is because an individual has the liberty to take action that is deemed efficacious. Meanwhile, there are four basic questions an individual needs to answer in a case of illness. For those underage, the question will be answered by caretakers. The questions include the "what, where, when, and how."

Determination of what is wrong and what measures should be applied are the two critical starting points. A person defines what is wrong by assessing the symptoms through the nature of illness experience and bodily indications. The feeling of pain and discomfort provides the cues for the individual to define what might be wrong or relate the experience to significant others or caregivers. The local or personal understanding forms the basis for the definition of the symptoms. Before contact with any caregiver, there are various personal appraisals which could determine the need to seek care from other domains or use certain measures at an informal level.

The foregoing leads us to the second question, which is *where* care can be obtained. When there are several options, an individual needs to weigh various possibilities and opportunities. Despite the availability of different providers, there are also opportunities at informal levels. In most developing countries, there is a possibility of informal consultation with significant others or agents (e.g., patent medicine sellers) at an informal level. It is also possible to obtain over-the-counter drugs. This shows that self-medication is still a possibility.

In Africa, certain illnesses are seen as amenable to treatment by modern medical practitioners, while others are considered best treated by traditional methods or a mixture of both (Beiersmann et al. 2007; Deressa 2007). It has been observed that a large proportion of malaria cases are treated outside the official health care system (Mukanga et al. 2012; Rutta et al. 2012). Mukanga et al. (2012) observed that, among the Iganga population (Uganda), there was awareness that the community health workers (CHWs) provide better treatment services for malaria, but a good proportion of respondents purchased drugs from medicine/drug stores for self-medication.

The next question deals with when the measure will be obtained. An individual needs to decide when to seek help from any caregiver. Early treatment is often advocated. Unfortunately, most disease conditions develop complications before many seek professional medical care. The question of "when" is often critical in chronic diseases. In the acute form or after an accident, a decision is often made very quickly. Some acute illnesses (e.g., medical emergencies) are thought to produce expedient care-seeking devoid of any prolonged social process (Alonzo 1980). The last question deals with "how" the measure will be applied or implemented. This involves various means of administering therapeutic measures and the interactional process involved (doctor-client interaction and consent and compliance). It may involve a selection of available options and therapeutic channels such as rectal, oral, intravenous, or surgical.

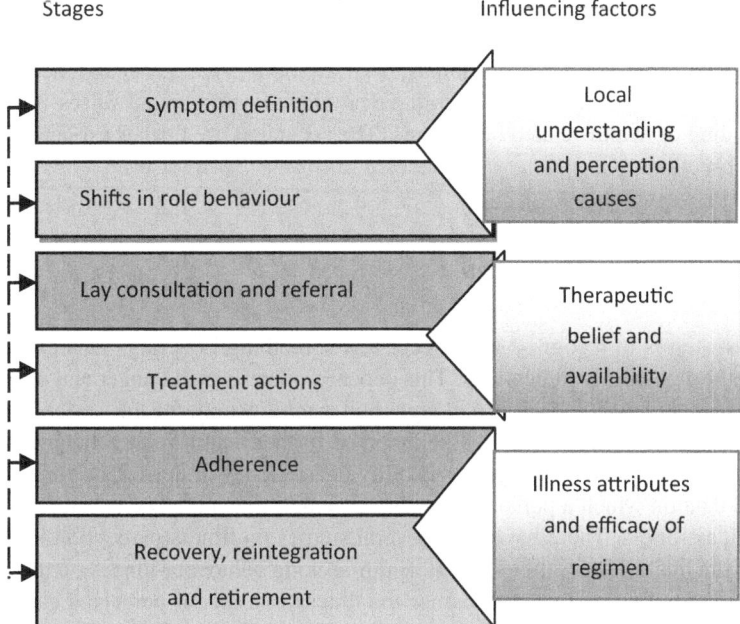

Fig. 3.1 Stages of illness behaviour

3.5 Stages of Illness Behaviour

There have been a number of suggestions on the trajectory of illness behaviour. Illness behaviour in this sense is synonymous with health-seeking behaviour. An ill person follows a number of steps in the quest for wellness. Chrisman (1977) identified five major stages while Igun (1979) recognised 11 stages. That of Igun is an expansion of the basic major steps. This section will explain Chrisman's (1977) five stages because his model is more concise, but one stage will be added to make it six stages. In 1977 Chrisman introduced a concept that he referred to as the health-seeking process, a model to conceptualise behaviour or the "steps taken by an individual who perceives a need for help as he/she attempts to solve a health problem" (Chrisman 1977, p. 353). He identifies five stages of health-seeking behaviour, which includes symptom definition, shifts in role behaviour, lay consultation and referral, treatment action, and adherence. Then, "recovery, reintegration, and retirement" is added as the last stage. Figure 3.1 presents the framework showing a downward movement from one stage to the next. Issues that may influence decisions are embedded.

This model shows the health-related actions that a sick person may exhibit, but they are not necessarily sequential as steps may be skipped (Chrisman 1977). It is also possible for some stages to occur simultaneously. As Chrisman (1977, p. 353) observed, "[I]f a sick person interacts with others at some point during the illness, he [or she] may be simultaneously receiving aid in categorising symptoms, bargaining for the legitimacy of avoiding role obligations, receiving support or information from peers, and obtaining treatment or practitioner suggestions." The stages or processes are from previous studies on illness behaviour (see Fabrega 1973; Kasl and Cobb 1966; Mechanic 1962; Suchman 1965; Twaddle 1969, 1974) and the sick role (Parsons 1951; Segall 1976), which have provided significant advances in the understanding of health-related behaviours. The six stages are further explained in the next subsections.

3.5.1 Symptom Definition

The first step is to recognise and accept that something is wrong. This can be observed through bodily indications. This depends on perceived danger and disability. Chrisman noted that the factors of *danger* and *disability* underlie this variable, which is significant in determining the likelihood of further health-related behaviours. In addition, factors such as symptom visibility or frequency of appearance are the perceptual data on which a person draws as the symptom experience is categorised, or defined, as illness. There have been several studies on illness perception in Africa. One of the major observations is that health-seeking behaviour hinges on the ability of an individual to correctly recognise the illness in terms of perceived causes and symptoms. Beliefs about the aetiology of illnesses also invariably dictate the type of therapies and healers to be consulted. General research in the area of treatment seeking has documented that this is related to sociocultural beliefs about the cause and cure of illness (Mwenesi et al. 1995).

3.5.2 Illness-Related Shift in Role Behaviour

Chrisman observed that relaxation or cessation of a person's social obligations because of illness-based restrictions or inabilities to fulfill obligations are part of the indicative factors. A gradual shift in role behaviour is more related to chronic diseases. Injuries or some acute diseases are often medically evaluated as emergent or urgent and have a high probability of producing death or disability if medical care is not expeditiously obtained (Alonzo 1980). In acute illness behaviour, there may be a sudden cessation of obligation due to hospitalisation or illness-imposed restrictions. On the other hand, chronic diseases often produce a gradual shift in role behaviour.

3.5.3 Lay Consultation and Social Referral

A person may call upon other individuals for aid in identifying an illness, for suggestions about treatment, and for recommendations of competent help (Chrisman 1977). Lay consultation involves communication with significant others about the nature and course of illness. During lay consultation, an individual may take certain treatment measures prescribed by the significant others. For instance, in managing childhood malaria, Afolabi et al. (2004), in a study conducted in Nigeria, observed that a majority of caregivers had given one form of treatment or the other before visiting official health centres. In a Tanzanian study among 652 caregivers, Nsimba et al. (2002) found that a total of 54 % of the mothers reported giving medication at home, 21 % had taken the children to other health facilities, and 3 % had visited traditional healers before referral to a modern health facility. More so, there may be a re-definition of illness based on the experience of the significant others. Generally, relatives and neighbours serve as the first contact and a source of social referrals. It has been reported that illness and pathology may not be reported if persons are able to *contain* its signs and symptoms of illness within socially defined situations and daily activities could not be interrupted (Alonzo 1979; Mechanic 1995). This signifies that illness will be reported if it is simply beyond containment, inflicts undesirable discomfort, or when the sufferer or significant others perceive dangers.

3.5.4 Treatment Actions/Initiation

For the purpose of assessing health care, treatment sources in Africa can be divided into three main categories: traditional, official, and self-treatment sources (McCombie 2002). The traditional treatment involves the use of traditional remedies or visits to traditional practitioners or faith-based healers. Use of official health facilities includes the use of hospitals, clinics, dispensaries, primary health care centres, and private care providers. Self-treatment, on the other hand, includes anything from home treatment with herbal remedies to the purchase and use of modern drugs. Home treatment or informal care refers to care, both affective and instrumental, provided in the domestic or private arena, mostly by women and often for family members, and mostly unpaid (Gabe et al. 2004). In an African setting, medical personnel can also provide informal care for relatives, friends and community members at a low cost. This has been part of the primary sources of treatment in Africa. The major issue is that treatment is initiated based on illness definition, availability of care providers, and other intervening variables. An individual, depending on the illness and available measures, may require one or more episode of treatment. If an illness has perceived mystical or supernatural causes, treatment would involve traditional methods of intervention (e.g., rituals, sacrifice, and other forms of spiritual interventions).

3.5.5 Adherence

Adherence or compliance encompasses the importance of continuing to follow the treatment plan as designed, including properly taking all medication(s) for the duration of the treatment, making and keeping follow-up appointments, and maintaining health behaviour (Crespo-fierro 1997). Treatment adherence means not only taking the medications but also following the dosing, scheduling, storage, and administration requirements necessary to obtain and maintain the clinical benefits from the treatment. Non-adherence occurs when (1) the patient fails to obtain the medication; (2) the patient fails to take the medication as prescribed; and (3) when the patient prematurely discontinues the medication (Lofholm and Katzung 2009). It is expected that the patient should comply with a therapeutic regimen as part of illness behaviour in order to get better. Non-compliance or non-adherence is a negative illness behaviour that has been implicated in the development, spread, and intensification of drug resistance, and, in particular, treatment failure (see Bloland et al. 2000).

3.5.6 Recovery, Re-integration, or Retirement

The last stage is recovery and reintegration or retirement (this is not in the original formulation by Chrisman). As Igun (1979, p. 450) opined, if treatment is having the desired effects the stage of "recovery and re-integration" is next. An individual may require one or more episodes of treatment, especially if the initial treatment does not lead to a desired result. This may even lead to the re-definition of the symptoms/illness. It is not uncommon in Africa to start treatment at home, and then move to other care providers in case of treatment failure (Amzat 2009). Igun (1979) also noted that a lack of recovery may lead to re-labeling the illness. For example, a condition previously perceived as malaria could be re-labeled as another disease or a mysterious illness inflicted by supernatural agents.

After recovery, the individual is re-integrated into the society where he/she continues with previous role obligations and other daily activities. It is important for the person to be accepted and defined as a healthy member of the social system. This is very important, especially in the case of mental illness. It may be difficult to resume obligations if an individual is not defined as being healthy. This indicates that the process of recovery and reintegration might continue indefinitely (especially in a case of chronic illness) or cut short by permanent retirement (mortality) from social roles. This implies that not all patients get well and not all that get well fully resume normal social roles. Hence, Fig. 3.1 shows that adherence, recovery, reintegration, and retirement are affected by illness attributes and efficacy of regimen; illness attributes in particular because many diseases are not curable, but manageable for a long time, or might lead to a terminal end.

3.6 Factors Affecting Health and Illness Behaviours

Several factors have been implicated in explaining health and illness behaviours. It is important to explain some of these factors. A number of factors may interact to produce a definite behaviour. Depending on its peculiarity and the individual, the same factor may limit or trigger the motivation for appropriate health or illness behaviour. In the next subsection, seven of these factors will be explained.

3.6.1 Illness Attributes/Perception

One major factor affecting health and illness behaviour is the attribute of the disease, especially whether it is acute, accident, chronic, or mental. Many acute illnesses are self-limiting and could be resolved with limited or even without any medical intervention, while some require urgent medical attention. Some injuries and accidents require emergency and intensive care. In chronic illness, most patients often delay contact with the physician. This is because some of its symptoms may be contained. This is often dangerous as early detection helps in proper management of the illness.

More so, the perceived aetiology of disease often determines the kind of therapy to be used. If the perceived cause of an illness includes mystical or supernatural forces, it may require spiritual or traditional intervention. Illness perceptions generally contain an identity component, which includes the local term for the illness and the range of symptoms that the patient believes are associated with the condition, including the perceived causes and modes of transmission of the illness condition (Petrie et al. 2007). A study of patients with TB in South Africa also revealed that stigma may influence decision in health-seeking behaviour and adherence to TB treatment. A full 95 % of those interviewed believe people with TB tend to hide their TB status out of fear of how others may react to them (Cramm et al. 2010). The situation of people living with HIV/AIDS (PLWHA) is also similar as they may conceal their status to prevent discrimination. This is often not a positive illness behaviour.

3.6.2 Class and Socioeconomic Status

A high poverty rate is a major problem in most developing nations. Unfortunately, most of the countries in Africa still do not have a functional insurance scheme. Hence health care is part of out-of-pocket expenditures. In a society entrenched in poverty, many people cannot afford to pay for such services. For instance, in Liberia, given that the majority of the population (up to 75 %) lives below the poverty line, the ability to pay for health services is very low. Generally, the poor utilise health services less often than individuals at higher economic levels (Young 2004). Poverty is a major factor responsible for low utilisation of health services (where available) in Africa. Basic needs such as food and shelter are grossly inadequate as well. Hence most poor households engage in self-treatment or use of herbal medicine that could be relatively less expensive. Self-diagnosis is practiced more by the poorer households while the least poor used patent medicine dealers and community health workers less often for the diagnosis of malaria in Africa (Uzochukwu and Onwujekwe 2004). Self-medication usually saves people treatment expenditures but sometimes is ineffective.

The effect of socioeconomic status is worse in chronic illness which often gulps a lot of resources and requires long-time management. For instance, most poor households cannot afford the cost of renal dialysis or a kidney transplant. Therefore, poverty prevents adequate prevention and proper management of both communicable and non-communicable diseases in SSA and elsewhere in the world.

3.6.3 Gender

It is important to note that sex and gender are not the same and should not be used interchangeably. Sex refers to the biological/physiological differences between men and women, while gender refers to the socially and culturally prescribed identities and differential roles played by the different sexes in the society. The distinct roles and behaviours often give rise to gender inequalities and unequal power relations, which can also translate to inequalities in health status and access to health care. More often than not, women bear the brunt of gender inequality. Gender affects exposure and vulnerability to health risks (see Sect. 4.2 for discussion of gender as a determinant of health). For instance, in most countries of the world women tend to be in charge of cooking. In Africa, women often cook over an open fire or traditional stove, exposing them to pollutants on a daily basis (WHO 2009). The WHO reported that indoor smoke is responsible for half a million of the 1.3 million annual deaths caused by chronic obstructive pulmonary disease (COPD) among women.

Gender influences health-seeking behaviour and access to health services. Most women in Africa require permission from their partners to access health care facilities. Men also bear the cost of spouses' health care and decide when to access health care and what form of health care. When such permission and monetary support are not granted, women may be unable to access health care. Most women in Africa do not enjoy reproductive autonomy as reproductive authority lies with men. This is why Amzat and Grandi (2011, p. 144) observed that it is often difficult for health professionals to advise married women, especially in developing countries, about untimely pregnancies because women are powerless in making such a decision. Unfortunately, untimely pregnancy is associated with a high rate of maternal morbidity and mortality. It is quite evident that gender affects health and illness behaviours in a variety of ways.

3.6.4 Education

Most African countries still have considerable levels of illiteracy. Access to education is being hindered among various groups due to structural constraints such as poverty and inadequate educational institutions. Education is used as a comparative term: a comparison among those who are educated and those who do not have a substantial level of education to enable them to read and write. Schooling or education leads to the acquisition of diverse knowledge and capacity that aids individual daily life choices and chances. Education creates understanding that aims to influence individual lifestyle decisions and raises awareness of the determinants and risk factors of health, and encourages individuals to adopt positive health and illness behaviours (see Sect. 4.4 for further discussion of education/health literacy as a determinant of health). Cutler and Lleras-Muney (2007) observed that education affects morbidity and mortality. They observed that education lowers the propensity of death by a considerable percentage. It was observed that the magnitude of the relationship between education and health varies across conditions, but it is generally large. Education promotes positive health behaviour, and improves knowledge of preventive measures, sources of health care, and general access to health information. Regions with a higher level of education often have better health indicators.

3.6.5 Age

Age is also correlated with both health and illness behaviour. It is part of the determinants of exposure and preventive behaviour. Most lifestyle-related medical conditions are relatively lower among children while some diseases are related to old age. The guardians take most decisions on health behaviour on behalf of the school-age children. The youth takes self-responsibility of health and often engage in risky behaviours like smoking and alcohol consumption. More so, health and illness behaviours have been observed to be socially and culturally acquired from childhood. Crane and Martins (2002) observed that patterns of illness behaviour are learned during childhood and have a significant impact on both the way that individuals respond to symptoms and their beliefs about personal health in adulthood.

3.6.6 Religion or Spiritual Worldview

Religion is both a personal and public phenomenon. The level of religiosity and spirituality is gradually improving in the face of multiple life challenges in Africa. There is a quest for divine intervention on all social problems. Generally, most Africans believe in a world filled with spirits and supernatural entities, most of which can harm an individual. Therefore, religion is a source of life protection and healing from all forms of illness and adversities. There are a growing number of faith-based healers (see Sect. 10.2.1.8) who often believe that there is no disease beyond the power of God to cure.

More so, religious prohibitions control some risk behaviours such as sexual, smoking, dietary behaviours, and alcohol consumption. Islam and Christianity forbid sexual relationship outside marriage. This controls sexual behaviour among committed adherents. In the same vein, the Seventh-Day Adventists often avoid meat and prefer to eat a diet low in saturated fat and high in nutrient density rather than other forms of food. Protestantism does not favour consumption of alcohol. Those who are committed adherents often follow these guidelines, which may positively affect morbidity from certain chronic diseases. Oman and Thoresen (2002) identified four other ways through which religion affects health behaviour:

1. In the case of illness, religion provides social support and improves health behaviours. It provides social meaning to life and raises personal connections with others. Visits on sickbed and other forms of support (including monetary) may come from religious groups. This social capital is important in human life/health.
2. Religion provides additional mechanisms such as "enhanced positive psychological states (e.g., faith, hope, inner peace) acting through psychoneuroimmunologic or psychoneuroendocrinologic pathways" (Oman and Thoresen 2002, p. 365). Religion enhances faith in divinity and the possibility of healing (through divine powers). It could promote a positive state of mind for the adherents.
3. Religion provides positive checks for extreme behaviours and provides a legitimate avenue for acquiring or maintaining positive health behaviours. Disciplinary and regulatory functions are fundamental in religion.
4. Religion also influences health by distant healing or intercessory prayer (Oman and Thoresen 2002). Generally, religious adherents do not doubt the power of divine intervention. Even though the connection between prayer and actual healing cannot be empirically verified, religious adherents often view spiritual power as the last resort.

3.6.7 Place and Space

"Place or space" is also a major determinant of health and illness-related behaviours. This may simply be explained as the location of an individual or the nature of the space for daily living. For instance, most people in rural Africa often use traditional medicine, more so than urban dwellers. This is because TM is the closest form of health care available to rural dwellers. Most rural areas are underserved with modern health care. This invariably affects the health and illness behaviours of the local population. A higher percentage of child and maternal mortalities in Africa takes place in the rural communities. Rapid population growth in the urban centers with the resultant problems of urban slums, degraded environment, unemployment, inadequate social amenities, poverty, and increasing urban social ills (e.g., drug use and transactional sex) across African countries can also explain urban health indicators (Harpham 1996; Vearey et al. 2010).

Spatial features and processes influence accessibility to some vital indices of patterns of livelihood. For example, types of food stores and restaurants influence food choices and, subsequently, diet-related health outcomes (Morland and Evenson 2009). The local food environment affects the prevalence of obesity. More so, the prevalence of infectious disease in the neighbourhood also put individuals at high risk of such diseases. Individuals in malaria-endemic areas are at a greatest risk of contracting malaria. In addition, the level of infrastructural facilities (leisure, water, transportation, power, and sanitation) in the locality can influence health indicators (Sarkar et al. 2013; Stoler et al. 2012). It is not all negative. The built environment of disadvantaged neighbourhoods, which account for limited access to motor vehicles, increases walking for transport and may reduce sedentary lifestyle, thereby reducing the risk of certain chronic disease (Turrell et al. 2013). In addition, another study shows that the existence of "social traps or dangers" in the neighbourhood also affects livelihood. Fear of crime and perception of neighbourhood safety can also influence social activities and propensity to certain injuries (physical and psychological) (Carver et al. 2008). Invariably, geographical space and associated spatial processes often influence access to basic facilities of life and exposure to health risks, which can influence the population health and health-seeking behaviours.

References

Adudans, M. K., Montandon, M., Kwena, Z., Bukusi, E. A., & Cohen, C. R. (2011). Prevalence of forced sex and associated factors among women and men in Kisumu, Kenya. *African Journal of Reproductive Health, 15*(4), 87–97.

Afolabi, B. M., Brieger, W. R., & Salako, L. A. (2004). Management of childhood febrile illness prior to clinic attendance in urban Nigeria. *Journal of Health and Population Nutrition, 22*(1), 46–51.

Alonzo, A. A. (1979). Everyday illness behaviour: A situational approach to health status Deviations. *Social Science & Medicine, 13A*, 397–404.

Alonzo, A. A. (1980). Acute illness behaviour: A conceptual exploration and specification. *Social Science & Medicine, 14A*, 515–526.

Alonzo, A. A. (1993). Health behaviour: Issues, contradictions and dilemmas. *Social Science & Medicine, 37*(8), 1019–1034.

Amzat, J. (2009). *Home management of childhood malaria and treatment failure among mothers of under-five children in Offa, Nigeria*. PhD Thesis submitted to the Department of Sociology, University of Ibadan, Nigeria.

Amzat, J. (2011). Assessing the progress of malaria control in Nigeria. *World Health and Population, 12*(3), 42–51.

Amzat, J., & Grandi, G. (2011). Gender context of personalism in bioethics. *Developing World Bioethics, 11*(3), 136–145.

Andersson, N., Paredes-Solís, S., Milne, D., Omer, K., Marokoane, N., Laetsang, D., & Cockcroft, A. (2012). Prevalence and risk factors for forced or coerced sex among school-going youth: National cross-sectional studies in 10 southern African countries in 2003 and 2007. *BMJ Open, 2*, e000754. doi:10.1136/bmjopen-2011-000754.

Băban, A., & Crăciun, C. (2007). Changing health-risk behaviour: A review of theory and evidence-based intervention in health psychology. *Journal of Cognitive and Behavioral Psychotherapies, VII*(1), 45–67.

Beiersmann, C., Sanou, A., Wladarsch, E., Allegri, M., Kouyaté, B., & Müller, O. (2007). Malaria in rural Burkina Faso: Local illness concepts, patterns of traditional treatment and influence on health-seeking behaviour. *Malaria Journal, 6*, 106. doi:10.1186/1475-2875-6-106.

Bloland, P. B., Ettling, M., & Meek, S. (2000). Combination therapy for malaria in Africa: Hype or hope. *Bulletin of the World Health Organization, 78*, 1378–1388.

Carver, A., Timperio, A., & Crawford, D. (2008). Playing it safe: The influence of neighbourhood safety on children's physical activity—a review. *Health & Place, 14*(2), 217–227.

Chrisman, N. J. (1977). The health seeking process: An analysis of the natural history of illness. *Culture, Medicine and Psychiatry, 1*, 351–377.

References

Clark, E. G., & Leavell, H. R. (1953). Levels of application of preventive medicine. In H. R. Leavell & E. G. Clark (Eds.), *Textbook of preventive medicine* (pp. 7–27). NY: McGraw-Hill.

Cramm, J. M., Finkenflügel, H. J., Møller, V., & Nieboer, A. P. (2010). TB treatment initiation and adherence in a South African community influenced more by perceptions than by knowledge of tuberculosis. *BMC Public Health, 10*, 72. doi:10.1186/1471-2458-10-72.

Crane, C., & Martin, M. (2002). Adult illness behaviour: The impact of childhood experience. *Personality and Individual Differences, 32*(5), 785–798.

Crespo-fierro, M. (1997). Compliance/adherence and care management of HIV disease. *J. Assoc Nurses in AIDS Care, 8*(4), 43–54.

Cutler, D. M., & Lleras-Muney, A. (2007). Education and health: A policy brief. National Poverty Centre. Michigan: USA.

Dake, J. A., Price, J. H., Maziarz, L., & Ward, B. (2012). Prevalence and correlates of sexting behaviour in adolescents. *American Journal of Sexuality Education, 7*(1), 1–15.

Deressa, W. (2007). Treatment-seeking behaviour for febrile illness in an area of seasonal malaria transmission in rural Ethiopia. *Malaria Journal, 6*, 49. doi:10.1186/1475-2875-6-49.

Derman, E. W., Patel, D. N., Nossel, C. J., & Schwellnus, M. P. (2008). Healthy lifestyle interventions in general practice. *SA Family Practice, 50*(4), 6–12.

Fabrega, H. (1973). Towards a model of illness behaviour. *Medical Care, 11*(6), 470–484.

Gabe, J., Bury, M., & Elston, M. A. (2004). *Key concepts in medical sociology*. London: Sage Publications.

Greif, M. J., Dodoo, F. N., & Jayaraman, A. (2011). Urbanisation, poverty and sexual behaviour: The tale of five African cities. *Urban Studies, 48*(5), 947-957.

Guttmacher Institute. (2012). In brief: Facts about abortions in Africa. http://www.guttmacher.org/pubs/IB_AWW-Africa.pdf. Accessed 20 Feb. 2013.

Harpham, T. (1996). Urban health in The Gambia: A review. *Health & Place, 2*(1), 45–49.

Harris, D. M., & Guten, S. (1979). Health-protective behaviour: An exploratory study. *Journal of Health and Social Behavior, 20*(1), 17–29.

Heinemann, L., Gottfried Enderlein, G., & Stark, H. (2012). The risk factor concept in cardiovascular disease. http://www.ilo.org/safework_bookshelf/english?content&nd=857170028. Accessed 6 May 2012.

Hulka, B. S., & Moorman, P. G. (2008). Breast cancer: Hormones and other risk factors. *Maturitas, 61*(1–2), 203–13.

Igun, U. A. (1979). Stages in health-seeking: A descriptive model. *Social Science & Medicine,13A*, 445–456.

Islam, S. M. S., & Johnson, C. A. (2007). Western media's influence on Egyptian adolescents' smoking behaviour: The mediating role of positive beliefs about smoking. *Nicotine and Tobacco Research, 9*(1), 57–64.

Jegede, A. S., Amzat, J., Salami, K. K., Adejumoh, P. O., & Oyetunde, M. O. (2006). What women do to prevent and treat malaria: Experiences from market women in Ibadan, Nigeria. *African Journal for the Psychological Study of Social Issues, 9*(1), 165–178.

Karanja, J., Wambari, E., Okumu, D., Odhaimbo, E., Karuri, I., Muthwii, S. M., Kibe, M., Osawa, N., & Osaki, Y. (2002). A study of awareness of malaria among Kibera population: Implication for community based intervention. *Journal of National Institute of Public Health, 51*(1), 51–55.

Kasl, S. U., & Cobb, S. (1966). Health behaviour, illness behaviour, and sick role behaviour. *Archives of Environmental Health, 12*, 246–266.

Khan, M., Rasolofomanana, J. R., McClamroch, K. J., Ralisimalala, A., Zafimanjaka, M., Behets, F., & Weir, S. S. (2008). High-risk sexual behaviour at social venues in Madagascar. *Sexually Transmitted Diseases, 35*(8), 738–745.

Levitt, N. (2008). Diabetes in Africa: Epidemiology, management and healthcare challenges. *Heart, 94*(11), 1376–1382.

Lofholm, P. W., & Katzung, B. G. (2009). Rational prescribing and prescription writing. In B. G. Katzung (Ed.), *Basic and clinical pharmacology* (11th ed., pp. 1127–1136). Appleton & Lange.

Lundberg, P., Johansson, E., Okello, E., Allebeck, P., & Thorson, A. (2012). Sexual risk behaviours and sexual abuse in persons with severe mental illness in Uganda: A qualitative study. *PLoS ONE, 7*(1), e29748.

Marmorstein, N. R. (2009). Longitudinal associations between alcohol problems and depressive symptoms: Early adolescence through early adulthood. *Alcohol Clin Exp Res, 33*(1), 49–59.

Martinez, P., Røislien, J., Naidoo, N., & Clausen, T. (2011). Alcohol abstinence and drinking among African women: Data from the world health Surveys. *BMC Public Health, 11,* 160. doi:10.1186/1471-2458-11-160.

Mashita, R. J., Themane, M. J., Monyeki, K. D., & Kemper, H. C. G. (2011). Current smoking behaviour among rural South African children: Ellisras longitudinal study. *BMC Pediatrics, 11,* 58. doi:10.1186/1471-2431-11-58.

Mbanya, J. C. N., Motala, A. A., Sobngwi, E., Assah, F. K., & Enoru, S. T. (2010). Diabetes in sub-Saharan Africa. *The Lancet, 375*(9733), 2254–2266.

McCombie, S. C. (2002). Self-treatment for malaria: The evidence and methodological issues. *Health Policy and Planning, 17*(4), 333–344.

Mechanic, D. (1995). Sociological dimensions of illness behaviour. *Social Science & Medicine, 41*(9), 1207–1216.

Mechanic, D. (1962). The concept of illness behaviour. *Journal of Chronic Diseases, 15,* 189–194.

Morland, K. B., & Evenson, K. R. (2009). Obesity prevalence and the local food environment. *Health & Place, 15*(2), 491–495.

Mpofu, E., Caldwell, L., Smith, E., Flisher, A. J., Mathews, C., Wegner, L., & Vergnani, T. (2006). Rasch modelling of the structure of health risk behaviour in South african adolescents. *Journal of Applied Measurement, 7*(3), 323–34.

Mukanga, D., Tibenderana, J. K., Peterson, S., Pariyo, G. W., Kiguli, J., Waiswa, P., Babirye, R., Ojiambo, G., Kasasa, S., Pagnoni, F., & Kallander, K. (2012). Access, acceptability and utilization of community health workers using diagnostics for case management of fever in Ugandan children: A cross-sectional study. *Malaria Journal, 11,* 121. doi:10.1186/1475-2875-11-121.

Mwenesi, H., Harpha, T., & Snow, R. W. (1995). Child malaria treatment practices among mothers in Kenya. *Social Science and Medicine, 40*(9), 1271–1277.

Nsimba, S. E. D., Massele, A. Y., Eriksen, J., Gustafsson, L. L., Tomson, G., & Warsame, M. (2002). Case management of malaria in under-fives at primary healthcare facilities in a Tanzanian District. *Tropical Medicine and International Health, 7*(3), 201–209.

Nuwaha, F. (2002). People's perception of malaria in Mbarara, Uganda. *Tropical Medicine and International Health, 7*(5), 462–470.

Oman, D., & Thoresen, C. E. (2002). 'Does religion cause health?': Differing interpretations and diverse meanings. *Journal of Health Psychology, 7*(4), 365–380.

Parsons, T. (1951). *The social system*. Glencoe: Free Press.

Peltzer, K. (2009). Health behaviour and protective factors among school children in four African countries. *International Journal of Behavioral Medicine, 16,* 172–180.

Petrie, K. J., Jago, L. A., & Devcich, D. A. (2007). The role of illness perceptions in patients with medical conditions. *Current Opinion in Psychiatry, 20,* 163–167.

Rutta, A. S. M., Francis, F., Mmbando, B. P., Ishengoma, D. S., Sembuche, S. H., Malecela, E. K., Sadi, J. Y., Kamugisha, M. L., & Lemnge, M. M. (2012). Using community-owned resource persons to provide early diagnosis and treatment and estimate malaria burden at community level in north-eastern Tanzania. *Malaria Journal, 11,* 152. doi:10.1186/1475-2875-11-152.

Sarkar, C., Gallacher, J., & Webster, C. (2013). Built environment configuration and change in body mass index: The Caerphilly Prospective Study (CaPS). *Health & Place, 19,* 33–44.

Segall, A. (1976). The sick role concept: Understanding illness behaviour. *Journal of Health and Social Behavior, 17,* 163–170.

Shuper, P. A., Neuman, M., Kanteres, F., Baliunas, D., Joharchi, N., & Rehm, J. (2010). Causal considerations on alcohol and HIV/AIDS—a systematic review. *Alcohol, 45*(2), 159–166.

References

Sosa-Estani, S., Colantonio, L., & Segura, E. L. (2012). Therapy of chagas disease: Implications for levels of prevention. *Journal of Tropical Medicine, 2012,* 10. doi:10.1155/2012/292138.

Steptoe, A., & Wardle, J. (2004). Health-related behaviour: Prevalence and links with disease. In A. Kaptein & J. Weinmen (Eds.), *Health psychology* (pp. 21–51). BPS: Blackwell.

Stoler, J., Fink, G., Weeks, J. R., Otoo, R. A., Ampofo, J. A., & Hill, A. G. (2012). When urban taps run dry: Sachet water consumption and health effects in low-income neighbourhood of Accra, Ghana. *Health & Place, 18*(2), 250–262.

Suchman, E. A. (1965). Stages of illness and medical care. *Journal of Health and Human Behavior, 6,* 114–128.

Szabo, C. P., & Allwood, C. W. (2004). A cross-cultural study of eating attitudes in adolescent South African females. *World Psychiatry, 3*(1), 41–44.

Szabo, C. P., & Allwood, C. W. (2006). Body figure preference in South African adolescent females: A cross cultural study. *African Health Science, 6*(4), 201–206.

Temple, J. R., Paul, J. A., van den Berg, P., Le, V. D., McElhany, A., & Temple, B. W. (2012). Teen sexting and its association with sexual behaviors. *Archives of Pediatrics & Adolescent Medicine, 166*(9), 828–833. doi:10.1001/archpediatrics.2012.835.

The Hunger Project. (2012). Empowering women and men to end their hunger. http://www.thp.org/africa. Accessed 19 May 2012.

Turrell, G., Haynes, M., Wilson, L., & Giles-Corti, B. (2013). Can the built environment reduce health inequalities? A study of neighbourhood socioeconomic disadvantage and walking for transport. *Health & Place, 19,* 89–98.

Twaddle, A. C. (1969). Health decisions and sick role variations: an exploration. *Journal of Health and Social Behavior, 10,* 105–115.

Twaddle, A. C. (1974). The concept of health status. *Social Science & Medicine, 8,* 29–28.

Uzochukwu, B. S. C., & Onwujekwe, O. E. (2004). Socio-economic differences and health seeking behaviour for the diagnosis and treatment of malaria: A case study of four local government areas operating the Bamako initiative programme in south-east Nigeria. International Journal for Equity in Health, 3, 6. doi:10.1186/1475-9276-3-6.

Vearey, J., Palmary, I., Thomas, L., Nunez, L., & Drimie, S. (2010). Urban health in Johannesburg: The importance of place in understanding intra-urban inequalities in a context of migration and HIV. *Health & Place, 16*(4), 694–702.

WHO. (2005). WHO multi-country study on women's health and domestic violence against women: Summary report of initial results on prevalence, health outcomes and women's responses. Geneva: WHO.

World Health Organization (WHO). (2009). 10 facts about women's health. http://www.who.int/gender/documents/10facts_womens_health_en.pdf. Assessed 21 May 2012.

World Health Organization (WHO). (2012). *World Malaria Report 2012.* Geneva: WHO.

Young, J. T. (2004). Illness behaviour: A selective review and synthesis. *Sociology of Health & Illness, 26*(1), 1–31.

Chapter 4
Social Determinants/Context of Health

4.1 Introduction

This chapter discusses the various social factors which determine human health and disease. In the preceding chapter, the roles of some social factors in health and illness behaviour were discussed. This chapter provides an elaboration of the social determinants of health, dwelling more on how social factors interact to produce health or illness. The notion that health has a social context is traced to the father of western medicine, Hippocrates (460 BC–370 BC). Fathalla (2000) observed that Hippocrates suggested the consideration of social issues in human health. Such factors play significant roles in human health, and (preventive) medicine in particular should note such significant roles. The notion of social aetiology of health or illness is synonymous with the consideration of social factors in human health and illness. The social context accounts for exposure and vulnerability to diseases. The roles of the social determinants are considerably important in the understanding of human health. For instance, if the world is able to ensure gender justice and improve standards of living, the disease burden will be significantly reduced.

It is possible to reduce these social determinants of health (SDH) to social position in the society which affects human health. Simply, SDH refers to the full set of social conditions and characteristics within which living and working take place that invariably account for human health (Tarlov 1996; CSDH 2007). Social position determines social status and roles while social condition determines individual place in a social stratification system. The concepts mentioned in the preceding sentence have the prefix "social" because they are created or constructed by the society. This means that they are not static, natural, or biological. Social roles are created, allocated, and performed by individuals in various social positions in the society. Social roles are duties and obligations assigned to individuals in a specific social position within social organisations such as family (parents, children), occupation (lecturer, physician, nurse), or associations/clubs (president, secretary, or member). All of these positions are socially stratified based on power relations. Social stratification is the manner in which social condition and positions are ranked in terms of power, prestige, or status and wealth.

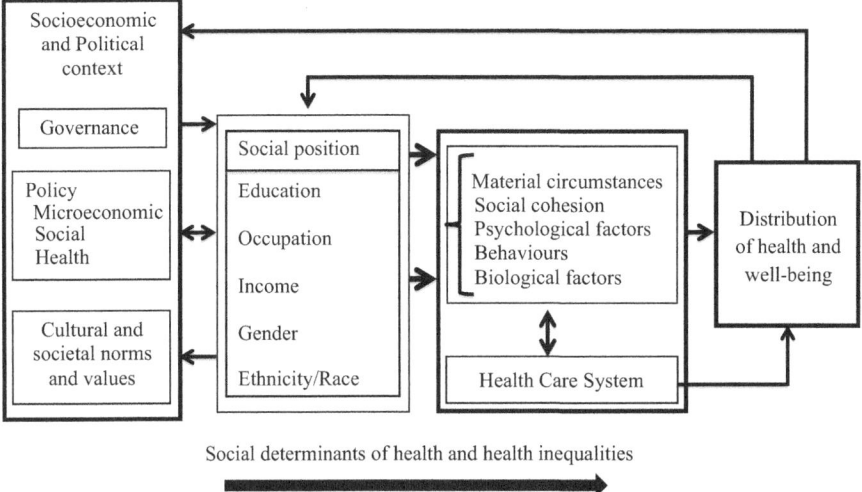

Fig. 4.1 Social determinant of health conceptual framework. (Source: CSDH (2008))

The differential social positions and roles generate unequal opportunities and vulnerabilities in human society. Such differential opportunities reflect in education, occupation, income, and other personal attributes, which also account for inequality in health. Thus the idea of differential social positions and conditions are summed as SDH because they lead to differential disease exposure and vulnerability and consequences of health conditions. Social condition may increase the possibility or probability that an individual will develop a particular illness condition because of (increased) frequency of contacts with pathogens or risk factors. For instance, a driver is more exposed to road accidents than other occupations. This is an example of how occupational status may increase exposure to injury. The social condition also contributes to differential consequences because they account for an individual's capability to access appropriate health care. While those with high socioeconomic status (SES) living in urban African cities may have access to numerous health services, their counterparts with low SES (in rural communities or in the slum) have access to limited health services (if available at all).

From the foregoing discussion, there is a very strong ground to discuss the roles of social factors in health and illness. Figure 4.1 shows the conceptual framework advanced by the WHO Commission on the SDH (CSDH). The figure shows the interplay of numerous social issues that influence human health, starting from the socioeconomic and political contexts. The various governmental policies and nature of political governance determine commitment to health care development. The political context depicts the level of development of the state and how resources are allocated. This affects various social positions in the society, such as level of educational achievement and income distribution. The sociocultural norms also determine the gender framework of the society and social positions. Individual attributes (e.g., income, education, and occupation) also affect behaviours, psychosocial factors, and material circumstances, which are modified by the nature of the health care system

Table 4.1 Gender discrimination throughout a woman's life. (Source: Updated from Heise et al. (1994, p. 5))

Prenatal	Prenatal sex selection, battering during pregnancy, coerced pregnancy (rape during war), sex-selective abortion
Infancy	Female infanticide, emotional and physical abuse, differential birth ceremony, and differential access to food and medical care
Childhood	Genital cutting; incest and sexual abuse; differential access to food, medical care, and education; child prostitution, child marriage, child labour
Adolescence	Dating and courtship violence, economically coerced sex, sexual abuse in the workplace, rape, sexual harassment, forced prostitution, honour killing
Reproductive	Abuse of women by intimate partners, marital rape, dowry abuse and murders, partner homicide, psychological abuse, sexual abuse in the workplace, sexual harassment, rape, abuse of women with disabilities, domestic/unpaid work, deprivation of reproductive autonomy, domestication of women, low autonomy in household/social interaction, economic insecurity, honour killing (especially by the partner)
Old age	Abuse of widows, elder abuse (which affects mostly women), deprivation of inheritance

and subsequently the distribution of health and well-being. The interplay of these issues and factors are complex.

The subsequent subsections will examine a number of social determinants of health. The list might not be exhaustive, but the examples should give a better understanding of how social factors function in the determination of human health.

4.2 Gender Inequality

Gender signifies the social construction of roles and obligations between the sexes. Gender inequality is a social creation and it places people in a position which affects their health. Simply put, gender also affects the nature, severity, and exposure to health problems. Women suffer more from gender inequality and inequities, thereby putting them at a disadvantaged position. Gender constitutes a fundamental basis for discrimination in most African societies where the gender gap is still very wide. There is socially entrenched gender division of labour and power within the household. Men are usually the breadwinners and most often women are confined to the private or domestic sphere where they only engage in unpaid labour.

Gender discrimination starts from the prenatal stage due to a preference for a particular sex—most times with more *social value* on male children. Advanced technology makes it possible to determine a female foetus, which may be aborted. Another extreme form of gender inequality is the practice of female infanticide due to male child preference (Sen 2003). This shows that a female child may not be given the chance to life. Women without at least a male child suffer psychological dissatisfaction and discrimination in the community. Exposure to health-damaging conditions runs throughout the life of women. Table 4.1 shows forms of gender discrimination at different stages of a woman's life, which are damaging to women's health and well-being. There are several countries with a higher risk of mortality for women (mostly due to gender inequities). Such countries in Africa include Angola, Chad, Somalia, Mali, Democratic Republic of the Congo, Nigeria, Sierra Leone, Guinea-Bissau, the Central African Republic, Burkina Faso, Niger, Burundi, and North African countries (World Bank 2011).

Table 4.1 shows a number of "social conditions" that are apparently disastrous for female health at different stages of life, which include female infanticide, genital mutilation, rape or gender-based domestic violence, forced prostitution, and differential access to food. Child marriage is also common in Africa—some girls are offered for marriage before the age of 10 (UNFPA 2004). A number of maternal health problems (e.g., vesicovaginal fistula [VVF] and mortality) are associated with pregnancies that come too early. CSDH (2007) also opined that there are widespread patterns of the underfeeding of female children, relative to their male siblings, which also undermines their health status.

Generally, most diseases relating to reproduction are more prevalent in women than men because of a woman's reproductive roles in pregnancy, childbirth, postpartum care, and abortion. In societies in which reproductive health services are not prioritised, women are at high risk of maternal-related morbidity and mortality. WHO (2009) reported that every day, 1,600 women die from preventable complications during pregnancy and childbirth—almost 99 % occurs in the developing world. It is further reported that one in every five women is sexually abused before the age of 15, putting them at high risk of contracting STDs, including HIV; unwanted pregnancies which account for a high number of abortions and related morbidity and mortality; and life-long psychological ordeal (WHO 2009).

CSDH (2007) further observed that *socially constructed models of masculinity* could have deleterious health consequences for men and boys, especially when those models encourage aggressive behaviour or alcohol abuse. This may push boys to engage in violent activities to demonstrate their strong masculinity. This is part of why men are more exposed to injuries violence, and tobacco-related diseases in Africa. Globally, the smoking rate among men tends to be 10 times higher than women, although tobacco use among younger females is rising (WHO 2010). In short, there is gender variation in the consideration of health, and closing the gender gap will impact positively on human health.

4.3 Socioeconomic Status

Socioeconomic status (SES) is often defined as the social standing or class of an individual within or relative to a social group. Generally, three major variables (among others) account for socioeconomic status—level of income, education, and occupation. Level of education could determine an individual's occupation and level of income. One of the major ways of classifying SES is to divide it into three levels: high, middle, and low SES. Those who have low SES are regarded as the poor or those living in poverty. Poverty has significant adverse effects on human health. Poverty is often described as a state of inability to procure basic necessities of life, such as food and shelter, due to limited resources. More often, it is a lack of monetary capacity to meet human needs. One critical issue is that SES and health have a reciprocal or bi-directional relationship. Socioeconomic status affects health and vice versa. Poor households usually have poor health indicators. The level of personal income positively affects the individual's position in the "social gradient ladder." These individuals in the upper social gradient generally enjoy better access to health care, nutrition, and often live longer than people on the lower rungs of the ladder (SACOSS 2008). In a similar vein, Irwin et al. (2006, p. 749) observed that "throughout the world, people who are socially disadvantaged have less access to health resources, get sicker, and die earlier than people in more privileged social positions."

For instance, malaria is often described as a disease of poverty, and contributes to growing poverty (Amzat 2011). Poor households in Africa have access to limited health information and basic preventive measures (e.g., ITN) for malaria. The poor often live in places infiltrated by mosquitoes and in neighbourhoods with poor drainage where mosquitoes breed. Hence, the poor have high vulnerability to malaria, and often spend substantial portion of their inadequate income in the treatment of malaria (WHO 2000; Yusuf et al. 2010). Most of those consider as poor constitute more than half of the population of Africa and they earn less than one US dollar a day (i.e., live below the poverty line). A majority of the poor dies of common preventable diseases.

Furthermore, Grant (2005) discussed six main dimensions through which poverty interacts with ill-health which include (1) poor nutrition, (2) poor shelter, (3) poor working conditions, (4) health care costs, (5) erosive livelihood strategies, and (6) coping strategies. Figure 4.2 diagrammatically presents the six dimensions. The first component is poor nutrition. Members of a poor household may die of hunger or obtain only poor nutrients, which may cause a low capacity for work resulting in low productivity and income. Poor nutrition weakens immunity to fight diseases. The second component is poor living condition. Poor households often reside in open spaces, slums, or overcrowded environments. For instance, there are a growing number of street households and street children across Africa, such as the *faseurs* of Congo (Brazaville), the *shegues* of Congo (Kinshasa), the *talibes* of Senegal and Egypt, the *tsotsis* of South of Africa, Kaponye of Zambia, *youthman* of Sierra-Leone, the *area-boys* of Lagos, and the *almajirai* of Northern Nigeria (Amzat 2008). They reside on the streets and are exposed to hazardous and harmful social conditions, which adversely affect their physical, emotional, and psychological well-being. In street livelihood, there are very limited infrastructures, such as water supply. This accounts for increased vulnerability to water-borne-related diseases, pollution, and other related adverse conditions.

Poor working condition is another major component. In SSA, it is not uncommon for the poor people to hawk along the streets, in heavy traffic or roadsides, or work in unventilated factories with hazardous machinery or substances. Poor working conditions also expose the poor to work injuries and other adversities. Unfortunately, poor health status also leads to reduction in productivity and employability. Poor income also leads to the inability to meet (quality) health care costs. As it has been

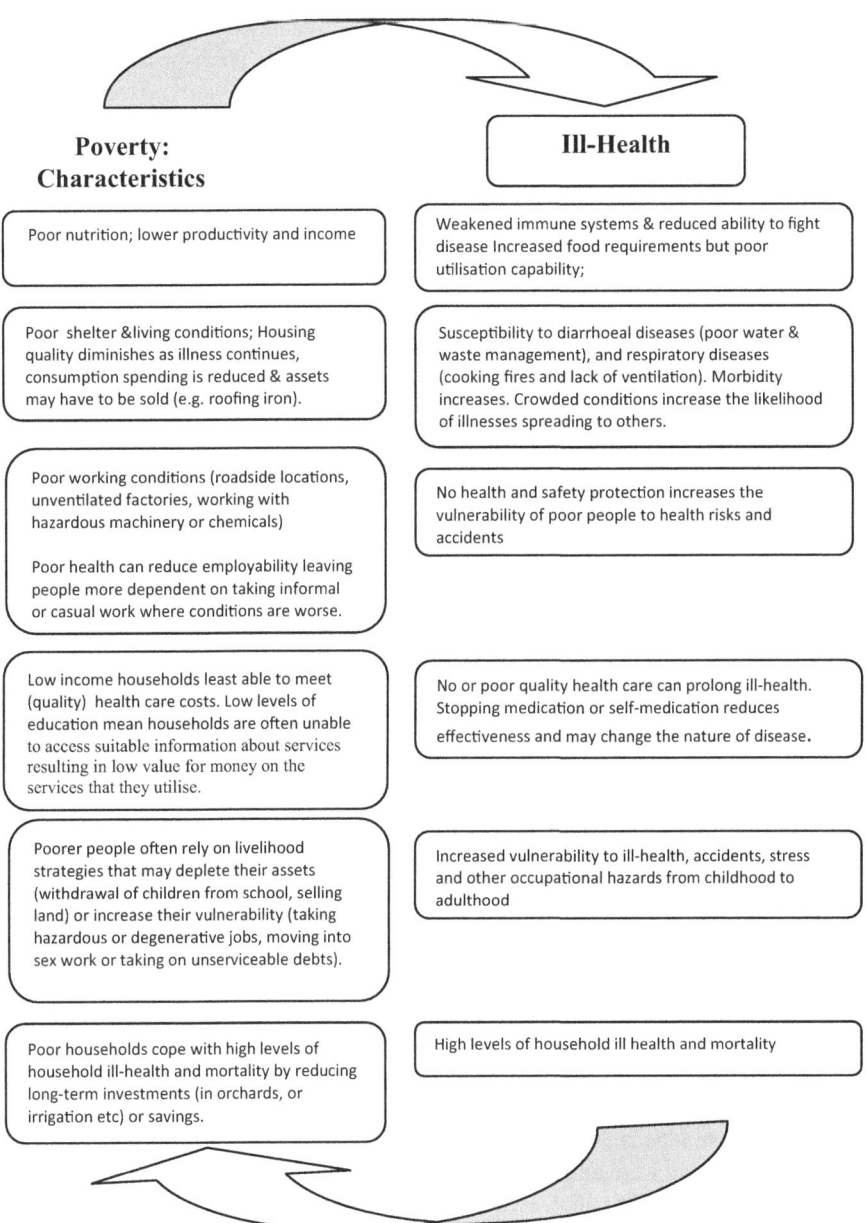

Fig. 4.2 Poverty and health: A bi-directional model. (Source: Grant (2005))

indicated previously, there is no functional insurance policy that covers a substantial majority of the poor in Africa. Hence most health care costs are covered out-of-pocket. Poor access to health care would also prolong the period of illness and might lead to poverty and eventual death.

The fifth and sixth components deal with erosive livelihood strategies and coping strategies. The culture of poverty itself directly or indirectly predisposes households to ill-health and ultimately accounts for the reproduction of poverty. A child from a poor household may be withdrawn from school; this leads to low levels of education and health literacy; a limited chance to get a well-paid job; engagement in degenerative works, thus leading to vulnerability to adverse health conditions and poverty itself. A poor household may also engage in self-medication without diagnosis, which may worsen the condition and lead to a higher treatment cost.

Furthermore, Fathalla (2000) averred that the socioeconomic conditions that had an adverse impact on the reproductive performance of women in the city of Aberdeen in the 1940s and 1950s still have that impact on the health and lives of hundreds of millions of women and their babies in developing countries. The impact of socioeconomic status is not only at the individual level but also across many countries of the world. Due to increasing poverty which accounts for a number of adversities, especially poor health indicators, life expectancy in African countries is very low—less than 40 years in Mozambique and Swaziland; around 43 years in Zimbabwe, Lesotho and Sierra Leone; and between 46 and 49 years in South Africa, Nigeria, Malawi, Somalia, and Rwanda, while most of the rich countries (e.g., Switzerland, Spain, Sweden, Italy, Norway, and France) have life expectancies of more than 80 years. One major determinant of low life expectancy in Africa is low SES. This is why Marmot (2005) submitted that to reduce health inequalities between individuals, groups, and countries, it is vital to take action on the social determinants of health, especially a relief of poverty.

4.4 Education and Health Literacy

Education also contributes to health in a number of other ways, whether in terms of morbidity, mortality, or health behaviour (Mackenbach et al. 2008; Albouy and Lequien 2009; Brunello et al. 2011). Unfortunately, there is relatively low educational development in Africa. Literacy level is less than 30 % in Mali, Chad, Guinea, and Niger (UNDP 2009). Figure 4.3 presents some ways through which education can affect human health outcomes. Education in this sense is often measured by the number of years in schools with emphasis on the ability to read and write. Education affects occupation and income. In SSA, one year of education is associated with a 3–14 % increase in wages and productivity (Appleton 2000). For example, people with higher education are more likely to be able to find "good" jobs with better wages (Cutler et al. 2006). This increases their chances for stable incomes, job security, and job satisfaction, which are preconditions for life satisfaction. This can enhance better mental stability and deter unnecessary life pressures and inadequacies. Higher income also allows an individual to easily pay for health care expenditures.

Education also promotes a healthy lifestyle and positive choices. Increasing levels of education lead to more rational thinking and decision-making patterns in life choices (Cutler and Lleras-Muney 2006; Mackenbach et al. 2008). It generally moderates the excesses of life. More often, people who are educated engage in physical activities—especially exercise, checking their weight, and completing medical

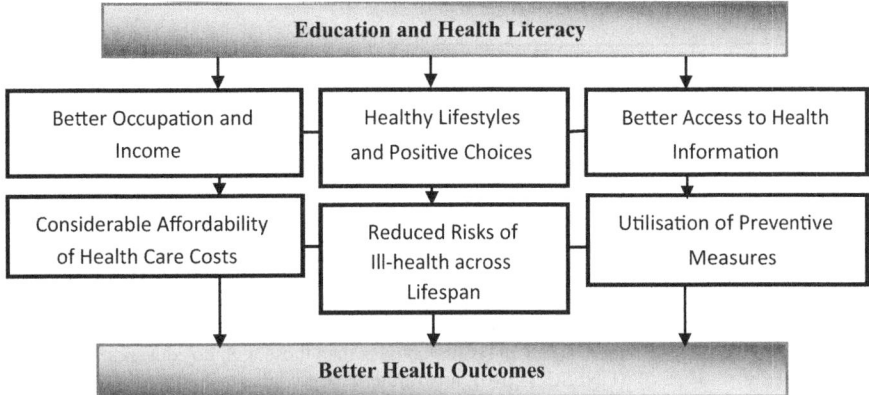

Fig. 4.3 Education and better health outcomes

checkups regularly. A healthy lifestyle considerably reduces the risk and vulnerability to diseases across an individual's lifespan. Those who engage in moderate exercise and have a well-balanced diet reduce their risk of obesity and other related risks. It has been observed that people who are more educated are less likely to suffer from hypertension, emphysema, or diabetes (Fonseca and Zheng 2011; Picker 2012). Physical and mental functioning is also better for the better educated. Among those with chronic conditions such as diabetes and hypertension, the better educated are more likely to have their condition under control (Cutler and Lleras-Muney 2006; Sánchez-Barriga 2012).

Figure 4.3 also shows that education provides access to health information. Education provides people with the knowledge and skills they need to solve problems and to cope with changing circumstances (Lochner 2011). This gives the educated a sense of control over their circumstances, which in turn contributes to psychological balance and better health. Education facilitates the attainment of health literacy, which refers "to the personal, cognitive and social skills which determine the ability of individuals to gain access to, understand and use information in ways which promote and maintain good health" (Nutbeam 2000, p. 263). Apart from access to health information, Kickbusch (2001) noted that education and health literacy enable individuals to:

1. Prioritise positive health and illness behaviours and minimise the influence of negative factors on health outcomes.
2. Read basic health information/instructions, including medicine labels, which helps improve regimen adherence.
3. Read and understand health promotion information to enhance rational understanding, which aids the initiation of preventive and treatment actions.
4. Comprehend and act upon necessary procedures and directions given by medical personnel as well as appointment schedules.

Education affects	
Knowledge of HIV	A study in Ghana showed that individuals with more education practiced more protective health behaviours against HIV/AIDS (Peters et al. 2010). This shows that education also reduces the chance of contracting HIV and other STDs. A study in Zambia found that HIV spreads twice as fast among uneducated girls, and women who remained in school after primary school were five times more likely to know basic facts about HIV than illiterate women (Vandemoortele and Delamonica 2002). Basic knowledge improves the use of preventive action
Maternal health	Education is also positively related to maternal health. In Burkina Faso, mothers with secondary education are twice as likely to give birth more safely in health facilities than those with no education (UNESCO 2010). It is further observed that a child born to a mother who can read is 50 % more likely to survive past the age of five than a child born to an illiterate woman (UNESCO 2010)
Life expectancy	Generally, as average education increases, life expectancy improves, and the returns appear to be larger in Africa (Appleton 2000)

Furthermore, the educated often report having lower morbidity from the most common acute and chronic diseases (heart condition, stroke hypertension, cholesterol, and diabetes) (Fonseca and Zheng 2011). Education differences are in part the result of differences in behaviour across education groups. Unfortunately, poor health has negative effects on schooling, as it results in school absenteeism and sometimes low intellectual capacity to cope with academic demands.

4.5 Living Conditions/Housing

In developing countries, suitable housing is often in short supply or not affordable. Hence many people live in places that are unfit and considerably below an acceptable standard of living condition. Millions of people are homeless; they sleep on the street without access to any basic amenities, while others live in slums or squalor. Houses in the slum, occupied by the poor or migrants seeking better opportunities or urban benefits, are usually self-built, mostly with substandard materials and without any technical input from building experts, and roofed with corrugated sheets and wooden boards with paper material as ceilings. Access to basic social amenities is grossly inadequate in places such as Kibera (Kenya), Ajegunle (Nigeria), Khayelitsha (Cape Town, South Africa), Kambwe (Zambia), Magadishu (Somalia), and Kisenyi (Kampala, Uganda). The slum is contaminated with human and animal faeces due to an open sewage system and the frequent use of "flying toilets" or "shot puts"—described as the act of defecating in a paper bag and throwing it to a nearby garbage site or bush. UN-HABITAT (2003) described a slum household as a group of individuals living under the same roof that lack one or more of the following conditions: access to clean water, access to sanitation, secure tenure, durability of housing, and sufficient living area. Unfortunately, as it is further observed, up to 70 % of urban dwellers in SSA live in slums/squalor.

Table 4.2 Components of poor living/housing conditions

Overcrowding and limited space	Increased transmission of airborne infections such as acute respiratory infectious diseases (e.g., pneumonia and tuberculosis);low food safety standards, frequent food spoilage and contamination, limited interior and external space
Poor garbage disposal	Indiscriminate garbage sites, air pollution; infiltrations of flies and other disease agents; open sewage system; pollution emanated from human refuse, garbage, soot, dust, and other wastes
Limited household facilities	Poor toilet and excretal disposal, open-space defecation, low standard bathroom or external bathroom (shared with a number of houses), lack of functional kitchens or cocking facilities
Poor sanitation and drainage	Unkempt environment, breeding sites for flies including mosquitoes, polluting environment, flooding, limited facilities for personal and domestic hygiene and sanitary food preparation; water pollutants; dust
Poor infrastructures	Limited or lack of water supply, limited power supply, lack of nearby health centre, the presence of indoor air pollution associated with fuels used for cooking and heating
Infiltrations of unwanted agents	Vectors and hosts of disease: mosquitoes, bed bugs, rodents, cockroaches, mice etc.
Poorly planned neighbourhoods	Flooding, poor ventilation, lack of emergency access (by ambulance or fire service vehicles), increased transmission of airborne infections (e.g., acute respiratory infectious diseases, pneumonia, and tuberculosis)
Substandard structures and housing materials	Houses usually self-built; poor wall, ceiling, and floor materials; non-permanent structure; substandard wiring
Neighbourhood violence	Limited access to safe play and recreation, frequent exposure to excessive noise, personal hazards and interpersonal violence (including rape and other forms of assault)

The slum is characterised with social ills such as poverty, crime, dirtiness, pollution, black spots, prostitution, drug trafficking, child labour, and abuse. There is no difficulty in associating poor living conditions with high prevalence and incidence of diseases. Table 4.2 presents a concise description of poor living conditions/housing. One dimension of poor living condition is overcrowding, a situation where many individuals live in a room that is relatively too small. A study by Govender et al. (2010) in Cape Town, South Africa, found that 59 % of the toilets were not in working order and blocked or overflowing drains were commonly observed (64 % of dwellings had pools of drain water outside the house). The number of persons per toilet ranged from two persons to 18 persons (Govender et al. 2010). The study describes a typical poor living condition. Evidence suggests that overcrowded dwellings are associated with a greater risk of infectious disease and poor mental health (Waters 2001).

Crowded living conditions have been associated with increased incidence of infectious disease, spread by the respiratory route, such as tuberculosis and meningococcal disease (Baker et al. 2000). A poor living condition is also linked with the lack of adequate and effective preventive health care (Kawachi and Wamala 2007). Bed bugs are found in the bedding, pillows, mattresses, carpets, upholstered furniture of homes, and clothes, where they feed on humans by sucking blood. In poor living conditions, cockroaches are co-occupants infiltrating many households, usually moving from dump sites or pit latrines contaminating food and posing risk to human health. Individuals living in dwellings that are damp, cold, or mouldy are at greater risk of respiratory conditions, meningococcal infection, and asthma (Waters 2001). Water-borne diseases are also common in areas with limited access to clean water.

Generally, people living in owner-occupied homes appear to have better health and longer life expectancy than those who live in rented accommodations (Waters 2001). A house and a "home" are required for a healthy living condition. People living in poor living conditions often suffer stigma and discrimination. It is often difficult for many individuals to disclose their residential area due to stigmatisation. This indicates that the lack of stable and decent housing also poses relational and psychological challenges. Worse still, poor neighbourhoods are often not well designed, restricting vehicular access during emergencies, which may lead to a high number of casualties in such cases. In short, living condition/housing is part of the SDH.

4.6 Individual Behaviour and Lifestyle Factors

There is relatively a new trend towards the formulation of a health lifestyle theory (see Cockerham 2013). "Health lifestyles are collective patterns of health-related behaviour based on choices from options available to people according to their life chances" (Cockerham 2013, p. 138). Two critical issues are apparent in health lifestyle : life chances and choices. While there are choices to be made, such choices are facilitated or constrained by life chances or class position. The class circumstances hold powerful influence on lifestyle forms, especially the components of lifestyles (see Fig. 4.4) (Cockerham 2013).

Life choices and decisions affect human health and well-being. In a previous chapter, risk behaviours were explained (see Sect. 3.3.1). The risk behaviours are part of the components of lifestyle and individual behaviour, which are constituents of SDH. Figure 4.4 shows basic components of individual behaviour and lifestyle, which include dietary, sexual, smoking, health and illness behaviours, alcohol and drug use, physical activities, health and illness behaviours, and lifestyle decisions and actions. These behaviours present life choices. This is part of self-accountability of health, a notion which depicts that individuals are also responsible for their health. Some individual factors play significant roles in smoking initiation, frequency of smoking, kind of tobacco (whether marijuana or light tobacco), and smoking cessation. For instance, marijuana smokers are more prone to drug-induced mental illness than cigarette smokers. In addition, the frequency of smoking (number of cigarettes smoked per day) is also associated with propensity to smoking-related health conditions.

Dietary behaviour is also linked to health condition. Dietary intake can reduce or increase risk to certain diseases. For instance, dietary fibre intake is inversely correlated with several diseases, including colorectal cancer, coronary heart diseases, stroke, hypertension, diabetes, obesity, and certain gastrointestinal and cardiovascular diseases (Anderson and Conley 2007; Anderson et al. 2009; Kranz et al. 2012;

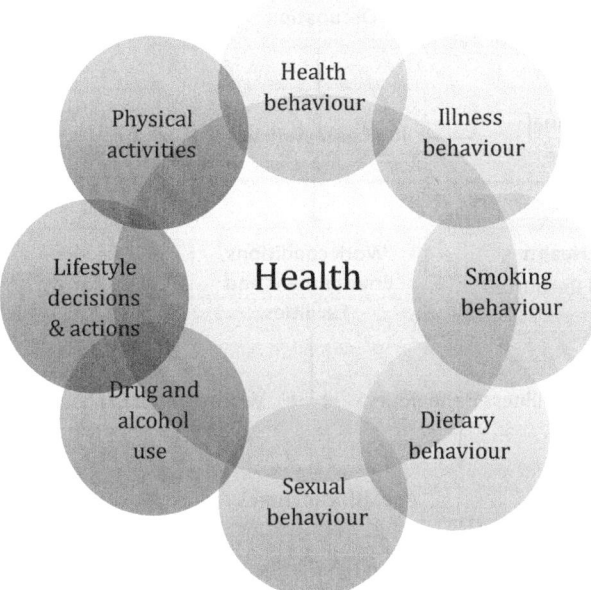

Fig. 4.4 Components of individual behaviours and lifestyle factors in health

Lairon et al. 2005; Whelton et al. 2005). These findings support the protective role of dietary fibre against certain diseases and recommendations for its increased consumption. On the other hand, excessive fat and carbohydrate intake poses significant health risks (Delisle et al. 2009; Lancaster et al. 2006; Mokhtar et al. 2001). Dietary behaviour is part of an individual's behaviour and lifestyle choices.

Furthermore, the patterns of health and illness behaviours are also part of the components of individual behaviour affecting health. Simple medical checkups and how individuals respond to bodily indications are part of life choices. While some individuals engage in appropriate protective behaviours, others may not. Additionally, some individuals follow normal and effective treatment regimens, whereas others may not. These are specific patterns of behaviour. More so, patterns of drug and alcohol consumption are also matters of lifestyle.

The level of an individual's control on excessive behaviour is part of the SDH. Behavioural patterns could be a strong indicator of health. Factors such as smoking, drinking, and using illicit drugs are obvious choices that individuals make that impact greatly on their health, both in the short and long term (SACOSS 2008). The decision to use tobacco, alcohol, and illicit drugs is often socially and personally patterned by an individual's dispositions and structural context. Those who manage to have proper hygiene, a balanced diet, adequate physical activities or exercise, relaxation and sleep, effective social networks or relationships, stress management, a non-violent lifestyle, and effective protective and treatment behaviours are more than likely to be of good health.

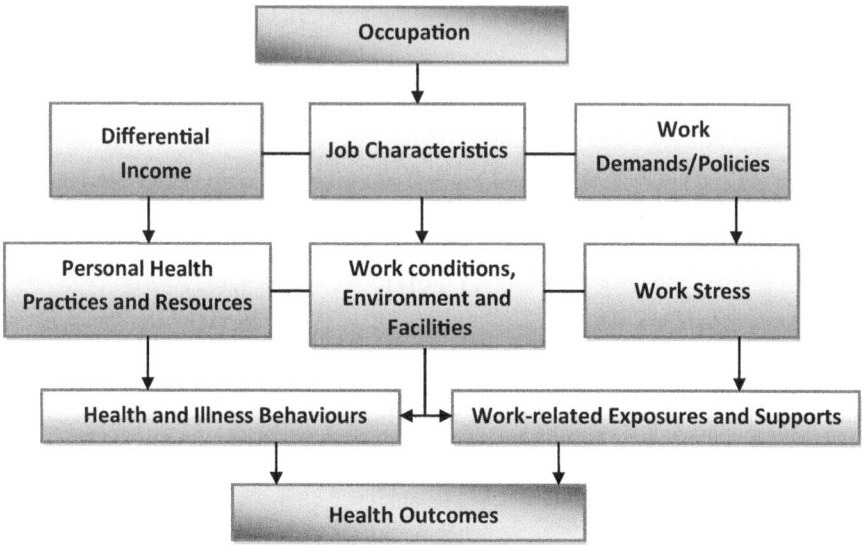

Fig. 4.5 Pathways by which occupation affects health outcomes

4.7 Employment or Occupation

Employment or occupational status affects individual health status in a number of ways. First, unemployment could have devastating effects on health. It leads to a low income and a lack of resources to manage health care, especially in a non-socialised health care system. Unemployment is strongly related to poverty and poor living condition. As it has been previously examined, low SES has ruinous effects on health care. Additionally, a transition into unemployment from employment undermines physical health, socioeconomic and psychological well-being, and could also account for grievous effects on an individual's health.

As shown in Fig. 4.5, an individual's occupation is related to health because it leads to a differential income. Invariably, this leads to differential capacity and resources to manage health. This could also be the case in terms of insurance coverage or personal income to pay for health care costs. People in low-paying jobs and occupational positions often have a limited capacity to manage their health and are more vulnerable to a number of health conditions. A study found that the risk of poor health gradually decreased in relation to higher occupational positions and that in comparison to people with the highest occupational positions, people with the lowest occupational positions were more likely to suffer from depression, diabetes, ischaemic heart disease, arthritis, muscle pain, and tension headache (Volkers 2007). Unfortunately, a greater percentage of populations in Africa is engaged in low-occupational positions. The employment situation is worse in Africa because most of the countries do not have social security system for the unemployed or underemployed. The ravaging unemployment rate puts individuals at a high risk of poverty and restricted access to health care services.

On the other hand, the nature of an occupation also affects an individual's health status. Some occupations could be health-threatening. Figure 4.5 shows that job characteristics, working environment, and condition influences work-related exposure to certain diseases. For instance, Li et al. (2008) studied traffic policemen, especially those who control traffic within the city. They found that the incidence of photosensitive dermatitis, eye diseases, heat stroke, chilblain, and noise-induced deafness in the outside-traffic policemen were higher than that of the policemen working indoors. The study also found that varicosis (problem relating to the veins of the leg) was higher in those who stood for over four hours every day, with the average period of the onset of the disease being 7–8 years (Li et al. 2008). Out-traffic policemen are common in Africa where there are inadequate traffic lights.

Another major issue is work-related safety. Construction workers often require personal protection such as gloves, goggles, masks, and footwear. Working on construction sites without such protective devices is highly hazardous. Such workers are also exposed to harmful substances from mixing cements and other work materials. Similarly, physicians and nurses sometimes experience accidents in the use of surgical instruments and needles, which might result in the transmission of diseases, including HIV. This is why appropriate work organisation and safety is necessary to protect workers as part of work-related supports.

Furthermore, it is important to discuss the links between agricultural work and health. This is because agriculture is a major occupation in Africa. Table 4.3 presents the major occupational health hazards of agricultural work in developing countries. It should be noted that a majority of the agricultural work in Africa is not mechanised as most farmers still rely on crude implements. Cole (2006) observed that the actual number of agricultural occupational morbidity and mortality is not documented. He observed that most farmers are exposed to vectors of disease and sharp tools, which might cause health hazards. It was further observed that parasitic diseases such as schistosomiasis, sleeping sickness, leishmaniasis, ascariasis, and hookworm are common among African farmers because of exposure to disease agents in soil, wastewater/sewage, dirty tools, and rudimentary housing (farm huts). Nomadic livelihood and the continuous shift in residency in the forest among the pastoralists (found in Mauritania, Senegal, Guinea, The Gambia, Mali, Nigeria, Sierra Leone, Burkina Faso, Benin, Guinea Bissau, Chad, Togo, and the Central African Republic) expose them to fatal or injurious bites and stings. Their close contact with animals through raising, sheltering, milking, and slaughtering also expose the pastoralists to animal-related diseases or zoonoses such as anthrax, bovine tuberculosis, and cowpox.

Finally, health status also affects productivity in all occupational spheres. For instance, ill-health arising from agricultural work has negative implications for agricultural productivity. Workers may take days off work because of ill-health. There are also long-term losses due to death, permanent injuries, and early retirement.

4.7 Employment or Occupation

Table 4.3 Occupational health hazards of agricultural work in developing countries. (Source: Cole (2006))

Exposure	Health effect	Specificity to agriculture
Weather, climate	Dehydration, heat cramps, heat exhaustion, heat stroke, skin cancer	Most agricultural operations are performed outdoors
Snakes, insects	Fatal or injurious bites and stings	Close proximity results in high incidence
Sharp tools, farm equipment	Injuries ranging from cuts to fatalities; hearing impairment from loud machinery	Most farm situations require a wide variety of skill levels for which workers have little formal training, and there are few hazard controls on tools and equipment
Physical labor, carrying loads	Numerous types of (largely unreported) musculoskeletal disorders, particularly soft-tissue disorders, e.g., back pain	Agricultural work involves awkward and uncomfortable conditions and sustained carrying of excessive loads
Pesticides	Acute poisonings, chronic effects such as neurotoxicity, reproductive effects, and cancer	More hazardous products are used in developing countries with minimal personal protective equipment (PPE)
Dusts, fumes, gases, particulates	Irritation of the eyes and respiratory tract, allergic reactions, respiratory diseases such as asthma, chronic obstructive pulmonary disease, and hypersensitivity pneumonitis	Agricultural workers are exposed to a wide range of dusts and gases from decomposition of organic materials in environments with few exposure controls and limited use of PPE use in hot climates
Biological agents and vectors of disease	Skin diseases such as fungal infections, allergic reactions, and dermatoses	Workers are in direct contact with environmental pathogens, fungi, infected animals, and allergenic plants
	Parasitic diseases such as schistosomiasis, malaria, sleeping sickness, leishmaniasis, ascariasis, and hookworm	Workers have intimate contact with parasites in soil, wastewater/sewage, dirty tools, and rudimentary housing
	Animal-related diseases or zoonoses such as anthrax, bovine tuberculosis, and rabies (at least 40 of the 250 zoonoses are occupational diseases in agriculture)	Workers have ongoing, close contact with animals through raising, sheltering, and slaughtering
	Cancers such as bladder cancer caused by urinary bilharzia contracted through working in flooded areas in North and sub-Saharan Africa	Agricultural workers are exposed to a mix of biological agents, pesticides, and diesel fumes, all linked with cancer

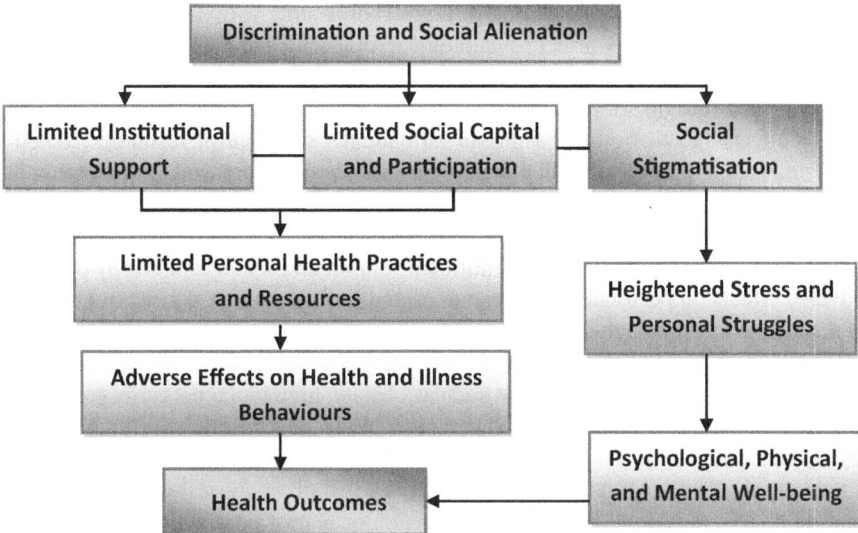

Fig. 4.6 Pathways by which discrimination and social alienation affect health outcomes

4.8 Social Alienation and Discrimination

Discrimination signifies a state of unequal treatment of an individual based on group or individual attributes such as gender, race, or ethnicity and class. It is a form of value judgment on an individual, which limits their social participation, rights, and privilege. Those who are discriminated against suffer from social alienation, a state in which people are distanced "from experiencing a crystallised totality in both the social world and in the self" (Kalekin-Fishman 2006, p. 6). Discrimination leads to inequalities in income, housing, education, and other factors and contributes significantly to disparities in mental and physical health. One critical form is when people are distanced from what is meaningful and relevant to them or their livelihood. This accounts for self-estrangement, low self-esteem, powerlessness, and, in particular, experience of inequity. Some of the aforementioned alienating practices are not apparent but manifested in unconscious acts, which have been entrenched within socio-spatial domains. Discrimination itself is a social stressor, which attracts responsive trajectories in daily life and systematically reflects in institutional patterns.

Figure 4.6 shows the pathways through which discrimination and social alienation (DSA) affect health outcomes. Discrimination and social alienation could adversely affect institutional support, social capital and participation, and social stigmatisation. Discrimination systematically limits the social relevance and value of an individual within social networks. Institutional discrimination creates social and structural boundaries that limit the opportunities, resources, and the standard of living of minorities. The individual then experiences heightened stress and devises personal strategies (coping styles and personal struggles) of dealing with daily experiences of social stressors. This may affect psychological, physical, and mental well-being and invariably affect health outcomes. Pascoe and Richman (2009) observed that apart from the fact that discrimination triggers sustained activation of stress responses, it also affects health by decreasing an individual's self-control resources, potentially increasing participation in unhealthy behaviours or decreasing participation in healthy behaviours. Extreme forms of discrimination may manifest in the form of interpersonal violence. An individual may be mentally and physically assaulted or even killed. More so, the limited institutional support and social capital may produce adverse effects on personal health resources and health and illness behaviour.

Evidence has shown the harmful health effects of discrimination and social alienation on mental health outcomes and well-being (Paradies 2006; Williams et al. 2003) and potential risk factors for disease such as obesity, high blood pressure, substance use (Williams and Mohammad 2009), and a lower health status (Williams et al. 2003; Haussman et al. 2008; Williams et al. 2008; Jackson et al. 2010; Copeland-Linder et al. 2011). All African countries (like western countries) are multi-ethnic and multi-religious, and there is always tension or fear of domination and discrimination manifesting in sociopolitical and economic activities. For instance, racial discrimination still exists in South Africa, and it is adversely consequential for health (Williams et al. 2008; Moomal et al. 2009). The minority groups are always at the receiving end. Such groups are usually in the lower rung of the society because of systematic social exclusion or discrimination in daily life. Social alienation adversely influences health status and health behaviour of minority groups. Discrimination is correlated with non-participation in behaviours that promote good health, such as cancer screening and safe sexual behaviour (Brodish et al. 2011).

4.9 Access to Health Care

Another SDH is access to health care. This is one of the critical determinants of health in Africa. Whether having or gaining access, both are required in the consideration of access to health care. Access to health care is a major health and development issue. Most governments want their citizens to enjoy universal and equitable access to good quality care (Obrist et al. 2007). But as Gulliford et al. (2002) observed, defining "access to health care" is a complex phenomenon. Access to health care refers to the ease with which an individual can obtain required health or medical services. It refers to opportunities to use health care facilities and obtain quality care without constraints. There are six dimensions of access which influence the course of the health-seeking process: availability, accessibility, affordability, adequacy, acceptability, and ability (Obrist et al. [2007]; see also Table 4.4).

The availability of facilities and services are important when discussing access to care. This is part of the spatial dimensions of access, which include accessibility and availability of services. This could also be termed as physical accessibility. Availability generally measures the number of services in comparison to the number

Table 4.4 Six dimensions of access to health care services[a]. (Source: Updated from Obrist et al. (2007), p. 1586)

Dimension	Questions
Availability: The existing health services and goods meet clients' needs.	What types of services exist? Which organizations offer these services? Is there enough skilled personnel? Do the offered products and services correspond with the needs of poor people? Do the supplies suffice to cover the demand?
Accessibility: The location of supply is in line with the location of clients.	What is the geographical distance between the services and the homes of the intended users? By what means of transport can they be reached? How much time does it take?
Affordability: The prices of services fit the clients' income and ability to pay.	What are the direct costs of the services and the products delivered through the services? What are the indirect costs in terms of transportation, lost time and income, bribes, and other "unofficial" charges?
Adequacy: The organization of health care meets the clients' expectations.	How are the services organized? Does the organizational setup meet the patients' expectations? Do the opening hours match with schedules of the clients, for instance the daily work schedule of small-scale farmers? Are the facilities clean and well kept?
Acceptability: The characteristics of providers match with those of the clients.	Does the information, explanation, and treatment provided take local illness concepts and social values into account? Do the patients feel welcome and cared for? Do the patients trust in the competence and personality of the health care providers? Are the service providers friendly?
Ability: The number, capacity, and skills of the providers and clients' needs.	Are there required numbers of personnel to meet clients' demands? What is the capacity of the facility in relation to the population of the clients? What are the various specialties available in the facility? Are there basic facilities to work with by the faculties?

[a] Obrist et al. (2007) identified the first five dimensions, we added the sixth dimension

of potential users of the service (Delamater et al. 2012). This concerns the supply of services. The idea is that health services should not be scarce (or competitive). They should be available as a basic amenity for all without discrimination or limitations. Accessibility in this sense can be measured from travel distance and time. Geographic accessibility is calculated by identifying the number of people residing more than 30 min from an acute care hospital (Delamater et al. 2012) or 5 km away from any health facility. Two major issues also surface: proximity to health facilities and the number of health facilities. Health facilities should be closer to the users. There is a problem of accessibility when the users have to travel more than 30 min or 5 km to access a health facility or when the location of a health facility is not accessible due to road network and related problems.

Affordability and adequacy of health care are also important measures or dimensions of access. Especially in poverty-ridden societies, inadequate monetary capacity is a major barrier to accessing health care. Complaints about fees and other associated costs (e.g., transportation) are usually frequent among people with low SES. If such costs are high, even where facilities are available, demand for health services may be low. Adequacy, on the other hand, deals with the organisation of health. It is important for providers to be cognisant of the peculiarities of their clients in terms of service schedules and appointments. Adequacy also has to do with the quality and level of services available. This should be adequate enough to meet the needs of the clients. In rural areas, there should be simple diagnostic tools.

Another dimension is acceptability of health care services. Some personal and sociocultural barriers may affect acceptability. The systems of care need to account for the social values and norms of the community. In Muslim-dominated parts of North Africa (see Fig. 12.1 for a map of Africa), gender concordance between caregivers and takers is often a preference. If such a social norm is not considered, health care may not be accepted by the community. In addition, to promote acceptability, it is necessary to mobilise the community and provide information that may encourage utilisation. More so, the ability of health care is part of access. This has to do with the availability of personnel: number of physicians, nurses, midwives, pharmacists, and other supportive staff. There will not be effective health care without adequate health workers. Shortage of personnel is a major problem confronting many countries, especially African countries.

These six dimensions of access to health care are critical in the determination of the health of the population. Facilitating access is concerned with helping people to command appropriate health care resources to preserve or improve their health (Gulliford et al. 2002). Without access to health care, especially based on the six (As) dimensions, the health indicators of the community may be very poor. This is why access to health care is a fundamental determinant of health.

So far, eight major social determinants of health have been discussed. There are other determinants of health, which include urbanisation and migration, globalisation, and health policies. All of these social conditions are fundamental in determining the health status of the community. It is therefore vital to address the social determinants of health in order to improve the health status of any population.

References

Albouy, V., & Lequien, L. (2009). Does compulsory education lower mortality? *Journal of Health Economics, 28*(1), 155–168.

Amzat, J. (2008). Lumpen childhood in Nigeria: A case of the Almajirai in northern Nigeria. *Hemispheres: Studies on Cultures and Societies, 23*, 54–66.

Amzat, J. (2011). Assessing the progress of malaria control in Nigeria. *World Health and Population, 12*(3), 42–51.

Anderson, J. W., & Conley, S. B. (2007). Whole grains and diabetes. In L Marquart, Jr. D. R. Jacobs, G. H. McIntosh, K. Poutanen, & M. Reicks (Eds.), *Whole Grains and Health* (pp. 29–45). Ames: Blackwell Publishing Professional.

Anderson, J. W., Baird, P., Davis, R. H. Jr., Ferreri, S., Knudtson, M., Koraym, A., Waters, V., & Williams, C. L. (2009). Health benefits of dietary fiber. *Nutrition Reviews, 67*(4), 188–205.

Appleton, S. (2000). Education and health at the household level in sub-Saharan Africa. CID Working Paper no. 33, Explaining African Economic Growth Performance Conference Series.

Baker, M., McNicholas, A., Garrett, N., Jones, N., Stewart, J., Koberstein, V., & Lennon, D. (2000). Household crowding a major risk factor for epidemic meningococcal disease in Auckland children. *The Pediatric Infectious Disease Journal, 19*, 983–990.

Brodish, A. B., Cogburn, C. D., Fuller-Rowell, T. E., Peck, S., Malanchuk, O., & Eccles, J. S. (2011). Perceived racial discrimination as a predictor of health behaviours: The moderating role of gender. *Race and Social Problems*. doi:10.1007/s12552-011-9050-6.

Brunello, G., Fort, G., Schneeweis, N., & Winter-Ebmer, R. (2011). The causal effect of education on health: What is the role of health behaviors? Discussion Paper Series, IZA DP No. 5944.

Cockerham, W. C. (2013). Bourdieu and an update of health lifestyle theory. In W. C. Cockerham (Ed.), *Medical sociology on the move: New directions in theory* (pp. 127–154). Dordrecht: Springer.

Cole, D. (2006). Understanding the links between agriculture and health: occupational health hazards of agriculture. International Food Policy Research Institute, Focus 13, Brief 8 of 16. Washington, D.C.: USA.

Copeland-Linder, N., Lambert, S. F., Chen, Y., & Ialongo, N. S. (2011). Contextual stress and health risk behaviours among African American adolescents. *Journal of Youth and Adolescence, 40*, 158–173.

CSDH. (2008). Closing the gap in a generation: Health equity through action on the social determinants of health. *Final Report of the Commission on Social Determinants of Health*. Geneva: World Health Organization.

Cutler D. M., & Lleras-Muney, A. (2006). Education and health: evaluating theories and evidence. NBER Working paper Series. http://www.nber.org/papers/w12352. Accessed 2 June 2012.

Cutler, D. M., Lleras-Muney, A., & Vogl, T. (2006). Socioeconomic status and health: Dimensions and mechanisms, National Bureau of Economic Research (NBER) Working Papers: 14333.

Delamater, P. L., Messina, J. P., Shortridge, A. M., & Grady, S. C. (2012). Measuring geographic access to health care: raster and network-based methods. *International Journal of Health Geographics, 11*, 15. doi:10.1186/1476-072X-11-15.

Delisle, H. F., Vioque, J., & Augusta, G. (2009). Dietary patterns and quality in West-African immigrants in Madrid. *Nutrition Journal, 23*(8), 3. doi:10.1186/1475-2891-8-3.

Fathalla, M. F. (2000). When medicine rediscovered its social roots. *Bull World Health Organ* [online], *78*(5), 677–678.

Fonseca, R., & Zheng, Y. (2011). The effect of education on health: Cross-country evidence. Working Paper, RAND WR–864.

Govender, T., Barnes, J. M., & Pieper, C. H. (2010). Living in low-cost housing settlements in Cape Town, South Africa—the epidemiological characteristics associated with increased health vulnerability. *Journal of Urban Health: Bulletin of the New York Academy of Medicine, 87*(6), 899–911.

Grant, U. (2005). *Health and poverty linkages: perspectives of the chronically poor*. Background paper for the chronic poverty report 2008–09. Manchester: Chronic Poverty Research Center.

Gulliford, M., Figueroa-Munoz, J., Morgan, M., Hughes, D., Gibson, B., Beech, R., & Hudson, M. (2002). What does 'access to health care' mean? *Journal of Health Services Research & Policy, 7*(3), 186–188.

Hausmann, L. R. M., Jeong, K., Bost, J. E., & Ibrahim, S. A. (2008). Perceived discrimination in health care and health status in a racially diverse sample. *Medical Care, 46*(9), 905–914.

Heise, L., Germain, A., & Pitanguy, J. (1994). Violence against women: The hidden health burden. World Bank Discussion Paper, No 255. Washington. D.C: The World Bank.

Irwin, A., Valentine, N., Brown, C., Loewenson, R., Solar, O., Brown, H., Koller, T., & Vega, J. (2006). The Commission on social determinants of health: Tackling the social roots of health inequities. *PLoS Medicine, 3*(6), e106.

Jackson, J. S., Knight, K. M., & Rafferty, J. A. (2010). Race and unhealthy behaviors: Chronic stress, the HPA axis, and physical and mental health disparities over the life course. *American Journal of Public Health, 100*, 933–939.

References

Kalekin-Fishman, D. (2006). Studying alienation: Toward a better society? *Kybernetes, 35*(3/4), 522–530.

Kawachi, I., & Wamala, S. (2007). *Globalization and health* (pp. 122–137). New York: Oxford University Press.

Kickbusch, I. S. (2001). Health literacy: Addressing the health and education divide. *Health Promotion International, 16*(3), 289–297.

Kranz, S., Brauchla, M., Slavin, J. L., & Miller, K. B. (2012). What do we know about dietary fiber intake in children and health? The effects of fiber intake on constipation, obesity, and diabetes in children. *Advances in Nutrition, 3*, 47–53.

Lairon, D., Arnault, N., Bertrais, S., Planells, R., Clero, E., Hercberg, S., & Boutron-Ruault, M. C. (2005). Dietary fiber intake and risk factors for cardiovascular disease in French adults. *The American Journal of Clinical Nutrition, 82*(6), 1185–1194.

Lancaster, K. J., Watts, S. O., & Dixon, L. B. (2006). Dietary intake and risk of coronary heart disease differ among ethnic subgroups of black Americans. *The Journal of Nutrition, 136*(2), 446–451.

Li, Y. C., Huang, H. J., Zhang, Z. L., & Qi, X. Y. (2008). Effects of occupation on health of traffic policemen in a city. *Chinese Journal of Industrial Hygiene and Occupational and Diseases, 26*(3), 165–7.

Lochner, L. (2011). Non-production benefits of education: Crime, health, and good citizenship, Working Paper 16722, National Bureau of Economic Research.

Mackenbach, J. P., Stirbu, I., Roskam, A. R., Schaap, M. M., Menvielle, G., Leinsalu, M., & Kunst, A. E. (2008). Socioeconomic inequalities in health in 22 European countries. *The New England Journal of Medicine, 358*(23), 2468–2481.

Marmot, M. (2005). Social determinants of health inequalities. *Lancet, 365*, 1099–1104.

Mokhtar, N., Elati, J., Chabir, R., Bour, A., Elkari, K., Schlossman, N. P., Caballero, B., & Aguenaou, H. (2001). Diet culture and obesity in northern Africa. *The Journal of Nutrition, 131*(3), 887S–892S.

Moomal, H., Jackson, P. B., Stein, D. J., Herman, A., Myer, L., Seedat, S., Madela-Mntla, E., & Williams, D. R. (2009). Perceived discrimination and mental health disorders: The South African stress and health study. *South African Medical Journal, 99*(5 Pt 2), 383–389.

Nutbeam, D. (2000). Health education as a public health goal: A challenge for health education and communication strategies into the 21st century. *Health Promotion International, 15*(3), 259–267.

Obrist, B., Iteba, N., Lengeler, C., Makemba, A., Mshana, C., Nathan, R., Alba, S., Dillip, A., Hetzel, M. W., Mayumana, I., Schulze, A., & Mshinda, H. (2007). Access to health care in contexts of livelihood insecurity: A framework for analysis and action *PLoS Medicine, 4*(10), e308. doi:10.1371/journal.pmed.0040308.

Paradies, Y. A. (2006). Systematic review of empirical research on self-reported racism and health. *International Journal of Epidemiology, 35*(4), 888–901.

Pascoe, E. A., & Richman, L. S. (2009). Perceived discrimination and health: A meta-analytic review. *Psychological Bulletin, 135*(4), 531–554.

Peters, E., Bakers, D. P., Dieckmann, N. F., Leon, J., & Collins, J. (2010). Explaining the effect of education on health: A field study in Ghana. *Psychological Science, 21*, 1369–1376.

Picker, L. (2012). The effects of education on health. http://www.nber.org/digest/mar07/w12352.html. Accessed 2 June 2012.

Sánchez-Barriga, J. J. (2012). Mortality trends from hypertension in Mexico by socioeconomic region and state, 2000–2008. *Revista panamericana de salud pública, 32*(2), 109–116.

Sen, A. (2003). Missing women—revisited: Reduction in female mortality has been counterbalanced by sex selective abortions. *BMJ, 327*, 1297–1298.

South Australian Council of Social Services (SACOSS). (2008). The social determinants of health. SACOSS Information Paper December 2008. Australia.

Tarlov, A. (1996). Social determinants of health: The sociobiological translation. In D. Blane, E. Brunner, & R. Wilkinson (Eds.), *Health and social organization* (pp. 71–93). London: Routledge.

UNESCO. (2010). *EFA Global monitoring report: reaching the marginalized*. Paris: Oxford University Press.

UNFPA. (2004). Child marriage advocacy programme: Fact sheet on child marriage and early union.

United Nations Development Programme (UNDP). (2009). *Overcoming barriers: Human mobility and development*. NY.

United Nations Human Settlements Programme (UN-HABITAT). (2003). *The challenge of slums: Global report on human settlements*. London: Earthscan Publications Ltd.

Vandemoortele, J., & Delamonica, E. (2002). Education vaccine against HIV/AIDS. *Current Issues in Comparative Education, 3*(1), 6–13.

Volkers, A. C., Westert, G. P., & Schellevis, F. G. (2007). Health disparities by occupation, modified by education: A cross-sectional population study. *BMC Public Health, 7*, 196.

Waters, A. (2001). Do housing conditions impact on health inequalities between Australia's Rich and Poor? Australian Housing and Urban Research Institute (AHURI) Positioning Paper No. 2.

Whelton, S. P., Hyre, A. D., Pedersen, B., Yi, Y., Whelton, P. K., & He, J. (2005). Effect of dietary fiber intake on blood pressure: A meta-analysis of randomized, Controlled Clinical Trials. *Journal of Hypertension, 23*, 475–481.

WHO. (2009). Ten facts on women's health. http://www.who.int/gender/documents/10facts_womens_health_en.pdf. Accessed 11 Feb. 2013.

WHO. (2010). Ten facts about tobacco and gender. http://www.who.int/gender/documents/10facts_gender_tobacco_en.pdf. Accessed 11 Feb. 2013.

WHO. (2000). African submit on roll back malaria. Geneva.

Williams, D. R., & Mohammed, S. A. (2009). Discrimination and racial disparities in health: Evidence and needed research. *Journal of Behavioral Medicine, 32*:20–47.

Williams, D. R., Gonzalez, H. M., Williams, S., Mohammed, S. A., Moomal, H., & Stein, D. J. (2008). Perceived discrimination, race and health in South Africa. *Social Science & Medicine, 67*(3), 441–452.

Williams, D. R., Neighbors, H. W., & Jackson, J. S. (2003). Racial/ethnic discrimination and health: findings from community studies. *American Journal of Public Health, 93*(2), 200–208.

World Bank. (2011). World Development Report 2012: Gender equality and development. Washington DC: World Bank.

Yusuf, O. B., Adeoye, B. W., Oladepo, O. O., Peters, D. H., & Bishai, D. (2010). Poverty and fever vulnerability in Nigeria: A multilevel analysis. *Malaria Journal, 9*, 235. doi:10.1186/1475-2875-9-235.

Chapter 5
Functionalist Perspective on Health

5.1 Introduction

The definition of medical sociology depicts the application of sociological theories in the understanding of human health and illness. This and the next three chapters are devoted to the examination of sociological perspectives or theories. Sociological theory is defined as a set of interrelated ideas that allow for the systemisation of knowledge of the social world (Ritzer 2010). Sociological perspectives or theories involve frameworks and insights derived from empirical observations and systematic reasoning about the social world. The theories focus on structural relationships and factors and consider individuals to be embodied (social) agents patterned to create and recreate the social world. Such perspectives are then used to understand, explain or interpret, control, and predict social phenomena and human society in general. Ritzer (2011) observed that a paradigm differentiates one scientific community from the other because there are usually many paradigms within a field of study. This is also true for sociology as a multi-paradigm social science discipline. Sociologists use different perspectives in the analysis of social issues.

Neuman (2011, p. 81) defines a paradigm as "a general organising framework for theory and research that includes basic assumptions, key issues, models of quality research, and methods for seeking answers." By implication, a paradigm may suggest what can be studied, how it will be studied, and how data will be interpreted. What is problematic for one paradigm may not be for another. The perspective used may also determine the results obtained. It is always important for sociologists to situate their studies within appropriate theoretical orientation. Since sociological research is a scientific endeavour, the assumptions and principles provided by a theory will structure the research ideas, data gathering, and interpretation of findings within a specific domain. Apart from theoretical explanations, sociologists also rely on observational explanations of events. In sum, sociologists produce a body of knowledge based on theoretical and empirical facts. The multiple paradigms in sociology add great scientific value to the discipline. One perspective may demonstrate intellectual superiority on one issue more than the other. Continuous empirical findings provide opportunities for modification of existing paradigms. This means that the perspectives are not static.

In sociology, there are three major perspectives or paradigms, which include functionalist, conflict, and interpretive perspectives. Each of the perspectives includes a number of substantive or middle-range theories. These also represent categories of theories usually invoked in sociology to explain social issues. It is important to note that theory and research are very key in sociological imagination or enterprising. Theories are usually tested and validated or debunked as adequate coherent ideas to explain social phenomena. Theories often show patterns and motivations of behaviour using various concepts. This helps sociologists in conceptual analysis and interpreting data based on the theoretical orientation. While there are a number of theories, there is no strict attachment to any particular theory or theoretical orientation. The selection of a perspective depends on the problem and the context from which the problem will be studied. In fact, the goal of research might be to test a particular theory—to know whether the theory is relevant in explaining a problem among certain groups.

While it has been argued that most sociological studies require a theory, it is important to note that a whole paradigm cannot form a theoretical framework of a particular research topic. A paradigm consists of a number of theories with each providing divergent explanations. That two theorists are functionalists does not mean that they have similar conceptual agreement or even point of view. Sociologists often apply middle-range theories or substantive theories in empirical investigations. These are particular models or explanations carved out of a broader perspective; some are specifically formulated to be applied in a subdiscipline such as medical sociology. For instance, Parsonian sick role is a good example of a substantive model or theory in medical sociology. The theory is derived from the functionalist perspective and from the numerous works of the American sociologist, Talcott Parsons. Apart from this, there are other various models (e.g., Suchman's illness behaviour model, Chrisman's or Igun's stages of the health-seeking process, and the health belief model) derived from empirical investigation that can be applied in medical sociology. Having provided this little background, discussion on the perspectives will start with functionalism.

5.2 The Functionalist Perspective: A General Overview

Functionalism (also known as the consensus paradigm) is a body of theories in social sciences in general. It is particularly the oldest theoretical tradition in sociology. It is dated to the works of August Comte (1798–1857), who coined sociology in 1838; *Positive Philosophy* (Comte 1896); *Rules of Sociological Methods* (Durkheim 1897); *Principles of Sociology* (Spencer 1896); and many other scholarly works. Functionalism is an approach that uses organismic analogy to explain human societies and social phenomena. The central concern of functionalism is how to maintain social order, equilibrium, or stability in human society. Social order means a state of normality in human society, especially when social institutions are functional and maintained for the continuous benefits and existence of the society (Amzat and

5.2 The Functionalist Perspective: A General Overview

Omololu 2012). It is important to understand the philosophical, epistemological, and intellectual foundations of functionalism. Functionalism grew with the rise of empiricism, rationalism, and, in general, the scientific revolution. First, functionalism is a realist tradition. The realists (also called essentialists or objectivists) believe in the reality of social existence and phenomena. To them, whatever exists is real and can be studied objectively and empirically. Health problems are a part of the realities of social existence. To study an event objectively implies that value detachment is possible. The researcher can always be objective and systematic in carrying out investigation. Realism promotes value-free science, which means that social research should be conducted in an objective manner based on empirical evidence without interference of moral and political values.

Functionalists also hold that social processes are determined, grounded on the principle of cause-effect (or deterministic) assumption that whatever happens has a cause. Science in general and empirical works in particular flow from the deterministic assumption. The primary endeavour of science is to understand causality. It is only when the cause is understood that scientists can understand the effects—without cause, there is no effect. Functionalism, like other approaches in science, believes in multiple causalities. A particular phenomenon can be attributed to many causal and intervening factors. The implication of this deterministic assumption in understanding human behaviour is that there are external and coercive factors responsible for human actions and behaviour. Particularly to the functionalists, the social norms, values and positions, and conditions greatly determine human behaviour. The social processes are fraught with expectations. Hence behaviour emerged in the process of meeting expectations and fulfilling social imperatives. Roles are randomly allocated, and all roles are functional for the survival of the society. Individuals cannot actually be held accountable for their own position. This distribution of social position is random without the influence of individuals. Sometimes, this deterministic approach is called the mechanical model of man.

Furthermore, functionalism is part of the perspective that signifies that sociology is a scientific endeavour because of the reliance on positivism. Comte (1896), Spencer (1896), and Durkheim (1897) recommended that the application of scientific methodology should be the *modus operandi* of sociology. The discipline must be based on systematic empirical understanding of social events and to produce a body of knowledge based on precise and verifiable evidence. This is why the primary task of sociology is to produce universal laws to explain human action and behaviour. Comte (1896) in *Positive Philosophy* advocated that sociology should employ experimental, observational, and comparative methods in the understanding of its subject matter. This positivist agenda illustrates the reliance of sociology on coherent and structured theoretical and empirical stance. The structured procedural approach further promotes the close association between medical sociology and medicine. This is because, like in medical sciences, empirical findings to a large extent can be verified, falsified, or refuted and replicated, mainly because sociology relies or adopts methods from the pure sciences.

As previously mentioned, sociologists tend to generate universal laws to explain human action and behaviour. It relies on generalisation often called the nomothetic

Table 5.1 Basic views of functionalism

View of the society	System, collective consciousness, harmony, integration or cooperation, shared values
Level of analysis	Macro, group or social aggregate
Key concepts	Structures, functions, roles, dysfunctions, social system, division of labour
View of the individual	People are shaped by norms and values or collective sentiments
View of the social order	Determined by collective values or consensus
View of social change	Evolutionary—gradual or in piecemeal or stages
View on disease or illness	It affects role allocation and performance, illness as a form of social deviance and leads to social vacuums, dysfunctional/immense consequences for social aggregate, health care institutions and other agents of the society can function to reduce disease burden

approach. With the use of scientific methods, it is possible for sociologists to generalise and provide a general basis for actions and interventions. Functionalism relies on nomothetic assumption, which is also made possible because of a macro level of analysis. Functionalists focus more on groups or the social aggregate. Data are obtained from a group with the use of random sampling and the findings are considered valid for the group or community. The macro or macroscopic level of analysis involves social phenomena that are relatively large in size, such as societies, groups, religion, culture, social class, organisation, and institutions. The sample size is often large to ensure validity and reliability. More so, the functionalists rely on objectivity and study events at the objective level. Objectivity implies value-neutrality. This is a major crux in science because without it, scientific knowledge will be largely biased and easily refutable. Objective level relates to the externality of events. Social events (human behaviour and society) can be studied and measured like "things" in the pure sciences.

What then are the methodological implications of these philosophical and epistemological foundations? A functionalist approach is closely linked with a quantitative approach, questionnaire design, experimentation, randomisation, probability sampling, objectivity, generalisation, large sample size, statistical analysis (both descriptive and inferential), and, generally, systematic research designs. The use of statistical models and analysis play a central role in generalisation. Probability sampling is usually used in quantitative research. There are various other specific methods from the positivist tradition used in sociology. These issues are easy to deduce because of functionalism's positivist orientation.

Functionalism has some specific views as shown in Table 5.1. It is important to understand some of these foundational features before explaining some substantive theories of functionalism. There are also divergent views in functionalism. The attempt here is to explain some of the general features of functionalism. It should be noted that there is no absolute consensus on some of the attributes. For instance, Robert K. Merton is a critical functionalist, who criticised most of the assumptions of functionalism. Despite that, there is a lot of common ground.

The first major feature of functionalism is organismic analogy. August Comte and Herbert Spencer observed that the human society is like a living organism. This perspective is borrowed from biology. The human society is thus a social organism which lives and functions like a biological organism. It is a social system with interrelated and interdependent parts. The parts of a biological organism—such as legs, hands, eyes, nose, ears, and mouth—function to make the whole body. They all contribute to the survival and existence of the biological organism. The parts of the social organism include institutions such as family, political, economic, religious, educational, and marriage institutions. All of these parts also function for the survival of the society. They play differential and specialised functions. If one part is malfunctioning, all other parts will be affected. If the family institution is not stable, it will adversely affect other institutions.

The essence of various parts is to fulfil the functional imperatives, prerequisites, or needs of the social systems (Ritzer 2011). Society has some needs that must be fulfilled. Society needs to regulate its affairs; that is why there is a political institution to do so. Society needs to produce goods and services for its members, which is the function of the economic institution. These functions are fundamental for the survival of the society. Problems in human society often manifest from inadequate adaptive processes and deviation of some members of the society. Such problems often suggest the need for adjustment within the system. Invariably, the problems are also functional even though the society must at all times keep them at the basic minimal level in order to prevent them from inflicting unbearable social burden. Events (e.g., health problems) that do not contribute positive function for the survival of the society are dysfunctional. Using the terms functionality and dysfunctionality, a health problem is functional because it suggests a task for the health institution and it is dysfunctional because it inflicts pain on some members of the society.

The society is held together by collective consciousness, sentiments, and shared values. Common morality and values explain the social bonding in human society. As health is a common value, it enables every individual to drive towards a common goal of ensuring a functional social system. There is mutual cooperation in human society. Therefore, functionalists assume that society consists of cooperating individuals who share common values.

Generally, the functionalists view health as a prerequisite for the smooth functioning of society while illness is a form of deviance. Health is a social value and every society needs it for survival and development. Illness is a form of infraction on the ability of the individual to carry out daily activities. Lupton (2003) observed that illness indicates a failure to conform to societal expectations and norms in some way. It is thus an unnatural state of the human body, causing both physical and social dysfunction, and therefore must be alleviated as soon as possible. The functional role of the medical practitioners or health care institution as a subsystem (in the whole social system) is to help in the control of disease, especially by helping people to get well and return to their normal roles in the society. Having highlighted some basic foundations of functionalism, the next subsection will discuss some functionalist substantive theories in medical sociology.

5.3 Functionalist Substantive Theories in Medical Sociology

The substantive theories are specific contributions within a perspective which can be applied in specialised areas. As noted in Chap. 1, most of the founding fathers of sociology were not particular about substantive areas of sociology but rather a general development of sociology as a discipline. This is why it took time to get the first major contribution directly related to medical sociology. It is important to start with the first acknowledged explicit sociological work in medical sociology which is the "sick role" developed by Talcott Parsons in 1951.

5.3.1 Parsons' Sick Role

Talcott Parsons (1902–1979) was an American sociologist and a structural functionalist. He analysed the works of Comte, Spencer, Durkheim, and Weber (among others), and he was particularly influenced by the ideas of these founding fathers of sociology. In his major work, *The Social System* published in 1951, Parsons introduced the concept of the sick role. The model of the sick role was the first theoretical concept that explicitly concerned medical sociology and enhanced the place of medical sociology in the mainstream of sociology. The model was primary designed to explain illness behaviour. Like other functionalists, Parsons was interested in value consensus and social order. His key focus is how social interaction/action produce social order. Parsons sought to analyse individual behaviour in the context of large-scale social systems (Bradby 2012). The individuals are primary units that contribute to the society in terms of the roles performed. Unfortunately, a high prevalence of illness is dysfunctional for society (Parsons 1951), preventing people from fulfilling their social roles. This influences the wider functioning of the society.

Bradby (2012) observed that the onset of illness was of interest to Parsons because it prevented the fulfilment of social roles, such as paid employment and parental duties. Illness is "one of the most important withdrawal behaviours in our society" (Parsons 1951, p. 31). Parsons argued that the ill take on a sick role, which (like all roles) provides them with a set of responsibilities and privileges (Emke 2002). Role constitutes socially recognised patterns of expectations of behaviour on the part of persons in certain positions. Like there are a number of roles attached to the position of a father, the sick role depicts the social position of the sick in the society and the expectations attached. There are expectations and obligations for them as well as for normal individuals in the society. This is why the concept is called the sick role or, put the other way around, the roles of the sick. Parsons (1951, pp. 436–437) identified four aspects of the institutionalised expectation system relative to the sick role. The first two aspects are rights of the patients while the last are duties.

1. An exemption from normal social role responsibilities relative to the nature and severity of the illness. The physician is usually the one to legitimise this right. At times, people are often resistant to admitting they are sick and it is not uncommon

for others to detect and inform them that they need medical help. Here, Parsons identified the critical roles of significant others in recognition of ill-health and social referral for appropriate care. Parsons observed that the essence of legitimation has the social function of protection against "malingering" a social pretence of being sick to claim excuse from roles and expectations. The implication is that it is possible for certain individual to avoid responsibilities and thus the sick role also serves as a mechanism of social control.
2. An exemption from responsibility to get well by one's own actions alone. In other words, the sick person cannot be expected to get better on her/his own but has the right to (medical) assistance. In Parsons' words, "... the sick person cannot be expected by 'pulling himself together' to get well by an act of decision or will." He or she needs support in the process of getting well. The importance of seeking medical and social assistance is stressed. This creates a state of dependence on social capital or significant others and health care institutions.
3. The sick should accept both that the state of being ill is not desirable and an accompanying obligation to *want* to get well. Sickness is dysfunctional to the social system. Hence, it is obligated that the sick should want to get well. This is required with the help of the physician, so that the patient can get out (of illness condition) as expeditiously as possible.
4. An obligation to seek *technically competent* help, normally from a physician and to *cooperate* with him/her in the process of trying to get well. Parsons stressed two major issues in the last aspect—technical competent help and cooperation. The patient has to seek for appropriate diagnosis from medical experts and submit to their directives, for instance, by providing required samples (e.g., blood or urine).

Parsons viewed health from the capability perspective. This is in line with the structural-functionalist principles that health is a functional prerequisite of society (William 2005). The first step is that an individual who is sick has to withdraw from his/her daily roles. For example, he or she might not be able to go to school or work. He is thus entitled to sick-leave. To Parsons, illness is a social deviance because it negates the value expectation of the society. As outlined in the four aspects of sick role, Parsons provided a discussion of illness behaviour as a description of a set of defined roles, norms, and expectations. It is highlighted that for the parties of the illness event, the phases create an avenue for resolution of the event and a return to normal roles in the society (Young 2004). This also accounts for the therapeutic legitimising function of the physician. It can be observed that the sick role is a socially prescribed mechanism for channelling and controlling this deviance called sickness (William 2005). It provides the channel an individual needs to follow in order to return to his/her functional capacity.

Furthermore, while individual entitlement to relief from duties is legitimate, it has to be sanctioned by a competent person, usually the physician. The model recognises the roles of physicians in helping the sick by first relieving their role burden and providing a safety net for their absenteeism (from usual roles). However, this should not promote malingering, as the next stage stipulates that an individual has to develop the motivation to get better and also seek competent help. Parsons (1951, p. 440) noted that "the urgency of the need of help will vary with the severity of the disability, suffering, and risk of death or serious, lengthy or permanent disablement." The fault of the illness is not placed on the patient, but he or she has the responsibility to seek the appropriate channels to get well and cooperate with the competent persons in the process. He/she has to keep appointments and comply with a therapeutic regimen.

Another major primary aim of Parsons for discussing medical practice and the sick role is the reflection on rational action and modern values. Parsons (1951, p. 432) observed that medical practice is a mechanism in the social system for coping with the illnesses of its members. It involves a set of institutionalised roles, which are guided by principles and values of the society. This is why a medical institution earns its place in the social structure, for its distinct contribution to the functional existence of every individual in the social system. Parsons (1951, p. 438) observed that by relating the sick role and the pattern of patient-practitioner relations to the pattern variables, some inherent values in the institutionalised roles of both the physicians and the patients are obvious.

1. "It [patient-practitioner relations] is inherently *universalistic*, in that generalized objective criteria determine whether one is or is not sick, how sick, and with what kind of sickness..." This is against *particularism*. Universal criteria are employed to determine whether an individual is sick and therefore entitled to exemption from duties. Invariably, the physician-patient relation is not based on a personal relationship, and diagnosis is objectively determined.
2. "It is also *functionally specific*, confined to the sphere of health, and particular 'complaints' and disabilities within that sphere." This relates to the increasing social differentiation of functions and specialisation. Seeking for competent help by the patient is thus confined to the medical sphere. The other side is *diffuseness* in contact based on varieties of personal attachments or reasons.
3. "It is furthermore *affectively neutral* in orientation in that the expected behaviour, 'trying to get well,' is focused on an objective problem not on the cathectic significance of persons." As Parsons observed, it should not be interpreted that the status of an individual does not play any role in illness behaviour. Professional roles should be based on value-neutrality. The other side of the coin is *affectivity*, based on emotional involvements.
4. The last pattern variable is that "the orientation of the sick role vis-à-vis the physician is also defined as *collectively oriented*." This orientation is beyond *self-interest* because of the involvement of various parties in the process of getting well. The act of seeking help goes beyond the self-interest of the patient to get better, but also the expectation of the society.

5.3.1.1 Criticisms of the Sick Role Theory

Since the conception of the theory in 1951, it has been heavily criticised. While Parsons provided a universal and ideal-type model of the sick role, the nature of illness, sociocultural attributes of the patients have more often than not regulated the role expectations of the sick (Segall 1976). For instance, a patient with chronic

5.3 Functionalist Substantive Theories in Medical Sociology

illness might not be exempted from roles because the illness might not present with disabling symptoms. Other criticisms include:

1. The sick role provides a one-way obligation by recommending that the patient needs to cooperate in the process of getting well. It is as if the patient is helpless and does not have any knowledge, competency, or aspirations in the process of care. This may defy the right to self-determination. The patients also have the right to reject certain treatments based on personal reasons. For instance, a Jehovah's Witness may reject blood transfusion for religious reasons. This cannot be regarded as a lack of cooperation. The physicians also have to cooperate with the patients.
2. Parsons assumes that recovery is always possible, but since the Twentieth century there has been a growing burden of chronic rather than acute conditions (Bilton et al. 2004). The model envisages that the sick role is temporary, but a chronic condition suggests that sickness experience might be lifelong and a person in such condition cannot be exempted from role obligation for life. Chronic conditions only require behavioural or lifestyle adjustment since patients may only be partially restricted in their capacity to perform certain roles.
3. The sick role model assumes that the physicians are there to serve the interest of the patients. However, in some cases, the interest of the physician may override that of the patients. This may also expose the patients to exploitation. For instance, it is possible for the physician to be interested in profit motive. This simply implies that the interests of doctor and patient might conflict, especially because of unequal power relations. Parsons (1951, p. 445) started the critique of the sick role himself when he opined that a combination of helplessness, lack of technical competence, and emotional disturbance (on the part of the patient) makes the patient a peculiarly vulnerable object for exploitation.
4. Patients could also face harassment from physicians. Patients are sometimes victims of sexual, verbal, and even physical abuse at health facilities (Lamont and Woodward 1994). Abuse negates the rights of the patients. As Parsons noted, it is essential for the physician to have access to the body of his/her patient in order to perform some procedures, some of which might be very sensitive, such as rectal, penile, breast, or vaginal examination. This indicates that the patient has to give away a high volume of trust, which sometimes could be defiled.
5. The model also depicts increasing medicalisation of various aspects of life (see Sect. 9.1). The physician is required to legitimise exception from duties. A number of behaviours, situations, and conditions are being interpreted in medical terms and this requires a medical certificate of clearance. It gives the medical professionals increased power in determining normal and abnormal behaviours—especially when it is appropriate to be exempted from normal duties (see Zola 1972 for more discussion on this).
6. For some illnesses (e.g., venereal diseases), the patient is not exempted from blame, and for others, he/she may suffer stigma (Levine and Kozloff 1978). Especially in most lifestyle-related diseases, patients take responsibility for smoking, sexual, and dietary behaviours. There is also a tendency to blame society for

various forms of injustices that may increase exposure of individuals. Therefore, Parsons is not completely correct to assume that patients should be exempted from fault of their conditions.

Despite these criticisms, the sick role is still relevant in the explanation of sickness trajectories. It is often regarded as a major step in the development of medical sociology.

5.3.2 *Emile Durkheim: Understanding Mortality through Suicide*

It is not common to read the elaboration of Emile Durkheim's theoretical dispositions on suicide in many texts in medical sociology. This is why Parsons' sick role is often the starting point and is commonly regarded as the first explicit contribution of one of the key sociological theorists in medical sociology. In fact, Durkheim did not actually aim to contribute to the field of medical sociology but to exercise the empirical relevance of sociology in studying various social phenomena—to develop a general theory of suicide and explicitly explain the "sociology" in suicidal currents. Other subdisciplines in sociology such as social deviance and criminology have extensively focused on the issue of suicide; perhaps suicide is a form of social deviance, and in many countries it is a crime. But more obviously, and as described by Durkheim, it is about morbidity and mortality—hence the significance of this contribution to the field of medical sociology. Durkheim presents a grand attempt to understand mortality through suicide. Like his other counterparts (Comte, Weber, Marx, and Spencer), he was interested in how to maintain social order in human society. An orderly society, at least to a large extent, is devoid of social and structural problems (including health problems) that can deny people access to good life.

Emile Durkheim (1858–1917), a French sociologist, conceived sociology as the scientific study of social facts. In *The Rules of Sociological Method* (first published in 1895 and later in 1982), Durkheim argued that sociology should concentrate on understanding social facts. He viewed social facts as forces and structures that are external to, and coercive of, the individual. Social facts are determinants of human behaviour and actions. As he noted, social facts exist *sui generis*— independent of human mind, as they are not abstractions but objective realities and, as he claimed, must be studied as *things*. Studying social facts is close to studying the social determinants of health, and such determinants are social facts that if understood could help in disease control and prevention. Ritzer (2011, p. 19) observed that Durkheim reasoned that if he could link an individual behaviour such as suicide to social causes (social facts), he would be able to demonstrate the positivist stance in sociology. Ritzer further noted that Durkheim did not examine why individual *A* or *B* committed suicide; rather, he was interested in the causes of differences in suicide rates among groups, regions, and countries. *Suicide*, first published in 1897 and later in 1951, presents an empirical application of sociological (scientific) methods in the study of a particular form of behaviour called suicide.

Table 5.2 The four types of suicide

Social fact	Level	Kind of suicide
Integration	Low	Egoistic suicide
	High	Altruistic suicide
Regulation	Low	Anomic suicide
	High	Fatalistic suicide

Suicide is the first major application of statistical methods in sociological investigation. It primarily involves an extensive explanation of social problems, focusing on social causes (independent and dependent variables). As noted in the editor's preface, "Durkheim has treated or touched on normal and abnormal psychology, social psychology, anthropology (especially the concept of race), meteorological and other 'cosmic' factors, religion, marriage, the family, divorce, primitive rites and customs, social and economic crises, crime (especially homicide) and law and jurisprudence, history, education, and occupational groups" (Durkheim 1897, p. 13). These variables were correlated with suicide rate. This could be translated to studying the role of social factors in human morbidity and mortality, of course in this case, mortality through suicide. Without much argument, suicide is death, and death is a health phenomenon.

Durkheim (1897, p. 44) defined suicide as "all cases of death resulting directly or indirectly from a positive or negative act of the victim himself [or herself], which he [or she] knows will produce this result [i.e., death]." Suicide exists when the victim, at the moment he/she commits the fatal act, is conscious of both the act and the outcome with certainty. After settling on a conceptual definition of suicide, Durkheim formulated a number of hypothetical ideas in order to establish the causes of suicide within the social system. He observed that the critical factors in differences in suicide rates were to be found in differences at the level of social facts (Ritzer 2011). Various societies have different levels of social fusion, which affects an individual's decision to commit suicide. Durkheim (1897, p. 43) argued that "the causes of death are outside rather than within us, and are effective only if humans venture into their sphere of activity." Durkheim then identified two major factors (social facts) which account for four different kinds of suicide (see Table 5.2). The factors include *integration* and *regulation*, and their fluctuations lead to the types of suicide that will be discussed.

Egoistic suicide occurs when an individual has little or no connectedness (cohesion) with others in the social system—the social string is weak or nonexistent. Such individuals are detached from others, sometimes as a result of rejection, inability to fit into any functional role, or, more importantly, the inability to adapt with others and the environment. Egoistic suicide is a manifestation of social alienation and a type of suicide springing from *excessive individualism*. This is why Durkheim observed that individual (selfish) thought and fewer shared practices may predispose individuals to egoistic suicide (i.e., weakening of common faith positively affects suicide rate). Hence the conclusion is that suicide varies inversely with the degree of integration of the social groups of which the individual forms a part (Durkheim 1897/1951).

On the other hand, a high level of integration (too strong a social string) will lead to *altruistic suicide*. Little wonder why this could also lead to suicide when it is previously argued that a low level of social integration leads to egoistic suicide. The response is simple: too little food is as dangerous as excessive food to human health. In life, no good is measureless: too little and too much are typical extremes that project negative effects. Hence Durkheim submitted that excessive individuation leads to suicide, and insufficient individuation has the same effects. Altruistic suicide could be optional or obligatory as a sign of group loyalty or when a social prestige is attached to suicide, a form of heroism or ultimate sacrifice in a struggle. This is done as a sign of a strong bond an individual has with a group. This form of suicide is mostly perpetuated by fanatics who seek to be martyrs (like terrorists), and among military with regimented life, mostly to save face from a failure or greater disgrace.

The pattern of social regulation or control also affects suicide rates. When the regulative role of the society is too feeble, a state of normlessness or anomy prevails. This accounts for *anomic suicide*. Weak regulation can reflect when the economic and political environment cannot ascertain the needs of the citizens or the traditional norms and values are dwindling. The fourth type of suicide is *fatalistic suicide*, which Durkheim mentioned and very briefly explained in a footnote (see Durkheim 1897, p. 276, footnote no. 25). Fatalistic suicide results from excessive regulations. Those who encounter oppressive regulation or discipline, such as the slaves, are more prone to fatalistic suicide. While slavery should be over, unfortunately, there is increasing sex slavery, human trafficking, forced labour, and other forms of exercise of coercion on others which puts them in slavery conditions. Therefore "fatalistic suicide" is still a relevant concept.

The major inference is that there are *social determinants of mortality through suicide* in human society. This inference was derived through a large amount of data from various countries and groups. Durkheim incriminated a number of variables or factors, particularly declining birth rates, increasing social discrimination, and exacerbated gender role tensions (Kushner 2005), which he believed had negative consequences for population health (as evidenced through *suicidogenic* behaviour). This is because, among groups, Durkheim found a number of what were often considered demographic variables affecting suicide rate. These variables include marital status, socioeconomic status, occupation and occupational status, and religious affiliation. Durkheim found that

1. Suicide was higher among Protestants than Catholics and lowest among Jews.
2. Suicide was higher among single people (including widows and widowers) than married people and lowest among married people with children.
3. Childless widows are more prone to suicide than their counterparts with children.
4. Divorced men have a higher suicide rate than the undivorced. Family life is inversely related to suicide.
5. Suicide is higher among whites than blacks, higher among men than among women, higher in urban areas than in rural areas, and suicide rate increases with age.

5.3 Functionalist Substantive Theories in Medical Sociology

6. Suicide rates were relatively high among the highest income groups than lower income groups.
7. Suicide was higher among soldiers than civilians.
8. The suicide rate was higher in times of economic depression and economic booms than during more stable periods.

Durkheim's theoretical explanation of suicide remains as relevant today as it was in the 1950s (Baller et al. 2010; Classen and Dunn 2010; Helmut 2010; Maimon et al. 2010; Marson and Powell 2011). Durkheim showed the importance of social capital or cohesion in population health. More recent works have found that social capital or cohesion is a protective factor in population health (Van Poppel and Day 1996; Kawachi et al. 1997; Muntaner and Lynch 1999; Hean et al. 2002; Brown and Day 2008). For instance, Brown and Day (2008) observed that prisoners who have less or no social support systems are at higher risk for egoistic suicide than their counterparts who are not lonely. Another study among the elderly observed that the death of friends, spouses, and family members can weaken the social ties the elderly have in the community, making them feel less integrated, which is consequential for suicide rate among them (Marson and Powell 2011).

Furthermore, more recent studies examined the influence of social ties and suicide among the elderly and submitted that suicide continues to be a major health issue among the elderly (Hooyman and Kiyak 2011). Elderly persons are more likely to die from suicide than any other age group (AAS 2012) and whites are more likely to commit suicide than blacks within a similar age bracket (NIMH 2012). An investigation of religion's effects on suicide rates in 1970 reveals that religion continues to affect suicide rates in the United States, with a lower rate among Catholics and a higher rate among Protestants (Pescosolido and Georgianna 1989). Durkheim is still correct when he observed that the suicide rate increases with age and that religious affiliation is one of the determinants of suicide rate.

Despite the high rate of poverty in Africa, the suicide rate is still relatively low when compared to western countries. Statistics compiled by the WHO (2012) attested to the low rate of suicide in Africa—0.1 and 15.5 per 100,000 inhabitants in Egypt and Austria in 2009, respectively. In the United States, Caucasian youth are twice as likely as African American youth to commit suicide (AAS 2012). This may support Durkheim's assertion that suicide tends to be higher among high-income groups. All available data also show that suicide rate is consistently higher among males than females (AAS 2012; Burrows and Laflamme 2008; WHO 2012). Moreover, on marital status, divorce, marital separation, and early widowhood are perpetuating risk factors (AAS 2012).

Despite this, Durkheim could be criticised for his total reliance on secondary data which might not be reliable or complete in some countries or among some groups. The findings could also be contested on the grounds that there could be underreporting of suicide among some groups due to social stigmatisation, among other factors. Of course, while Durkheim identified that some psychological dispositions can also account for suicide, he did not explore such factors adequately since that would transcend the focus of sociology. Therefore, his theory cannot explain why a specific individual might commit suicide, but it does explore suicide rates among various groups.

5.3.3 Social Capital Theory of Health

The idea of "social capital" is one of the major sociological contributions to health social sciences and health studies in general. Social capital is a major factor in social patterning of health. In sociology, the intellectual origin of the concept of social capital can be traced to the works of a number of classical scholars including Emile Durkheim, George Simmel, Karl Marx, Max Weber, and Talcott Parsons (Portes 1998; Song et al. 2010; Song 2013). The concern for social order and cohesion were predominant in the works of these early sociologists. Durkheim (1897/1951) discussed suicide in relation to social cohesion/integration noting that suicide rates vary according to the level of social bond in human society. Simmel is the proponent of sociation—by which he claimed that human society is an intricate web of multiple relations of individuals in constant interaction with one another (Coser 2004). Simmel observed that the formation of groups: dyad, triad, small or large, is imperative in the society with resultant consequences. Karl Marx argued that men must enter into social relationships in the social production of their existence—by implications, mutual dependence is a vital component of human existence. Parsons (1951) explained that the sick must seek assistance in order to get well. This creates a state of dependence on social capital or significant others and health care institutions.

While it is possible to derive the notions of social capital from the works of the classical sociological theorists, it was not until 1900 that John Dewey, a philosopher, laid the foundation of, and mentioned the concept of social capital (Farr 2004). Farr claimed that Dewey defined society as a form of associational life towards a realisation of any form of experience. From another perspective, some scholars argued that it was in 1916 that Lyda Judson Hanifan (1879–1932) formally mentioned the concept in his paper: *The Rural School Community Center* (see Hanifan 1916; Farr 2004; Song 2013). Generally, a more formalised conception of social capital began in the 1980s and 1990s with the works of some sociologists, Nan Lin (1982), Pierre Bourdieu (1986), and James S. Coleman (1988, 1990), and one political scientist, Robert D. Putnam (1993) (Song 2013). The next subsection will discuss some conceptions of social capital and it forms.

5.3.3.1 Defining Social Capital and its Forms

The most fundamental stance about the concept of social capital is to view it as "social resources"—it implies the links and support that individuals can access at a particular time. But it should be acknowledged that the concept is not as simple as primarily described. The concept has generated multiple definitions, conceptualisations, and empirical measurements (Lin 2008). Where capital is often defined in

5.3 Functionalist Substantive Theories in Medical Sociology

terms of property and cash in economic terms, Hanifan (1916, p. 130) explained that social capital on the other hand, refers to "... good-will, fellowship, mutual sympathy and social intercourse among a group of individuals and families who make up a social unit, the rural community, whose logical center is the school. In community building as in business organization and expansion there must be an accumulation of capital before constructive work can be done."

Hanifan (1916) expatiated that social contacts beyond the family are essential ingredients in human wellbeing not just because people meet face-to-face, but a lot of sociological processes both tangible and intangible social exchanges take place. Mutual social support is a reflection of accumulation of social capital, essential in community building and general living condition. Hanifan (1916, p. 130) further asserted that

> [t]he individual is helpless socially, if left entirely to himself[/herself]. Even the association of the members of one's own family fails to satisfy that desire which every normal individual has of being with his[/her] fellows, of being a part of a larger group than the family. If he[/she] may come into contact with his[/her] neighbor, and they with other neighbors, there will be an accumulation of social capital, which may immediately satisfy his[/her] social needs and which may bear a social potentiality sufficient to the substantial improvement of living conditions in the whole community.

Lin (1982) formulated a notion of social capital based on instrumental action—an action that requires the use of network tie to achieve its goal. Lin advanced a theoretical notion of social capital by arguing that social resources are embedded in one's social networks, and because the resources are social in nature, they can only be accessible through one's direct and indirect ties. Precisely, Lin conceived social capital as resources embedded in one's social networks. Lin (2008) identified a number of sources for social capital including structural sources (an actor's characteristics [SES, race, family origin etc.], position and roles in the social hierarchy); and networking sources (strength of tie and network location) (see also Song 2013). Mobilisation of, and accessibility to the resources are, however, also influenced by individual structural position and the strength of network ties (strong or weak) (see Lin 1982, 2008). Lin (1982, p. 133) argued that "frequency of interaction and intensity of relationship are more likely to occur among individuals who share similar characteristics"—Islam et al. (2006) operationalised this as horizontal social capital. In accessing social resources people tend to direct attention to people of higher status—this implies the use of vertical social capital (see Fig. 5.1). The vertical social capital depicts a weak tie, but which is often more beneficial. "Weak ties rather than strong ties tend to lead to better social resources" (Lin 1982, p. 134). Since level of resources possessed is directly related to the individual position in the social hierarchy, individuals in high positions have more social resources and reaching out to individuals in higher positions might be highly beneficial in terms of influence and information.

Bourdieu (1986, p. 248) defines social capital as "the aggregate of the actual or potential resources which are linked to possession of a durable network of more or less institutionalized relationships of mutual acquaintance or recognition." Bourdieu stressed on social connections, which are geared towards the recognition of some

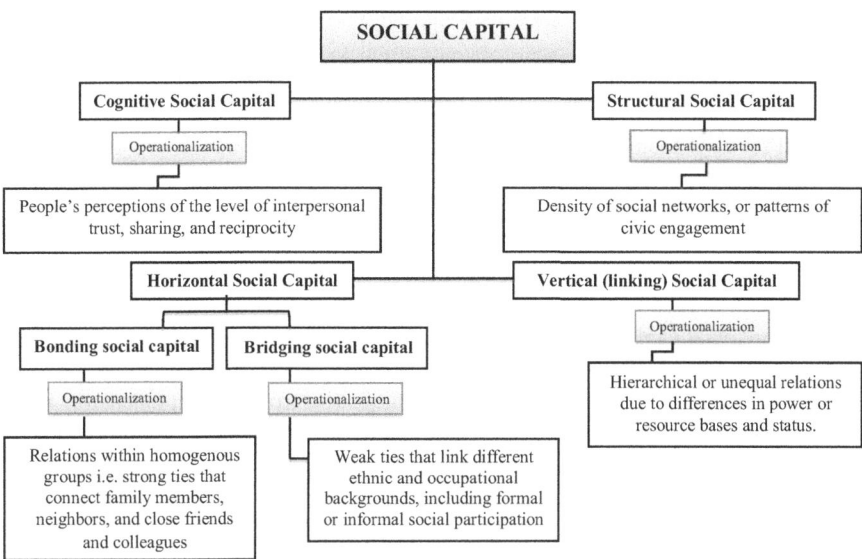

Fig. 5.1 Forms and dimensions of social capital with operationalization. (Source: Islam et al. 2006)

individual potential that can contribute to a common good. Coleman (1990) reiterated that social capital is the set of resources that inhere in family and community relations from which the notions of authority, trust and norms develop, which are forms of social capital. According to Coleman, social capital helps in the development of human capital throughout lifetime—this, invariably, is an extension of the argument that the society makes us human through inculcation of values and norms. Societal values are not independently created and imbibed; it takes the efforts of others. So also, individual goal cannot be independently arrived at, it is interdependently achieved. Coleman described social capital as social-structural resources, which can be defined by their functions. Social capital facilitates certain actions of individuals who are within the structure; and it is productive by enabling the achievement of certain ends.

Apart from social capital, which is embodied in the relations among persons, Coleman (1990, p. 304) mentioned other kinds of social capital: physical capital which is in material form and tangible; and human capital which "is less tangible, being embodied in the skills and knowledge acquired by an individual" as a member of a family and community. This is why Islam et al. (2006) opined that social capital may generate material/market and non-material/non-market returns to the individual.

In addition, Putnam (1993, p. 167) described social capital as "features of social organization, such as trust, norms, and networks, that can improve the efficiency of society by facilitating coordinated actions" towards the achievement of certain ends. Therefore, the features of social capital include trust, norms, and networks (cf. Coleman 1990), and thus social capital is "ordinarily a public good, unlike conventional capital, which is ordinarily a private good" (Putnam 1993, p. 170).

Mutual trust leads to proliferation of social networks of individual who believe in common good. In a similar vein, social capital is "complexly conceptualised as the network of associations, activities, or relations that bind people together as a community via certain norms and psychological capacities, notably trust, which are essential for civil society and production of future collective action or goods, in the manner of other forms of capital" (Farr 2004, p. 9).

Furthermore, Portes (1998, p. 12) conceived social capital as "the capacity of individuals to command scare resources by virtue of their membership in networks or broader social structure." While Link and Phelan (1995) observed these social connectedness as part of the resources embedded in socioeconomic status, most scholars of social capital view it as a social and natural good: sometimes inevitable as a result of human social existence. This is why Coleman (1990, p. 300) noted, "social interdependence and systemic functioning arise from the fact that actors have interests in events that are fully or partially under the control of other actors."

For Bourdieu, Coleman, Lin and other scholars, there are varieties of ways of conceptualising social capital and it forms. In simplifying the concept of social capital, four main theoretical ingredients can be identified: **social trust/reciprocity, collective efficacy, voluntary social participation and social cohesion (or sense of belonging)** (see Lochner et al. 1999; Islam et al. 2006). A study on social capital should focus on how to operationalise these ingredients, and the dimensions of social capital (see Fig. 5.1). Participation involves some level of sociability and both formally and informally organised activities in schools, religious gatherings and social clubs. Sense of belonging implies a considerable social acceptance devoid of discrimination. Social cohesion starts from the level of family and neighbourhood. Lochner et al. (1999, p. 265) observed that neighbouring "involves social interactions, by which residents establish social connections that are either personal or at the neighborhood level." One major aspect of social cohesion is social support i.e., the use of personal resources for collective wellbeing. Social support could also signify the level at which individuals can access or count on others for various resources, especially in terms of need. Such support could include emotional, financial, moral, and information supports—these are invaluable within any social network.

In some cases, social cohesion manifest in the formation of social groupings comprising individuals who come in contact (from time to time) as a result of such group membership and share both tangible and intangible resources. For instance, age-grade associations are important social organisations in Africa (see Kottak 2013; Haviland et al. 2013). Age grades are organised by certain age intervals (e.g., 10 or 15 years). The age-grade is a kind of cooperative group, which performs public duties and various self-help activities for the wellbeing of members and community at large. More importantly, African societies are still dominated by the extended family structure. Even when some individuals form a nuclear family system, they still have wide range of responsibilities for close and distance relations. In African context, where social safety nets are inadequate, many families rely on a network of reciprocal assistance provided by members of a larger group: the men support the women or vice versa, the young support the aged, and the employed support the unemployed. Also, there are landlords' associations in many communities, organised to discuss issues (e.g., sanitation, security, terms of tenancy, and social amenities) affecting the community.

On social trust and reciprocity, Lochner et al. (1999) observed that mutual dependence often grows out of trust, a kind of social reliability. This is a form of interpersonal trust, which creates a sense of openness. Community competence or collective efficacy involves the development of problem-solving abilities, which grows out of collective efforts—when resources are pooled through concerted efforts in response to specific matters (Lochner et al. 1999). Having defined the concept of social capital, it is important to turn to its various dimensions and other forms.

Following some review of previous works, Islam et al. (2006) observed that social capital has two major aspects: cognitive and structural social capital (see Fig. 5.1). Cognitive social capital signifies a micro aspect including norms, values, attitudes and trust, and specifically, it refers to what people think of the level of interpersonal cooperation with others in any community. Structural social capital is the macro aspect, which refers to externally observable aspects of such social connection, such as the density of social involvement, and institutional arrangements that facilitate cooperation.

Islam et al. (2006) further identified two types of social capital : horizontal and vertical social capital. The authors also divided horizontal social capital into two including bonding and bridging social capital. Bonding refers to social connectedness with primary groups such as the family members, friends, neighbours, and co-workers. Bridging social capital signifies weak ties involving informal and formal social groupings with some secondary groups. On the other hand, vertical social capital depicts ties with people of different hierarchies in terms of status, power or prestige. In a traditional/rural African community, which is a reflection of what Tönnies (1957) described as *Gemeinschaft* (i.e., a community with high level of integration), both horizontal and vertical social capitals are abundant—individuals often feel an obligation to assist others (family members) and those in need (in general). This assistance might be material or nonmaterial. In cases where there are discrimination based on a disease condition, it is often as a result of inadequate knowledge about communicability or some misconceptions resulting from cultural beliefs.

In modern/urban African societies, there is relatively some level of individualism, which has reduced but not totally nullified the sense of social support, extended familial bonding and communal relations. African societies are still largely traditional and rural, imbued with what the French Sociologist, Emile Durkheim described as mechanical solidarity. Social capital is an abundant resource that is often tapped to counterbalance the inadequacy of the formal support systems (e.g., pension, health insurance, paid employment, and public provision of infrastructures). In other words, informal social support or networks often mitigate government failure by promoting welfare in the absence of public services. For instance, because of high rate of unemployment in many African countries, the dependency ratio is often high. The dependents (the aged, underage and unemployed) are actually reliant on the working class for survival. This kind of social bonding holds a lot of implications for health and general wellbeing.

5.3.3.2 Social Capital and Health

Social capital has been described as a major determinant of health (Kawachi et al. 1997; De Silva et al. 2005; Carpiano 2006, 2007; Lynch et al. 2000). While many studies have shown the positive effects of social capital on health in both developed and developing worlds (see Ramlagan et al. 2013; Chola and Alaba 2013; Islam et al. 2006), such effects should be larger in developing countries where a majority of populations is living with low socioeconomic status, and (formal) health resources are grossly inadequate. A study in South Africa found that self-reported good health among the elderly was associated with age, education and higher social capital (being married or cohabiting, high trust and solidarity and greater psychological resources) (Ramlagan et al. 2013). Also, Campbell et al. (1999) have argued that high levels of social capital may act as a buffer in deprived communities, serving to shield them from some of the worst effects of deprivation. Generally, group solidarity and memberships often provide some support, which will invariably facilitate access to valued resources. For instance, network contacts might provide health information, which is crucial to disease control and prevention. Also, informal health care and support can be provided in case of illness. Reciprocal support and assistance are part of the bedrock of extended family and communal relationships in African societies. For instance, in case of illness, hospital bills might be contributed; baby-siting assistance can be provided; and cooking, washing and other supportive care might be provided by other family or community members.

Social capital in most health studies is often operationalised in terms of civic engagement or grassroots participation, neighbourliness, social networks, social support, informal social control and perception of the local area. It is practically beneficial for individuals to feel some level of social connection with others—such sense of belonging is crucial in mediating state of physical and mental health. Pearce and Smith (2003, p. 125) observed that indicators of social capital, such as trust and sense of belonging are strongly related to mortality rates.

Figure 5.2 shows a framework indicating the links between social capital and health. Carpiano (2006, 2007) presented a more elaborate version of the framework which guided his empirical work. The Figure shows that structural antecedents, which are structural characteristics of a neighborhood or locality, have implications for the type and strength of social ties and resources accessible to individuals (Carpiano 2007). The structural antecedents include socioeconomic condition of the area and residential stability (length of stay), which invariably affects the level of social connection. The individual confounders or characteristics also affect some structural antecedents—for instance, it determines the area of residence (urban or rural; low or high income area; and the nature of friends). Lin (1982, p. 132) previously argued that the influence of personal cofounders is obvious in the manner of access to social resources, an individuals occupying a higher position, has greater command of social resources.

The individual confounders also affect the level of social capital in terms of social support, leverage and civic participation. For instance, in most Muslim-dominated parts of Africa (including the region of North Africa, Mali, Sudan, Niger, Chad),

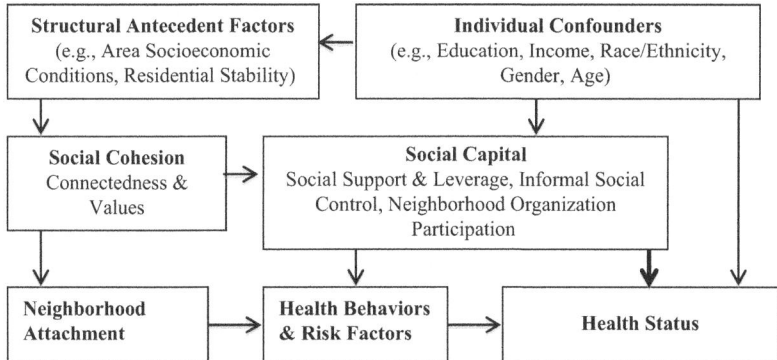

Fig. 5.2 Social Capital and Health. (Source Modified from: Carpiano 2007, p. 640)

there are a number of cultural barriers stymieing the presence of women in the public sphere or their (especially married ones) free mingling with the opposite sex. Such condition will limit their civic participation, but which is only one aspect of social capital. Women could receive more support because they are more likely to share their health concerns than men. Men could be disadvantaged in information sharing because of culture of masculinity, which prescribes that men should be strong. In general, Campbell and McLean (2004) argued that social capital is not a homogenous resource equally available to all members of a geographical community, but is shaped and constrained by factors such as gender, ethnicity and social class.

Social capital also involves social leverage, which means the use network ties (especially social influence) for social gains including access to information and social mobility. Informal social control is the ability of individuals or groups (with some form of social links) to ensure conformity to the norms and values of the society—this implies informal measures of behaviour control. Both social leverage and informal social control can exert some influence on health behaviour and risk factors (such as smoking, sedimentary lifestyle and indiscriminate sexual behaviour). For instance, those who belong to some religious networks might desist from some "immoral" practices, which could adversely impact their health status.

5.3.3.3 Some Criticisms of Social Capital Theory of Health

1. Social capital is often difficult to operationalise or measure in empirical work (see Tlili and Obsiye 2013). It is possible to measure social capital at the individual (micro) level and structural/community (macro) level. In most empirical studies, there is still lack of uniform indicators in measuring social capital. De Silva et al. (2005, p. 619) observed that the theory of social capital emphasises multiple dimensions within the concept: it can be divided into a behavioural/activity component (e.g., participation) and a cognitive/perceptual component (e.g., trust).
2. There is still the need to spell out "whether good health is the result of social capital or whether social capital is the result of good health" while controlling

for the roles of personal characteristics (Kawachi 2006, p. 992). This implies that the pathways of causality between social capital and health are still ambiguous.
3. The outputs of social capital are usually unstable, and cannot be obligated. The gains are probable that are possible: difficult to envisage or calculate. For policy issues, it will be uneasy to count on resources that cannot be authoritatively ascertained as constant. Although, a number of policies or activities rely on volunteering, when other aspects of social capitals (e.g., social, emotional and material supports, and some cognitive aspects [such as trust]) are considered, it could be difficult to implement health policies based on social capital. By implication, there is still a gap between the theory's propositions and health implementation research.
4. The theory of social capital of heath over assumes that individuals or group always work for the good of others. Either manifestly or latently, the outputs of social network are not always positive. This takes account of the dysfunctions of social networks. An individual can actually start smoking or engage in other risk behaviours as a result of the nature of his/her social network. This point assents to the argument that social capital is context specific: it is neither inherently good nor inherently bad (Bruegel 2005, p. 4).
5. There is still a contentious issue of whether SES plays more important intervening roles in the link between social capital and health. This is why Lynch et al. (2000) observed the influence of social capital on health might have been exaggerated above material factors. Kawachi (2006) also highlighted a number of reports, which indicated that social capital might not be so functional for the health of people in comparatively egalitarian societies, in contrast to highly unequal societies with inadequate safety nets.

References

AAS (American Association of Suicidology). (2012). Risk factors for suicide: Fact sheet. http://www.suicidology.org/stats-and-tools/suicide-fact-sheets. Accessed 15 June 2012.
Amzat, J., & Omololu, F. (2012). Basics of sociological paradigms. In I. S. Ogundiya & J. Amzat (Eds.), *Basics of the social sciences* (pp. 115–134). Lagos: Malthouse.
Baller, R. D., Levchak, P., & Schultz, M. (2010). The great transformation and suicide: Local and long-lasting effects of 1930 bank suspensions. *Suicide and Life-Threatening Behavior, 40*(6), 574–586.
Bilton, T., Bommett, K., Jones, P., Lawson, T., Skinner, D., Stanworth, M., & Webster, A. (2004). *Introductory sociology* (4th Ed.). London: Palgrave Macmillan.
Bourdieu, P. (1986). The forms of capital. In J. G. Richardson (Ed.), *The handbook of theory: Research for the sociology of education* (pp. 241–258). New York: Greenwood.
Bradby, H. (2012). *Medicine, health and society*. London: Sage.
Brown, S., & Day, A. (2008). The role of loneliness in suicide prevention and management. *Journal of Offender Rehabilitation, 47*(4), 433–449.
Bruegel, I. (2005). Social capital and feminist critique. In J. Franklin (Ed.), Women and social capital (pp. 4–17). Families & Social Capital ESRC Research Group Working Paper No. 12, London South Bank University.

Burrows, S., & Laflamme, L. (2008). Suicide among urban South African adolescents. *International Journal of Adolescent Medicine and Health, 20*(4), 519–528.

Campbell, C., & McLean, C. (2004). Social capital, social exclusion and health: Factors shaping African-Caribbean participation in local community networks. In C. Swann & A. Morgan (Eds.), *Social capital for health: Insights from qualitative research* (pp. 29–46). London: NHS, Health Development Agency.

Campbell, C., Wood, R., & Kelly, M. (1999). *Social capital and health*. London: Health Education Authority.

Carpiano, R. M. (2006). Toward a neighborhood resource—based theory of social capital for health: Can Bourdieu and sociology help? *Social Science and Medicine, 62,* 165–175.

Carpiano, R. M. (2007). Neighborhood social capital and adult health: An empirical test of a Bourdieu-Based Model. *Health and Place, 13*(3), 639–655.

Chola, L., & Alaba, O. (2013). Association of neighbourhood and individual social capital, neighbourhood economic deprivation and self-rated health in South Africa—a multi-level analysis. *PLoS ONE, 8*(7), e71085.

Classen, T. J., & Dunn, R. A. (2010). The politics of hope and despair: The effect of presidential election outcomes on suicide rates. *Social Science Quarterly, 91*(3), 593–612.

Coleman, J. S. (1988). Social capital in the creation of human capital. American Journal of Sociology, 94, 95–121.

Coleman, J. S. (1990). *Foundations of social theory*. Cambridge: Belknap Press of Harvard University Press.

Comte, A. (1896). *The positive philosophy. Vol II & III, Trans Version by Harriet Martineau*. London: George Bell.

Coser, L. A. (2004). *Masters of sociological thought: Ideas in historical and social context* (2nd ed.). New Delhi: Rawat.

De Silva, M. J., McKenzie, K., Harpham, T., & Huttly, S. R. A. (2005). Social capital and mental illness: A systematic review. *Journal of Epidemiology and Community Health, 59,* 619–627.

Durkheim, E. (1895/1982). *The rules of sociological method*. New York: Free.

Durkheim, E. (1897/1951). *Suicide: A study in sociology*. New York: Free.

Emke, I. (2002). Patients in the new economy: The "sick role" in a time of economic discipline. *Animus, 7,* 81–93.

Farr, J. (2004). Social capital: A conceptual history. *Political Theory 32,* 6–33.

Hanifan, L. J. (1916). The rural school community center. *Annals of The Academy of Political and Social Science, 67,* 130–138.

Haviland, W. A., Prins, H. E. L., McBride, B., & Walrath, D. (2013). *Cultural anthropology: The human challenge*. (14th edn.). Belmonth: Wadsworth, Cengage Learning.

Hean, S., Cowley, S., Forbes, A., Griffith, P., & Maben, J. (2002). The M-C-M cycle and social capital. *Social Science Medicine, 56,* 1061–1072.

Helmut, T. (2010). Violent crime (and suicide) in imperial Germany, 1883-1902: Quantitative analyses and a Durkheimian interpretation. *International Criminal Justice Review, 20*(1), 5–34.

Hooyman, N., & Kiyak, H. (2011). *Social gerontology: A multidisciplinary perspective*. Boston: Prentice-Hall.

Islam, M. K., J. Merlo, I. Kawachi, M. Lindstrom, & U-G. Gerdtham. (2006). Social capital and health: Does egalitarianism matter? A literature review. *International Journal of Equity in Health, 5*(1), 3.

Kawachi, I. (2006). Commentary: Social capital and health—making the connections one step at a time. *International Journal of Epidemiology, 35*(4), 989–993.

Kawachi, I., Kennedy, B. P., & Lochner, K. (1997). Long live community: Social capital as public health. *The American prospect, 8*(35), 56–59.

Kottack, C. P. (2013). Mirror for humanity: A concise introduction to cultural anthropology (9th ed.). New York: McGraw-Hill.

Kushner, H. I. (2005). The limits of social capital: Durkheim, suicide, and social cohesion. *American Journal of Public Health, 95*(7), 1139–1143.

References

Lamont, J. A., & Woodward, C. (1994). Patient-physician sexual involvement: A Canadian survey of obstetrician-Gynecologists. *Canadian Medical Association Journal, 150,* 1433–1439.

Levine S., & Kozloff, M. A. (1978). The sick role: assessment and overview Ann. *Review of Sociology, 4,* 317–343.

Lin, N. (1982). Social resources and instrumental action. In P. V. Marsden & N. Lin (Eds.), *Social structure and network analysis* (pp. 13–45). Beverly Hills: Sage.

Lin, N. (2008). A network theory of social capital. In D. Castiglione, J. van Deth, & G. Wolleb (Eds.), *The handbook of Social Capital* (pp. 50–69). Oxford: Oxford University Press.

Link, B. G., & Phelan, J. (1995). Social conditions as fundamental causes of disease. *Journal of Health and Social Behavior, 35* (extra issue), 80–94.

Lochner K, Kawachi I, & Kennedy, B. P. (1999). Social capital: A guide to its measurement. *Health & Place, 5,* 259–270.

Lupton, D. (2003). *Medicine as culture: Illness, disease and the body in western societies.* London: Sage.

Lynch, J., Due, P., Muntaner, C., & Smith, C. D. (2000). Social capital—Is it a good investment strategy for public health? *Journal of Epidemiology Community Health, 54,* 404–408.

Maimon, D., Browning, C. R., & Brooks-Gunn, J. (2010). Collective efficacy, family attachment, and urban adolescent suicide attempts. *Journal of Health and Social Behavior, 51*(3), 307–324.

Marson, S. M., & Powell, R. M. (2011). Suicide among elders: A Durkheimian proposal. *International Journal of Ageing and Later Life, 6*(1), 59–79.

Muntaner, C., & Lynch, J. (1999). Income inequality and social coercion versus class relations: a critique of Wilkinson's neo-Durkheimian research program. International Journal of Health Services, 29, 59–81.

Neumam, W. L. (2011). Social research methods: Qualitative and quantitative approaches. Boston: Pearson.

NIMH (National Institute of Mental Health). (2012). Older adults: Depression and suicide Facts. Factsheet. http://www.nimh.nih.gov/health/publications/older-adults-depression-and-suicide-facts-factsheet/index.shtml. Accessed 15 June 2012.

Parsons, T. (1951). *The social system.* Glencoe: Free.

Pearce, N., & Smith, G. D. (2003). Is social capital the key to inequalities in health? *American Journal of Public Health, 93*(1), 122–129.

Pescosolido, B. A., & Georgianna, S. (1989). Durkheim, suicide, and religion: Toward a network theory of suicide. *American Sociological Review, 54*(1), 33–48.

Portes, A. (1998). Social capital: Its origins and applications in modern sociology. *The Annual Review of Sociology, 24,* 1–24.

Putnam R. (1993). Making democracy work: Civic traditions in modern Italy. Princeton, NJ: Princeton University Press.

Ramlagan, S., Peltzer, K., & Phaswana-Mafuya, N. (2013). Social capital and health among older adults in South Africa. *BMC Geriatrics, 13,* 100. doi:10.1186/1471-2318-13-100.

Ritzer, G. (2010). *Contemporary sociological theory and its classical roots: The basics* (3rd edn.). St. Louis: McGraw-Hill.

Ritzer, G. (2011). *Sociological theory* (8th edn.). New York: McGraw-Hill.

Segall, A. (1976). The sick role concept: Understanding illness behaviour. *Journal of Health and Social Behavior, 17*(2), 162–169.

Song, L. (2013). Social capital and health. In W. C. Cockerham (Ed.), *Medical sociology on the move: New directions in theory* (pp. 233–257). Dordrecht: Springer.

Song, L., Son, J., & Lin, N. (2010). Social capital and health. In W. C. Cockerham (Ed.), *The new blackwell companion to medical sociology.* Oxford: Wiley-Blackwell.

Spencer, H. (1896). *The principles of sociology.* New York: D. Appleton & Co.

Tlili, A., & Obsiye M. (2013). What is Coleman's social capital the name of? A critique of a not very social capital. *Critical Sociology, 39*(2), 1–24.

Tönnies, F. (1957). Community and society. Translated by Charles Price Loomis. East Lansing: Michigan State University Press.

Van Poppel, F., & Day, L. H. (1996). A test of Durkheim's theory of suicide—without committing the ecological fallacy. *American sociological review, 61,* 500–507.

WHO. (2012). Suicide rates per 100,000 by country, year and sex. http://www.who.int/mental_health/prevention/suicide_rates/en/. Accessed 15 June 2012.

William, S. J. (2005). Parsons revisited: From the sick role to...? Health: An Interdisciplinary Journal for the Social Study of Health, Illness and *Medicine, 9*(2), 123–144.

Young, J. T. (2004). Illness Behaviour: A selective review and synthesis. *Sociology of Health & Illness, 26*(1), 1–31.

Zola, I. K. (1972). Medicine as an institution of social control. *Sociological Review, 20*(4), 487–504.

Chapter 6
Social Production of Health

6.1 Introduction

In the previous chapter, functionalism was discussed. This chapter will focus on the social production of health (SPH) with particular reference to Marxist analysis or political economy of health and feminist analysis of health. The two theoretical analyses flow from the notion of social inequality in the society system. They have been part of the dominant conceptual analysis of health in recent times. Like functionalism, Marxist and feminist perspectives are also realist and positivist traditions. While there are many versions of feminism, a majority stem from these traditions. The structures and organisations of human society determine the position of an individual in the society, which also affects population health. Refer to the previous chapter for a more elaborate discussion of positivism, realism, determinism, nomothetic approach, and macro analysis (see Sect. 5.2 for a discussion of the philosophical foundations of the social production of health).

Social production of health/disease refers to theoretical frameworks that explicitly address socioeconomic and political determinants of health and distributions of disease within and across groups and societies (Krieger 1994, 2001). It focuses on structural barriers that predispose individuals to diseases. The basic argument is that there are structural inherent characters of human society, especially social and economic conditions, which are fundamental causes of health inequalities (Link and Phelan 1995, 1996). The Marxist and feminist analyses focus on class and gender relations, respectively. Therefore, the idea of the social production of health shows how institutional arrangement and an individual's position within the social system engender his/her health.

6.2 Marxist or Conflict Perspective: A General Overview

In sociology, Marxist theory (often called conflict theory) is a major perspective. It is traced back to the works of Karl Marx, Vilfredo Pareto, Georg Simmel, Lewis Coser, Randal Collins, C. Wright Mills, W. E. B. Du Bois, and Immanuel Wallerstein, among others. In the field of medical sociology, this perspective is more prominent in the works of Vicente Navarro, Hans A. Baer, and Howard Waitzkin, among others. The perspective derived its other name, Marxism, from Karl Marx, who devoted most of his works to the elaboration of conflict and its implications for societal arrangements. In terms of features, conflict perspective is a direct opposite of functionalism. Table 6.1 shows some basic views from the conflict perspective. While functionalism recognises the existence of cooperation and consensus in human society, Marxists argue that conflict is inherent in social life. Marx observed that the history of all hitherto existing societies is the history of class struggle. This indicates that there are various groups in human society based on social inequality. There is also tension between these groups. Basically, there are bourgeoisie (those who occupy the upper class) and proletariat (consisting of those in the lower class of the society). A class refers to a group of people who share similar relations with the means of production. In other words, Gabe et al. (2004, p. 3) defined a social class as a segment of the population distinguished from others by similarities in labour market position and property relations. The bourgeoisie are the owners, employers, or the rich; and proletariats are the non-owners, employees, and the poor.

The proponents admit that production of material life is a basic historical and fundamental act of man. There are historical changes in human society with transformations from previous economic systems up to capitalism, which is now a dominant economic system. Capitalism allows for the private accumulation of wealth, which explains the differences in economic position of various individuals in the society. Economic status exacts great influence on an individual's behaviour and general position in the society. Conflict paradigm, because of its radical stance and strictures of capitalism, is widely influential (Amzat and Omololu 2012). The perspective focuses more on the contradictions (e.g., exploitation, alienation, capital accumulation, and pauperisation) in capitalist societies. In all social considerations, the lower class is always at the receiving end, bearing the brunt of all social problems.

Furthermore, socioeconomic decisions, transformations, and reforms are exercised by the dominant class. Such reforms are mostly unfavourable to the lower class. The conflict perspective notes that the power of the dominant class holds the society together. Health politics and policies are enacted and implemented by the dominant class. There is continuous unequal access to and allocation of resources, which account for the poverty of the lower class. The lower class experiences social alienation and is often at the margin of the society. Keeping all this in mind, how are these Marxist arguments used in explaining the distribution of health/diseases in human societies?

6.3 Marxist Analysis/Political Economy of Health

The Marxist framework examines health from the nature of political and economic systems of the society. Janzen (1978) defined the political economy of health (PEH) as a macro-level analysis that addresses the impact of power, resource allocation, and

6.3 Marxist Analysis/Political Economy of Health

Table 6.1 Basic views of Marxism

View of the society	Class struggle and conflict, divisions, tension
Level of analysis	Macro, group or social aggregate
Key concepts	Inequality, stratification, alienation, domination, capitalism, materialism, class, material life
View of individual	Determined by material life, power, status, and authority
View of the social order	Maintained by dominant forces or class
View of social change	Revolutionary—by force or coercion
View on population health	Diseases as well as risk factors are unequally distributed
	Material condition of the society reflects its health status
	The lower class bears the brunt of diseases
	Limited access to health care by the less privileged
	The medical institution portrays the agenda of the capitalist class

organisation on population health. The major reactions of political economists started with a critical examination of capitalism. This is why Baer (1982) observed that PEH is a multidisciplinary and critical endeavour which attempts to explain health-related issues within the context of class and imperialist relations inherent in the capitalist world-system. While Baer's definition of PEH is appropriate because of the domination of capitalism in the world economy, it should be noted that the perspective can be applied to all forms of economic systems. The perspective has some inherent features, such as dialectical and historical analysis. A more comprehensive definition therefore relates that PEH is "a macroanalytic, critical, and historical perspective for analyzing disease distribution and health services under a variety of economic systems, with particular emphasis on the effects of stratified social, political, and economic relations within the world economic system" (Morgan 1987, p. 132). Morgan's definition shows that PEH involves critical analysis and examination of objective conditions (as a macroanalysis or structuralist theory). All analysis in a political economic perspective always assesses the impact of socioeconomic and political inequality on any *explanandum* (i.e., whatever needs to be explained).

Baer (1982) further observed that the PEH is divided into two aspects:

1. **The political economy of illness:** this is often expressed in the social production of health, disease, or illness—an attempt to understand what is often called historical materialist epidemiology. This is generally concerned with the structural factors, constraints, or conditions responsible for unequal burden of disease among various groups in the society. In another words, political economy of illness refers to the holistic understanding of fundamental causes of diseases and the distribution of risk behaviours as well as the incidence of morbidity and mortality in human society. The bottom line in this aspect is the tracing of health status to socioeconomic condition and class relations in the society.
2. **The political economy of health care:** this aspect is largely concerned with the fundamental influence of structural inequality in the organisation of the health care system. Baer noted that this aspect examines the impact of (capitalist) modes of production on the production, distribution, and consumption of health services and the influence of class relations within which medical institutions are embedded.

While these two aspects are recognised, the *explanans* on either of the sides is based on class relations. This is why the aspects will not be discussed separately, but a simultaneous discussion stressing on the basic polemics of this perspective will be provided. Waitzkin (1978) and Baer (1982) traced the history of the Marxist analysis of health to Engels' *The Condition of the Working Class in England in 1844*, published in 1845, which described the dangerous working and housing conditions that created ill-health. Waitzkin observed that Engels linked diseases such as tuberculosis, typhoid, and typhus to malnutrition, inadequate housing, contaminated water supplies, and overcrowding. Engels (1845) described a poor working condition as social murder. Engels (1845, pp. 96–101) observed that

> it [i.e., a poor working condition] has placed the workers under conditions in which they can neither retain health nor live long; that it undermines the vital force of these workers gradually, little by little, and so hurries them to the grave before their time... Society knows how injurious such conditions are to the health and the life of the workers... And if life in large cities is, in itself, injurious to health, how great must be the harmful influence of an abnormal atmosphere in the working-people's quarters... Another category of diseases arises directly from the food rather than the dwellings of the workers. The food of the labourer, indigestible enough in itself, is utterly unfit for young children...

Engels explained how and why working conditions and poor income account for bad health among the working class. He explained that the urban conditions in terms of pollution and congestion are also detrimental to human health. The increasing alcohol consumption among the working class is related to their search for recreation. All of these actions and conditions happen as a result of societal injustice against a segment of the population and have adverse consequences for population health. More importantly, Engels observed that the mortality rate is based on class difference, as there was a higher mortality rate in the poor quarters. It was further observed that there was a wide gap in the life expectancy of the rich and the poor. Engels (1845) specifically noted that more than 57 % of the children of the working class perish before the fifth year compared to 20 % of that of the upper class. Engels' observations show that the idea that there are social determinants of health is not new, and the world is still confronted with such determinants.

The ideas of Engels marked the beginning of historical materialist epidemiology. Simply defined, historical materialist epidemiology deals with patterns, incidence, and distribution of death and disease based on the political, economic, and social structures of society (Schnall 1977). The inference shows that the prevalence of disease and death reflects transition in material circumstances, and, consequently, the analysis of the health of a group depends on its material condition. This indicates that improving standards and conditions of living are likely to impact positively on population health. The basic argument is that access to health care and the population health are determined by the level of socioeconomic development. Engels was able to prove this assertion in England from various data in 1844, with a conclusion that the health indicators of the working class were worse off. The health condition of the working class or the lower class reflects the vicious cycle of socioeconomic inequality and poor health. Figure 6.1 shows that there is a wheeled connection of

6.3 Marxist Analysis/Political Economy of Health

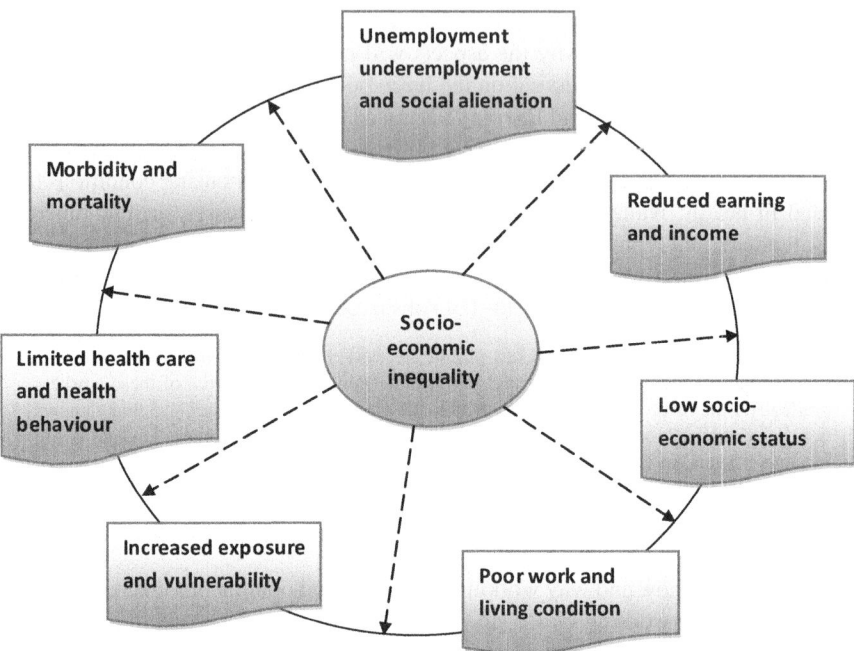

Fig. 6.1 Vicious cycle of socioeconomic inequality and poor health

socioeconomic inequality with various conditions producing ill-health. Such conditions are responsible for the reproduction of socioeconomic inequality itself and subsequent exposure to adverse health risks.

Engels and Marx published the *Communist Manifestoes*, which was not directly related to medical care but expanded the polemics about the adverse effects of structural inequalities and barriers on social condition and recommended a sociopolitical revolution in order to resolve the challenges facing the world. In addition, in *Capital: A Critique of Political Economy*, Marx (1887) explained the contribution of occupational status and class relation in welfare and well-being. Marx (1887, p. 176) observed that the working class requires some level of subsistence in order to maintain their health without which the consequences will be deleterious. The notion that health is linked to fundamental economic, political, and social conditions can also be found in the work of Rudolf Virchow (Holtz et al. 2006; Waitzkin 1978). Virchow traced the social origin of morbidity and mortality to economic deprivation and political inequity among the masses and recommended social transformation such as better wage packages, increased employment, and other forms of socioeconomic improvement as control measures (Baer 1982; Waitzkin 1981).

From the forgoing discussion, the major character of human society reflects in class division, especially between the proletariat and bourgeoisie. The proletariats have to work endlessly for their survival. Hence, in the process of offering their labour, they are open to exploitation, alienation, and pauperisation. They are exploited because the primary goal of the bourgeoisie is to acquire surplus value at the expense of the working class. Therefore, the working class does not really get the value of their labour. This continuous exploitation leads to pauperisation. Poverty is a critical determinant of health because it leads to a condition of inability to attain good nutrients and other materials for healthy living.

In general, the Marxist analysis of health is a departure from "blame-the-victim" perspectives such as functionalism and the health belief model. It looks deep at the social fabrics of the society to uncover the structural barriers, especially social inequality responsible for ill-health. The economic and political institutions create and reinforce social inequality, which is a fundamental cause of health inequalities (Krieger 2001). The sustainability of social inequality is responsible for the reproduction or vicious cycle of poor health among the less privileged. While the perspective agrees that individual lifestyle has an effect on health condition, it stresses that economic inequality pushes people to unhealthy lifestyles. The *push factors* should be the primary priority in disease control. For instance, the growing commercial sex work among the underprivileged population is not a choice but a function of structural preconditions. More so, Singer (1986) averred that alcoholism or drunkenness (like other risk factors) is a result of social condition and class relations. In a critical conclusion, while assessing the WHO report on social determinants of health, Navarro (2009) observed that the document highlights a number of social determinants of health without acknowledging the power relations responsible for such determinants. Navarro (2009, p. 15) concluded that it is fundamental to understand that inequalities do not kill people, but "it is those who are responsible for these inequalities that kill people." Therefore, any socioeconomic system that produces, maintains, and reproduces social inequalities will generate adverse determinants of health, especially among the lower rung of the society.

Furthermore, as earlier observed in Engels' work, the capitalist system might not provide an appropriate work environment for the majority of the underprivileged. Thus the proletarians work in hazardous conditions that are injurious to their health. The worker might not have the minimum standard of care in their work environment. More so, as a result of working with heavy machinery and with dangerous chemicals, the proletarians are exposed to various forms of injuries. This accounts for poor health among the lower class. The capitalist state also undermines the health of the citizen through poor wages. The standard wage crisis is a major point of agitation in the world today. The labour class often complains of insufficient wages in the face of growing inflation. Especially in the third world countries, the situation is often worse. Low wage is a reality that holds negative influence for the social existence of the workers.

As shown in the works of Navarro (1974, 1975a, 2009), the configuration of public institutions support economic systems based on private ownership of the means of production in a capitalist economy. The health institution is also configured to serve the interest of the capitalist class. This is why there is commodification of health in capitalist societies. Health becomes a commodity that can be procured by those who have the means. The provision of health care is not based on needs but on the ability

6.3 Marxist Analysis/Political Economy of Health

to pay for health services in open markets either by paying out-of-pocket or by paying premiums to health insurance companies. Those who do not have the means to pay or secure health insurance might not be able to access health care. Invariably, not all of the proletariats are able to access health care due to monetary limitation. The health indicators are often worse among those categorised as unfit to contribute to the capitalist economy. Lupton (2003) observed that ill, aged, or physically disabled people experience a greater social alienation because they do not contribute to the production and consumption of commodities. This category is often referred to as the lumpen-proletariat, classless, or under-class.

In addition, the allocation of health resources is determined by the power of the dominant class. The bourgeoisie determines who gets what, why, and when in terms of health care resources. There is often class bias in the distribution of health facilities, usually with the concentration of such facilities in urban centres where the bourgeoisie often reside. Navarro (1974, 1976) observed that the structures of power and the distribution of resources in health and medicine simply mirror the capitalist system as a whole. The upper class predominates on the governing boards of health care institutions, including private and state medical teaching institutions (Waitzkin 1978). The bourgeoisie of insurance companies determine which ailments are covered and which are not. Prioritisation of health care or coverage is based on internal market and profit maximisation. This explains systematic discrimination against individuals with a history of a certain illness or who are at greater risk of a certain illness which might undermine the profit motives.

More so, medicine and health services are determined by the power position of health professionals. Another underlying measure in determining the role of the professionals is profit accumulation. Not only does exploitation take place at the societal level, it also takes place during the social exchange in health care. Health professionals are part of those who concentrate on the development of those goods and services that are the preconditions for the functioning of the capitalist system— nurturing the working class. They both provide supportive services for the capitalist economy and also partake in the exploitation. Activities of health professionals often lead to what Illich (1974, p. 920, 2003, p. 921) described as indirect iatrogenesis— a situation in which health policies and practices reinforce industrial organisation, which generates ill-health. Navarro (1976) observed that the state replicates the class hierarchy that characterises capitalist societies within the health sector. The health labour force follows class division in the society with the physician often being from the elite class.

Health inequalities also exist between countries of the world, mainly because there is socioeconomic exploitation between countries. For instance, Baer (1986, p. 130) observed that "the process of capital accumulation initiated under European colonialism and continued by multinational corporations [and now global linkages] results in the overall economic underdevelopment of Third-World nations which in turn has various health consequences, including low levels of general health, commerciogenic malnutrition, and exposure to hazardous industries and products." While the advanced capitalist region is responsible for a greater percentage of world industrial pollution, it is hesitant to take responsibility of climate protection.

Countries with a high concentration of poor people or higher levels of inequalities also do worse on a range of health indicators, while the rich countries consistently possess better health indicators. There are unequal political and economic relations between the core and the periphery in the world system, resulting in unequal trade, power relations, and greater flow of capital to the highly industrialised countries. The pharmaceuticals and other medical bodies sometimes promote unethical clinical trials and medical experimentation among vulnerable populations, as well as the sales of expensive drugs (see Baer 1982, p. 15; Geissler and Molyneux 2011; Jegede 2009; Washington 2006).

The political economists advocate for state intervention by ensuring equity in health resource allocation irrespective of social class. Access to health care should be based on needs rather than ability. The gradual movement to a socialised health care system in many industrialised countries is part of a vital response to conflict perspective. Countries such as France, England, and Cuba have now adopted socialised medical care where there is egalitarian access to care irrespective of class or monetary capacity among various social groups. Also in the developing countries, there is a growing provision of free medical care for the underprivileged, apart from the concerted efforts to make health care available to all, regardless of any personal attribute.

6.3.1 Criticisms of the Marxist Analysis of Health

Some scholars prefer conflict perspective to functionalism because it emphasises the role of structural factors in the generation of health problems and stresses the significance of conflicts of interest between collectivities with differing amounts of power (Gabe et al. 2004). The Marxist analysis revolves around the explanation of social determinants of health such as living condition, inequity in health policies, and SES. While there is a tendency to explain health from these fundamental causes, the perspective over-stresses that the dominant class could be held responsible for the generation of health problems and unequal distribution of health services in the society. This is why the perspective often recommends a revolutionary reconstitution of the society, a form of detotalisation, as a solution to health care problems (see Doyal and Pennell 1979; Onoge 1975). Many strictures of the PEH start with its tendency for violent or drastic social change, but there are some other criticisms of the political economy of health.

1. Conflict perspective is tautological and monotonous because it over-emphasises class division and conflict of interest in explaining all aspects of health care. The same explanations are repeated on divergent issues such as distribution of illness, access, risk factors, health policies, and so forth. It is as if there are no other intervening factors or peculiarities from society to society. The perspective thus becomes monotonous as an intellectual and practical endeavour in explaining the situation of health and illness in human society. It is a one-way perspective

leading to one single conclusion and solution. Navarro is widely criticised for this monotonous and stack recycling of the same explanation (see Reidy 1984).
2. The perspective also underestimates global efforts (e.g., flow of aid and humanitarian efforts) across societies and countries. There are subsidised drugs, the flow of global funds, and the exchange or transfer of medical technologies to poorer regions. This has really alleviated the suffering of many individuals and creates some level of access to services which otherwise might not be available. The argument is that motives of the social exchange are not always based on self-aggrandisement, profit maximisation, and exploitation.
3. The PEH frees individuals from self-accountability for health. It does not provide an adequate explanation for lifestyle issues and how they are related to health conditions. To what extent can an individual blame structural factors for smoking, sexual, and consumption behaviours? It is difficult to argue that there is no element of free will in engaging in unprotected sex, the initiation of smoking, and a high consumption of alcohol. There are some measures of responsibility in many risk factors.
4. In the sociopolitical arena, there is gradual equity as more societies become less class-conscious. The distinction between classes is gradually dissipating, especially in advanced countries. There is also recognition of equal access and right to care. This is the bedrock of modern society, based on free and rational choices backed with equal rights. Most advanced capitalist societies (to a large extent) have these features and, consequently, their health indicators are better. If the Marxist arguments are true, one would expect that the more capitalism advances, the more the disparities in health care and even health problems will persist. The realities show that the burden of health problems in Africa is (mostly) a result of poor political leadership, not capitalism.
5. Efficiency in health care could easily be undermined if services are served by needs only. Even though health could be a right, there is a need for people to take responsibility in care and cure. There could be less control on risk factors if health care resources were distributed according to needs only. The argument does not mean that in capitalist societies needs are not considered at all, as there are sometimes health care programmes for the less privileged.
6. The political economists cannot account for the explanatory models of illness (see Sect. 8.2). The perspective cannot explain individual experiences of illness because it treats cultural and symbolic aspects of illness experience as marginal and negligible. The perspective stems from a macroscopic level of analysis; therefore, it cannot be used to explain micro-phenomena such as construction and perception of illness. Functionalism also shares this criticism.
7. The perspective undermines the functional roles of health institutions and professionals merely viewing them as part of the capitalist tools. Worse still, it completely undermines the contribution of capitalist industrialism in the development of medical technology and in particular medical institutions. Industrialism is a global force shaping and advancing all aspects of societies, including medical practices and institutions. As Hart (1982) observed, the Marxists often consciously refuse to acknowledge and confront the very real material progress in health and other spheres of existence achieved in capitalist societies.

6.4 Fundamental Cause Theory

In various parts of the book, the influence of socioeconomic status (SES) on health has been discussed (see Sects. 3.6.2, 4.3, and 6.3). In Sect. 6.3, the idea of health inequalities was discussed largely from a structural perspective—how social system engenders health and diseases through unequal distribution of resources. Some Marxist scholars also discussed the influence of SES on health (see Singer 1986; Navarro 1974, 1976; Onoge 1975). The Marxist idea is more concerned with how social inequality is produced and reproduced, and how it invariably translates to health inequalities. The fundamental cause theory is interested in how certain social conditions form essential explanations for health inequalities. The theory is largely credited to Bruce G. Link and Jo Phelan (1995, 2010) who also acknowledged several previous studies that linked social conditions and health. Link and Phelan (1995) particularly acknowledged that the works of House et al. (1990, 1994) influence the development of the theory.

House et al. (1994) observed that health varies with age, but it is, importantly, stratified by SES, with lower SES persons bearing a greater burden—higher health risks and early onset of diseases during the life course. House et al. (1990) also indicated that the roles played by biomedical, psychosocial, and other factors are less important than age and SES in determining the duration of morbidity and disability over the life course. The study concluded that a major intervention in improving wellbeing in our society should focus on reducing socioeconomic inequalities. House et al. (2005) observed that that the flow of causality is much greater from socioeconomic position to health than vice versa. The study also reaffirmed a previous finding that education and income (which are variables of SES) play great roles in the onset of functional limitations and particularly, income has much stronger effects on progression or course of functional limitations. These studies by House et al. exalted the significance of SES as a cause of morbidity and mortality, and this invariable led to the idea of irreducible fundamental nature of social conditions (especially SES) in the theory of Link and Phelan (1995, 2010).

Link and Phelan (1995) developed a relatively new framework called "fundamental cause theory or theory of fundamental causes," which further explains the connection between social condition and health. The theory is worth discussing because of the reasonably new dimension introduced, and systematic approach used in unloading the concept of SES beyond the common variables such as income, occupation and level of education. Fundamental cause theory is "a theory of the middle range that helps us understand the social patterning of disease and death from a distinctly sociological vantage point (Link and Phelan 2010, p. 15). The central approach is the use of specific sociological concepts, which can provide a contextual and historical explanation of the prevalence or distribution of disease among groups. The theory normally "identifies a relatively specific phenomenon it seeks to explain—i.e there exists connections between health and social factors" such as SES, discrimination, social capital (Link and Phelan 2010, p. 14). For instance,"... fundamental-cause theory provides an explanation for why SES might be related to many diseases and

6.4 Fundamental Cause Theory

why such an association might be reproduced in multiple contexts and at different times" (Link and Phelan 2010, p. 14). The theory tends to identify a factor that has persisted, which is fundamental or central despite changing circumstances, which can explain distribution of disease among groups in the society.

Link and Phelan (1995) admitted that there are a number of risk factors that predispose individuals to diseases. Various sections have discussed such risk factors that predispose individuals to diseases. Inadequate exercise or physical activities is connected to risk of cardiovascular diseases, obesity and a host of other conditions (see Sect. 3.3.1.1). Consumption of alcohol and use of drugs are also related to a lot of morbidities including substance dependence, liver diseases and HIV infection (see Sect. 3.3.1.2). Smokers and tobacco users are also highly vulnerable to a number of disease conditions (see Sect. 3.3.1.3). Individual choices in terms of diet and sexual behaviour can also influence health risks (see Sect. 3.3.1.4 and 3.3.1.5). Apart from these risk factors, there are other social determinants of health (see Chap. 4).

Furthermore, Phelan and Link (2013) inferred strong relationships between health and housing circumstances, poor sanitation, inadequate nutrition, and horrendous work conditions. But, over the years, there have been important improvement in health condition across the globe, especially in the developed countries such as the US and Canada, which are the major focus of Phelan and Link. Such improvement in health is owed to the changes in broad socioeconomic conditions than to specific medical advances. However, this is not to underestimate the impacts of medical technological advancement. Phelan et al. (2004, p. 266) maintained that

> ... the effect of socioeconomic status on mortality cannot be properly understood by reducing our explanations to behavioral, environmental, psychological, and biological mechanisms linking the two and that the effect of socioeconomic status on mortality cannot be eliminated by addressing the mechanisms that happen to link the two at a particular moment in time ... we have seen instances in which major proximal risk factors have been eliminated, yet socioeconomic disparities in mortality remain as strong as ever.

The general argument is that social conditions are fundamental causes, but Link and Phelan (1995) used SES to exemplify the theory of fundamental causes. They, however, observed that the idea of fundamental causes might also pertain to circumstances such as social capital, social stigma, and racism. The first major proposition of the fundamental cause theory is that despite the improvement in housing, sanitation, nutrition and work condition, the disparity in SES remains, and is majorly responsible for health disparities. In other words, the strong association between SES and health inequalities has persisted over time, and it is the fundamental cause of health inequality. The theory advances that social determinants are not mere correlates of risk factors; they are the causes of disease in human society. Among the social determinants, Link and Phelan (1995) explained that a fundamental cause has four major components:

1. It is a core or central factor, which exert influence on multiple disease outcomes. For instance, in Africa, SES is related to cholera, poliomyelitis, HIV, malaria, tuberculosis, and a host of other conditions. A fundamental cause forms a central

factor in explaining the high prevalence of numerous illness conditions among a social group.
2. A fundamental cause operates through multiple risk factors. It embodies a web of influences that greatly affect health condition. For instance, SES influences individual health behaviours, access to health care, kind of housing facility, access to basic amenities and so on. A person with low SES might engage in menial and hazardous occupation, live in a neighbourhood where sanitation is poor, and eat food that are short of essential minerals. All these constitute various conditions that could expose individual to a number of health risks. The realities of poor living condition is glaring among many communities in Africa.
3. The association between a fundamental cause and health persists and is reproduced over time and space through replacement of intervening mechanism. When certain risk factors are curtailed, other intervening mechanisms would surface to sustain the effects of a fundamental cause. Despite the improvement in living conditions in the highly industrialised countries, the SES-mortality association still persists. By implications, the effects of a fundamental cause will survive even when some proximate risk factors and intervening mechanisms are eliminated.
4. A fundamental cause involves access to resources (e.g., money and knowledge) that are necessary to minimise risk of diseases or disease outcomes. Such resources can enhance the use of preventive measures and general avoidance of risks. When a disease occurs, the resource can help to minimise the consequences of disease. For instance, it might enhance access to health care and required medication.

Still using SES to exemplify the fundamental cause theory, Link and Phelan (1995) observed that SES embodies a wide range of resources—including money, knowledge, prestige, power, and social connectedness (i.e., social support or capital), which can influence health outcomes. Link and Phelan (1995), and Phelan and Link (2013) averred that resources shape access to broad contexts such as neighbourhoods, occupations, and social networks that vary considerably in associated risk profiles and protective factors. Because of these context and reproduction of social inequalities, despite changes over time in knowledge of risk factors and treatments, the effects of SES persist. Link and Phelan (1995, p. 87) observed that in a static situation, where no new diseases, risks or knowledge of risks and treatments emerge, fundamental causes would not apply. But "[i]n the context of a dynamic system with changes in diseases, risks and knowledge of risks, and treatments, fundamental causes are likely to emerge." The argument is that "change" is a prerequisite for a fundamental cause to emerge. Those who have serviceable resources earlier mentioned would be able to transport them to the new situation. Therefore, "... those who command the most resources [i.e., persons with high SES] are best able to avoid risks, diseases and consequences of disease" (Link and Phelan 1995, p. 87). They would have more access to latest information regarding any new conditions and how to avoid it, have access to new treatments, and get more support when a disease occurs (Phelan et al. 2004).

On the other hand, life circumstances and poor resources might stymie those with low SES from having adequate knowledge, access to effective treatment or supportive network that is beneficial to health. Phelan et al. (2004, p. 269) observed that HIV/AIDS was not associated with SES in the very early years of the pandemic, but as scientist gained and spread more knowledge about the risk factors, followed by treatment possibility, the disease "has increasingly become concentrated in poor regions of the world and among poor and marginalised people of the richer regions of the world". Other diseases that hold a strong link with SES include malaria (Ricci 2012); VVF (Capes et al. 2011; Ijaya et al. 2010); TB (Ukwaja et al. 2013; Bati et al. 2013); and diahorrea (Alexander and Blackburn 2013) among others. Most of these diseases are often called diseases of poverty.

Ricci (2012) observed that the discovery of an effective vaccine might not eradicate malaria, but a fundamental understanding of mechanisms related to poverty that causes malaria, which will help communities affected and individuals to have improved knowledge, prevent and cure properly. Ricci's submission might not be viewed as pessimistic if the issue of polio vaccine is examined. Despite an effective vaccine, the world is still battling with several cases predominantly among the poor in developing countries. Poverty does not only influence prevalence of fever at the macro level but also at the individual and household levels in SSA (Novignon and Novignon 2012). VVF affects the most marginalised members of society: young, poor, illiterate women who live in remote areas (Capes et al. 2011). Poverty is both a cause and consequence of tuberculosis (Ukwaja et al. 2013). This is because TB patients are mostly from poor households, the (associated) costs to access care are potentially catastrophic even where treatments are provided free-of-charge. So also, child and maternal mortality can be explained by a fundamental cause—in this case, SES. Tragically, these preventable diseases of poverty are highly prevalent in Africa and account for millions of death each year.

6.4.1 *A Compounded Fundamental Cause*

Having exemplified the relevance of the fundamental cause theory by examining the SES-disease link, it is important to note that the situation in African is that of a "compounded fundamental cause." Most data used for the theory of fundamental causes were obtained in the developed countries. For instance, Phelan et al. (2004) tested a major hypothesis derived from the theory using data from population survey in the United States. Relatively, most of the proximate factors such as sanitation and basic social amenities have been improved, and it was easy to isolate the roles of SES in the distribution of disease in the developed countries. The situation in most African countries is far less desirable as basic infrastructures are still deficient in both urban and rural areas. The implication is that there are still intricate proximal factors that could compound any fundamental cause. In this case, individuals face multifactorial tragedies, which intensify the deleterious consequences of a fundamental cause such as SES. In the African scenario, it is difficult to isolate other proximal risk factors such as sanitation and condition of work. This is why the vicious cycle of socio-economic inequality and poor health (see Fig. 6.1) is still applicable.

Phelan and Link (2013) observed that a fundamental cause operates at individual and contextual levels. In African scenario, the contextual level in terms of life circumstances is still highly unfavourable for many individuals. For a little percentage of the African population with high SES, they have innovative ways of using their serviceable resources (such as money, power and knowledge) to their health advantage. For the majority, who are less privileged, they face the multifactorial tragedies which exert negative impact on their risk exposure, risk behaviour and disease outcomes. There is still high rate of poverty-induced commercial sex work, poor social amenities (e.g., water and power supplies, housing), inadequate social security, and high prevalence of social exclusion (e.g., gender discrimination and ethnoreligious intolerance). The high prevalence of these specific problems would definitely compound SES in accounting for disease prevalence—it is a case of compounded fundamental cause!

6.5 Feminist Analysis of Health

There is growing attention on the gender differences in human health. In Chap. 4, gender was discussed as a major social determinant of health. This section will discuss feminism as a major perspective in medical sociology. Before then, it is important to present some classical arguments in feminism, especially as conceived in some classical texts including *Sexual Politics* by Kate Millett, *The Second Sex* by Simone de Beauvoir, *The Dialectic of Sex* by Shulamith Firestone, and *The Sociology of Housework* by Ann Oakley. While Marxist analysis is configured on dialectic materialism based on class, feminism is a form of dialectic (materialism) based on sex. Haslanger et al. (2012) observed that the term "feminism" was used to refer to "the qualities of females" in the mid-1800s, but after the First International Women's Conference in Paris in 1892, the word, derived from the French term *féministe*, was used frequently in English in the advocacy of gender equality and equity. Haslanger et al. noted that feminism was then rooted in the mobilisation for women's suffrage in the early 20th century. Later, feminism became a philosophical and theoretical perspective in the analysis of human society. During the expansionist period, many feminists engaged a number of discourses bordering on the body, class, work, the family, globalisation, human rights, ethics, popular culture, poverty, racism, reproduction, science, the self, sex work, human/women trafficking, sexuality, and, especially, on several health-related topics.

In general, "feminist theory is a generalised, wide-ranging system of ideas about social life and human experience developed from a woman-centred perspective" (Lengermann and Niebrugge 2011, p. 454). In the first instance, the existence of gender stratification laid the foundation for the advocacy. As Beauvoir (1972) observed, defining the relation of master to slave is synonymous to the relation of man to woman. Feminism is grounded on the tenet that women are illegitimately oppressed or disadvantaged by comparison to men. There are many versions of these interpretations of feminist-grounded tenet. There are liberal, radical, and socialist feminisms, among others. In fact, Chafetz (1997) observed that there is little consensus among feminist sociologists about the basic theoretical questions because of the proliferation of so many versions of feminism. Here, feminism is presented from a structuralist tradition. While there could be a measure of common belief in structural feminism, its arguments and solutions are often divergent. The liberal ones are analytical and the radical are so critical. Irrespective of the different versions, the common distinct feature is the presentation of gender as a ubiquitous and fundamental feature of social life.

Firestone (1970) observed that unlike the arguments of Marx and Engels, gender stratification preceded class stratification. Gender division of labour is the first form of social differentiation with men in the public sphere and women mostly in the domestic realm. This division of labour is part of the causes of gender inequality. Firestone (1970, p. 6) averred that the original division of labour was "between man and woman for the purposes of child-rearing and within the family, the husband was the owner, the wife the means of production, the children the labour." According to Firestone, the division is a "whole sexual substratum of the historical dialectic that Engels at times dimly perceived" because he was so immersed in material life. To Firestone (1970, p. 6), it was wrong to explain the oppression of women strictly from an economic interpretation. Gender inequality is thus a fundamental social construction. In discussing how society generates gender stratification, Beauvoir (1972) noted that "human society is an antiphysis—in a sense, it is against nature; it does not passively submit to the presence of nature, but rather takes over the control of nature on its own behalf" by creating and recreating gender roles, thereby allocating more power to men than women.

The major social precept implicated in gender analysis is patriarchy. For instance, within most traditions, patriarchy grants the father nearly total control and ownership over his wife or wives and children, and such power could include that of physical abuse and other forms of violation (Millett 1969). The female body belongs to the male partner and is used in serving him in the form of procreation and domestic duties. Oakley (1974, 1980) extensively discussed the domestication of women and how it shapes the social value of women in human society. The biology of women also shapes the social construction of gender. This is why Firestone (1970) specifically explained that "women throughout history before the advent of birth control were at the continual mercy of their biology—menstruation, menopause, 'female ills,' constant painful childbirth, wet-nursing and care of infants, all of which made them dependent on males (whether brother, father, husband, lover, or clan, government, community-at-large) for physical survival." Due to their biology, women were then confined within the domestic domain and the dependency generated therefore promoted a massive gender gap.

While the Marxist will explain every issue from material circumstances, the feminist argument often stems from gender consideration (see Table 6.2 for a feminist view on society). Gender inequality is a major form of social problem on which most other life challenges (e.g., health problems, crime, poverty, racism, sexuality, and

Table 6.2 Basic views of feminism

View of the society	Gender stratification, gender division of labour, and gender conflict
Level of analysis	Macro, group, or social aggregate
Key concepts	Sex, gender, gender inequality, alienation, domination, material life
View of the individual	Determined by gendered material life, power, status, and authority
View of the social order	Maintained by male dominance or patriarchy
View of social change	Revolutionary—by force or coercion or evolutionary
View on disease or illness	Gender roles generate differential health risk between the sexes
	Health care access among women is limited due to discrimination
	Low social position of women affects their health and illness behaviour

more broadly social, political, and economic underdevelopment) can be explained. For this, the feminist agenda has been a critical factor in global affairs. From the foregoing discussion, the ultimate goal of most feminists is apparent. According to Millett (1969), feminism aims to end not just male privilege but sex distinction itself so that genital differences between human beings would no longer matter culturally.

The cultural manifestations of sex differences reflect in:

1. **Equity between men and women:** women often suffer from all forms of oppression and subjugation. Injustice, in whatever form it takes, should not be a part of any modern society.
2. **Human choices:** gender inequality imposes limits and boundaries in life choices and chances. A limited life choice is a form of violence imposed specifically on women.
3. **Sexual freedom:** the constraints on sexuality and contested ownership of the female body are detrimental to the women in particular and society at large.
4. **Equality:** there should not be discrimination based on a person's sex. Social fairness in daily life should be paramount. Inequality undermines life chances and opportunities.
5. **Autonomy and self-determination:** sex distinction gives room for gender oppression and slavery. This is evident in forced sex, marriage, and deliberate denial of life opportunities such as education and paid employment.
6. **Sociopolitical and economic progress:** sex discrimination sets limits to human progress in general. A situation in which a segment of the society is confined to a domestic space prevents their meaningful contribution to societal development.

There is an extension of feminist analysis in medical sociology because the aforementioned reflection of sex differences has enormous implications for human health and well-being. More worrisome, gender inequality not only extends to all spheres of life but it particularly reflects in health, prevalence and distribution of diseases, and access to health care.

The theoretical stance of the feminist analysis of health inherits a legacy of polarising men and women, male and female, and masculine and feminine from the broader discipline (Annandale and Hunt 1990). Apart from some classical works previously mentioned, the discourse on the feminist analysis of health in sociology

6.5 Feminist Analysis of Health

started with some groundbreaking works in the 1970s (see Nathanson 1975, 1977, 1984; Navarro 1975a, b; Stacey and Thorne 1985; Verbrugge 1976, 1985). Most of the literature that emerged shows the persistence of women's poor health relative to men; the acquisition of differential risks due to social roles, lifestyles, and health behaviours between the sexes; and that women's higher morbidity is firmly rooted in engendered circumstances and experiences (Verbrugge 1985; Annandale and Hunt 1990; Annandale 2013). These differences emerged as a result of the social construction of gender roles and consideration in daily life, or what Doyal (2000) described as inequalities inherent in the social definitions of femaleness and maleness. Such a consideration forms the lived experiences of both men and women. It is often argued that nobody is born a woman, but a person becomes one as a member of the society (Beauvoir 1972). Role orientation is acquired, reproduced, and sustained during the process of socialisation. Due to feminist advocacy, there is a gradually changing role of women in human societies. Traditional boundaries and differentiation of roles have long been broken in many societies in work, sexuality, leisure, family, parenthood, and so on. However, the gender gap is still a reality in many human societies, especially in the developing world.

Traditional masculine and feminine characteristics present conceptualisations of gender with divergent expectations, obligations, circumstances, and experiences of men and women. The differential gender-role socialisation accounts for unbalanced risk accumulation and predisposes the sexes towards different health-related behaviours and responses to symptoms. In other words, Verbrugge (1985) summarised the central theoretical viewpoint in the feminist analysis of health that sex differences in health are principally the outcome of differential risks acquired from roles, stress, lifestyles, and preventive health practices which are determined by the gender framework of the society. Following a review of some works (Nathanson 1975, 1977, 1984; Verbrugge 1976, 1985; Clarke 1983; Annandale and Hunt 1990; Nettleton 1996; Vlassoff 1994; Zaidi et al. 1996; Doyal 1996, 2000; Read and Gorman 2010 among others), there are some distinct and critical theoretical prepositions raised in the feminist analysis of health.

1. Gender role orientation has significant effects on health. Gender role differentiation is unnatural because biological differentiation is not a conclusive proof of gender identity. Due to patriarchy, some women's heath priorities (reproductive and maternal health services, including medical research) are undermined.
2. Traditional representation of masculinity and femininity is associated with positive or negative health. Societies often portray a picture of adventurous, strong, and functional men, and passive, submissive, and less functional women. Some forms of masculinity (e.g., aggressive behaviour, sexual experimentation, and poor health-reporting behaviour) also increase the exposure of men to health risks.
3. The lived experiences of women coupled with their social position with regard to social value/prestige, power, and wealth affect their health and response to illness. More specifically, gender-based oppression exists in all aspects of women's lives

irrespective of culture, sociopolitical arrangements and economic systems, and even health care services.
4. The differential access to life opportunities (e.g., education and paid employment) has a profound influence on women's health. Access to health care is undermined by the subjugated position of women in human society. There is systematically constructed unequal treatment/representation in the public domain (especially in economy, politics, and health institution), which accounts for the limited participation of women, which is also consequential for their health.
5. There are considerable forms of violence (e.g., physical, sexual, and mental) against women in the society, which also account for increasing exposure and, eventually, higher morbidity.
6. There are inherent sexist medical practices (e.g., sex determination and sex-selective abortion) in human society. There are also considerable unethical practices (in medical practices) which also compromise the woman's rights to autonomy and self-determination.
7. Due to the systematic alienation of women, there is increasing feminisation of social problems (e.g., poverty, unemployment, commercialisation of sex, etc.) which hold adverse outcomes for women's health.
8. In general, women constitute a vulnerable segment (or sociological group) of the population whose health needs should be prioritised.

Feminists do not overlook health disparities in men and women on the basis of physiology (Read and Gorman 2010). For instance, Verbrugge (1989, p. 283) observed that there are "biological risks—the intrinsic differences between males and females based on their genes or hormones," which confer differential risks of morbidity. Moreover, the medicalisation of pregnancy, childbirth, and other reproductive roles has generated a great deal of doctoring of women (Clarke 1983). While biological/physiological condition is held constant, social-structural, psychosocial, and behavioural characteristics and conditions greatly affect exposure and vulnerability between the sexes (Read and Gorman 2010; Rieker and Bird 2000; Verbrugge 1985).

The fact that those with a higher social standing have better health is a reality. The depreciated social standing/value of women starts from childbirth because of the preference for a male child in many societies. Such preference leads to natality inequality and subsequent relative care (medical, material, and non-material) (Sen 2001, 2003). Following these assertions, there is often a similar conclusion from the feminist sociologists on how to address gender-based differential morbidity and mortality. For instance, Verbrugge (1989, p. 295) concluded that

> [w]omen's excess morbidity in contemporary life is influenced by social factors especially by risks stemming from lesser employment, greater felt stress and unhappiness, stronger feelings of vulnerability to illness, fewer formal time constraints (related to fewer job hours), and less physically strenuous leisure activities. If these risks are reduced—by promoting engagement in productive roles, blunting stress and fostering happiness, and encouraging aerobic activity—women are likely to feel better physically and to suffer fewer daily symptoms and chronic health problems.

Promotion of gender equality and equity through unbiased access to life chances and opportunities in all spheres of life constitute a vital antidote for improving health indicators of women. Increased access to education, employment, and participation in policy formulation and implementation are central in uplifting the status of women in human society. This will eventually reduce the unnatural distribution of diseases and disabilities. This is why Nathanson (1984) asserted that sociological health research should also focus on a more complex model of causality that takes account of gender differences in the nature of morbidity and mortality risks.

6.5.1 Criticisms of the Feminist Perspective

There are also a number of criticisms against feminism and the feminist analysis of health. It is evident that there is differential exposure and risk, but it is never a deliberate imposition by men. Feminists have the tendency to hold men responsible for all social problems. This is an exaggeration of patriarchy. Apart from the stress on social perspectives, some feminists want to reorder natural occurrences. For instance, some feminists advocate a change in women's biological roles to secure freedom from pregnancy and childbirth. More so, feminists often ignore situations that are favourable to women. Overall, women have longer life expectancy than men (Read and Gorman 2010). There are underlying social influences which are responsible for poor health reporting despite risky adventures among men. Feminists do not often criticise areas in which women hold considerable advantages (e.g., to create a balance in life expectancy between the sexes).

References

Alexander, K., & Blackburn, J. (2013). Overcoming barriers in evaluating outbreaks of diarrheal disease in resource poor settings: Assessment of recurrent outbreaks in Chobe District, Botswana. *BMC Public Health, 13,* 775. doi:10.1186/1471-2458-13-775.

Amzat, J., & Omololu, F. (2012). Basics of sociological paradigms. In I. S. Ogundiya & J. Amzat (Eds.), *The basics of social sciences* (pp. 115–134). Lagos: Malthouse Press.

Annandale, E. (2013). Gender theory and health. In W. C. Cockerham (Ed.), *Medical sociology on the move: New directions in theory* (pp. 145–171). Dordrecht: Springer.

Annandale, E., & Hunt, K. (1990). Masculinity, femininity and sex: An exploration of their relative contribution to explaining gender differences in health. *Sociology of Health & Illness, 12*(1), 24–46.

Baer, H. A. (1982). On the political economy of health. *Medical Anthropology Newsletter, 14*(1), 1–17.

Baer, H. A. (1986). Sociological contributions to the political economy of health: Lessons for medical anthropologists. *Medical Anthropology Quarterly, 17*(5), 129–131.

Bati, J., Legesse, M., & Medhin, G. (2013). Community's knowledge, attitudes and practices about tuberculosis in Itang Special District, Gambella Region, South Western Ethiopia. *BMC Public Health, 13,* 734. doi:10.1186/1471-2458-13-734.

Beauvoir, Simone de (1972). *The second sex* (translated by H. M. Parshley). Penguin.

Capes, T., Ascher-Walsh, C., Abdoulaye, I., & Brodman, M. (2011). Obstetric fistula in low and middle income countries. *Mount Sinai Journal of Medicine, 78*(3), 352–361. doi: 10.1002/msj.20265.

Chafet, J. S. (1997). Feminist theory and sociology: Underutilized contributions for mainstream theory. *Annual Review of Sociology, 23,* 97–120.

Clarke, J. N. (1983). Sexism, feminism and medicalism: A decade review of literature on gender and illness. *Sociology of Health & Illness, 5,* 62–82.

Doyal, L. (1996). The *politics of women's health*: Setting a global agenda. *International Journal of Health Services, 26*(1), 47–65.

Doyal, L. (2000). Gender equity in health: Debates and dilemmas. *Social Science & Medicine, 51,* 931–939.

Doyal, L., & Pennell, I. (1979). *The political economy of health.* London: Pluto Press.

Engels, F. (1845). *The condition of the working-class in England in 1844* (translated by Florence K. Wischnewetzky). London: George Allen & Unwin LTD.

Firestone, S. (1970). *The dialectic of sex: The case for feminist revolution.* NY: Farrar Straus and Giroux.

Gabe, J., Bury, M., & Elston, M. A. (2004). *Key concepts in medical sociology.* London: Sage Publications.

Geissler, P. W., & Molyneux, C. (Eds.), (2011). *Evidence, ethos and experiment: The anthropology and history of medical research in Africa.* NY: Berghahn Books.

Hart, N. (1982). Is capitalism bad for your health? *The British Journal of Sociology, 33*(3), 435–443.

Haslanger, S., Tuana, N., & O'Connor, P. (2012). Topics in feminism. In E. N. Zalta (Ed.), *The Stanford encyclopedia of philosophy (Summer 2012 Edition).* Url: http://plato.stanford.edu/archives/sum2012/entries/feminism-topics/. Accessed 28 June 2012.

Holtz, T. H., Holmes, S., Stonington, S., & Eisenberg, L. (2006). Health is still social: Contemporary examples in the age of the genome. *PLoS Medicine, 3*(10), e419. doi:10.1371/journal.pmed.0030419.

House, J. S., Kessler, R. C., & Herzog, A. R. (1990). Age, socioeconomic status, and health. *The Milbank Memorial Fund, 68,* 383–411.

House, J. S., Lepkowski, J. M., Kinney, A. M., Mero, R. P., Kessler, R. C., & Herzog, A. R. (1994). The social stratification of aging and health. *Journal of Health and Social Behavior, 35,* 213–34.

House, J. S., Lantz, P. M., & Herd, P. (2005). Continuity and change in the social stratification of aging and health over the life course: Evidence from a nationally representative longitudinal study from 1986 to 2001/2002 (Americans' Changing Lives Study). *The Journals of Gerontology Series B: Psychological Sciences and Social Sciences, 60*(Spec. No. 2), 15–26.

Ijaiya, M. A., Rahman, A. G., Aboyeji, A. P., Olatinwo, A. W., Esuga S. A., Ogah, O. K., Raji, H. O., Adebara, I. O., Akintobi, A. O., Adeniran, A. S., & Adewole, A. A. (2010). Vesicovaginal fistula: A review of Nigerian experience. *West African Journal of Medicine, 29*(5), 293–298.

Illich, I. (1974). Medical nemesis. *The Lancet, 303*(7863), 918–921.

Illich, I. (2003). Medical nemesis. *Journal of Epidemiology and Community Health, 57,* 919–922.

Janzen, J. M. (1978). The comparative study of medical systems as changing social systems. *Social Science & Medicine, 12,* 121–129.

Jegede, A. S. (2009). Understanding informed consent for participation in international health research. *Developing World Bioethics, 9*(2), 81–87.

Krieger, N. (1994). Epidemiology and the web of causation: Has anyone seen the Spider? *Social Science & Medicine, 39,* 887–903.

Krieger, N. (2001). Emerging theories for social epidemiology in the 21st century: An ecosocial perspective. *International Journal of Epidemiology, 30,* 668–677.

Lengermann, P. M., & Niebrugge, G. (2011). Contemporary feminist theory. In G. Ritzer *Sociological theory.* NY: McGraw-Hill.

Link, B. G., & Phelan, J. (1995). Social conditions as fundamental causes of disease. *Journal of Health and Social Behavior* (extra issue), 80–94.

Link, B. G., & Phelan, J. C. (1996). Editorial: Understanding sociodemographic differences in health—The role of fundamental social causes. *American Journal of Public Health, 86*, 471–3.

Link, B. G., & Phelan, J. (2010). Social conditions as fundamental causes of health inequalities. In C. E. Bird, P. Conrad, A. M. Freemont, & S. Timmermans (Eds.), *Handbook of medical sociology* (6th ed.). Nashville: Vanderbilt University Press.

Lupton, D. (2003). *Medicine as culture: Illness, disease and the body in Western Societies*. London: Sage Publications.

Marx, K. (1887). *Capital: A critique of political economy*. (Translated by Samuel Moore and Edward Aveling, edited by Frederick Engels). Moscow: Progress Publishers.

Millett, K. (1969). *Sexual politics*. Granada Publishing.

Morgan, L. M. (1987). Dependency theory in the political economy of health: An anthropological critique. *Medical Anthropology Quarterly* (New Series), *1*(2), 131–154.

Nathanson, C. A. (1975). Illness and the feminine role: A theoretical review. *Social Science & Medicine, 9*, 57–62.

Nathanson, C. A. (1977). Sex, illness and medical care: A review of data, theory and method. *Social Science & Medicine, 11*, 13–25.

Nathanson, C. A. (1984). Sex differences in mortality. *Annual Review of Sociology, 10*, 191–213.

Navarro, V. (1974). A critique of the present and proposed strategies for redistributing resources in the health sector and a discussion of alternatives. *Medical Care, 12*, 721–742.

Navarro, V. (1975a). The political economy of medical care: An explanation of the composition, nature, and functions of the present health sector of the United States. *International Journal of Health Services, 5*(1), 65–94.

Navarro, V. (1975b). Women in health care. *New England Journal of Medicine, 292*, 398–402.

Navarro, V. (1976). Social class, political power and the state and their implications in medicine. *Social Science & Medicine, 10*, 437–457.

Navarro, V. (2009). What we mean by social determinants of health. *Global Health Promotion, 16*(1), 5–16.

Nettleton, S. (1996). Women and the new paradigm of health and medicine. *Critical Social Policy, 16*, 33–53.

Novignon, J., & Novignon, J. (2012). Socioeconomic status and the prevalence of fever in children under age five: Evidence from four sub-Saharan African countries. *BMC Research Notes, 5*, 380. doi:10.1186/1756-0500-5-380.

Oakley, A. (1974). *The sociology of housework*. London: Martin Robertson.

Oakley, A. (1980). *Women confined: Towards a sociology of childbirth*. Oxford: Martin Robertson.

Onoge, O. F. (1975) Capitalism and public health: A neglected theme in the medical anthropology of Africa. In S. R. Ingman & A. E. Thomas (Eds.), *Topias and utopias in health* (pp. 219–232). The Hague: Mouton.

Phelan, J., & Link, B. G. (2013) Fundamental cause theory. In W. C. Cockerham (Ed.), *Medical sociology on the move: New directions in theory*. Dordrecht: Springer.

Phelan, J., Link, B. G., Diez-Roux, A., Kawachi, I., & Levin, B. (2004). "Fundamental causes" of social inequalities in mortality: A test of the theory. *Journal of Health and Social Behavior, 45*, 265–285.

Read, J. G., & Gorman, B. K. (2010). Gender and health inequality. *Annual Review of Sociology, 36*, 371–386.

Reidy, A. (1984). Marxist functionalism in medicine: A critique of the work of Vicente Navarro on health and medicine. *Social Science & Medicine, 19*(9), 897–910.

Ricci, F. (2012). Social implications of malaria and their relationships with poverty. *Mediterranean Journal of Hematology and Infectious Diseases, 4*(1), e2012048. doi: 10.4084/MJHID.2012.048.

Rieker P. P., & Bird, C. E. (2000). Sociological explanations of gender differences in mental and physical health. In C. E. Bird, P. Conrad, & A. M. Fremont (Eds.), *Handbook of medical sociology* (pp. 98–113). Upper Saddle River, NJ: Prentice Hall

Schnall, P. (1977). An introduction to historical materialist epidemiology. *Health Movement Organization, 2,* 1–9.

Sen, A. (2001). When misogyny becomes a problem: Many faces of gender inequality. *The New Republic, 17* (September), 37–40.

Sen, A. (2003). Missing women—revisited: Reduction in female mortality has been counterbalanced by sex selective abortions. *British Medical Journal, 327,* 1297–1298.

Singer, M. (1986). Toward a political-economy of alcoholism: The missing link in the anthropology of drinking. *Social Science & Medicine, 23*(2), 113–130.

Stacey, J., & Thorne, B. (1985). The missing feminist revolution in sociology. *Social Problems, 32*(4), 301–316.

Ukwaja, K. N., Alobu, I., Lgwenyi, C., & Hopewell, P. C. (2013). The high cost of free tuberculosis services: Patient and household costs associated with tuberculosis care in Ebonyi state, Nigeria. *PloS One, 8*(8), e73134. doi: 10.1371/journal.pone.0073134.

Verbrugge, L. M. (1976). Females and illness: Recent trends in sex differences in the United States. *Journal of Health & Social Behavior, 17,* 387–403.

Verbrugge, L. M. (1985). Gender and health: An update on hypotheses and evidence. *Journal of Health & Social Behaviour, 26,* 156–82.

Verbrugge, L. M. (1989). The twain meet: Empirical explanations of sex differences in health and mortality. *Journal of Health & Social Behavior, 30*(3), 282–304.

Vlassoff, C. (1994). Gender inequalities in health in the Third World: Uncharted ground. *Social Science & Medicine, 39*(9), 1249–1259.

Waitzkin, H. (1978). A Marxist view of medical care. *Annals of Internal Medicine, 89*(2), 264–278.

Waitzkin, H. (1981). The social origins of illness: A neglected history. *International Journal of Health Services, 11,* 77–103.

Washington, H. A. (2006). *Medical apartheid: The dark history of medical experimentation on Black Americans from colonial times to the present.* NY: Doubleday.

Zaidi, S. A. (1996). Gender perspectives and quality of care in underdeveloped countries: Disease, gender and contextuality. *Social Science & Medicine, 43*(5), 721–730.

Chapter 7
The Interpretive Perspective in Medical Sociology: Part I

7.1 Introduction

The interpretive paradigm presents a microsociological approach in the study of health. In this first part, a number of microsociological models will be presented. In this approach, most of the substantive theories are presented in microsociological areas of social psychology and sociocultural research (Young 2004). Therefore, some of these substantive theories include:

Weber's Classical Theories

1. **Weberian Social Action Theory**: this is an application of the classical sociological theory of social action to explain care and support.
2. **Weber's Bureaucratic Rationality**: this also represents the application of the classical theory of Weber to the explanation of the organisation of health care.

Health and Illness Behaviour Models

3. **Health Belief Model**: a model developed from social psychology to explain health-related behaviours.
4. **Theory of Planned Behaviour**: a theory also developed from social psychology to predict behaviour in general but now consistently used for health-related behaviour.
5. **Suchman's Stages of Illness Behaviour**: a microsociological approach of illness behaviour built on the sick role model.
6. **Andersen's Model of Health Services Utilisation**: more of micro but includes a number of macro issues influencing health services utilisation.

7.2 The Interpretive Perspective: A Brief Overview

The interpretive perspective has been called various names including (symbolic) interactionism, social constructionism, social contructivism, social action perspective, and social definition perspective, and it is also a broad theoretical standpoint

Table 7.1 Basic views from the interpretive perspective

View of the society	Web or domain of social interaction or exchange, social action
Level of analysis	Micro—individual, action, interaction
Key concepts	Interaction, symbols, meaning, self, subjectivity, roles
View of individual	People create social worlds through the process of interaction; social actions are voluntary
View of the social order	Maintained by mutual understanding and reciprocal relationship
View of social change	Reflect in the level and nature of social interaction
View on disease or illness	Illness categories are socially constructed
	Illness is experienced within a sociocultural context
	Response to illness is socioculturally determined and legitimised
	The patient-caregiver relationship is a vital aspect of the social system
	Professional model of illness/disease is often different from the lay model

consisting of a number of small theories including symbolic interactionism, phenomenology, ethnomethodology, and dramaturgical and social exchange theories. The interpretive perspective is an alternative to the structuralist perspectives such as functionalism, Marxist, and the feminist analysis of health. Table 7.1 shows some of the basic views of the interpretive perspective. To the interpretivists, human society only consists of individuals bound by constant interactions facilitated by social interpretation and representation of events in the social world. The key philosophical foundation is based on idealism or nominalism, a framework that holds a strong belief in the social abstraction of realities. It exposes that the human society and social phenomena are not real like *things*, as claimed by the structuralists, or that society exists *sui generis* (as an external social fact), as proposed by Emile Durkheim. The argument is that what the structuralists called social realities/facts are subjective and immersed in social interpretations and representations.

The interpretivists/interactionists argued that the so-called objective facts are not external or coercive of human action or behaviour. The subjective conditions are nonstructures and do not have a deterministic impact on social existence. Therefore, human action and behaviours are not effects of certain deterministic conditions; rather they are hinged on voluntary volition based on understanding, meaning, and interpretation attached to social events. Specifically, while the structuralists believe in determinism, the interpretivists favour voluntarism. This explains relativism in human responses to similar conditions. This is a seemingly opposing view to the notion of the *mechanical man* who plays a passive role in the society. The implication is that individuals are actively involved in the social construction of social realities whether there are social constraints or opportunities.

In addition, the interactionists focus on the microscopic level of analysis. The microscopic level consists of social processes at the subjective level which are relatively small in size, such as individual actors, actions, behaviour, attitude, motives, gestures, perception, thoughts, and interaction. The *subjective* occurs solely in the realm of ideas (Foucault 1970; Ritzer 2011). The focus is not on the social group or social aggregate but on the individual. Due to this microanalysis, the interpretive perspective is also inclined to idiographic approach, a kind of mini-narrative. The

7.2 The Interpretive Perspective: A Brief Overview

proponents do not really have the motive to generalise or provide a universal explanation that is applicable to all individuals. Since reality is socially constructed, it is highly relative and therefore the idea of grand narrative (universal laws governing human nature) is greatly contestable and most times infeasible. What, then, are the methodological implications of this nominalist philosophical foundation?

If social facts are not viewed as *things* that are external and have determining effects, this negates the cause-effect assumption in science. Hence the nominalists employ a methodology that is less scientifically rigorous. In fact, they are often referred to as anti-positivists. It should be noted that anti-positivism does not mean a total opposition to science. The nominalists are more flexible in their approach. The major method is rooted in what Weber (1949, 1978) called *verstehen* (i.e., understanding). It involves getting a deeper understanding of human action by examining actors' motives, course, and consequences of actions. This is why the interpretivists mostly rely on qualitative research design, an approach that is more appropriate in studying micro or subjective realities such as action, behaviour, motives, gestures, interaction, and other microsocial realities. The qualitative approach, and by implication the nominalist perspective, also depend on non-probability sampling. In general, this is a non-experimental approach. Some of the groundbreaking theoretical works in medical sociology—such as the social construction of illness or the explanatory model of illness, Goffman's theories of stigma and total institutions, Glaser and Strauss' trajectory of dying, including contributions from Michel Foucault and Pierre Bourdieu (among others)—were developed using a qualitative methodology. Glaser and Strauss (1967) specifically elaborated the grounded theory approach in qualitative methodology as a major way of theoretical construction.

In general, interpretivists agree that actions are not mediated by external forces but by subjective thinking (Amzat and Omololu 2012). An individual in the society has a capacity for thought that is shaped by social interaction. In fact, social interaction is the real essence of life. Social interaction explains the connection individuals have in society and the capacity to interact, interpret, and make meanings to define the social nature of human beings. People reach a common understanding through language and other symbolic systems (Babbie 2005). Labels or appellations are created for easy understanding and therefore to facilitate interaction (Ritzer 2011). Social positions are not fixed but rather are fluid and changeable. Through interaction, people are involved in the process of negotiation and renegotiation of social events and, consequently, role taking.

The interpretivists view illness experience as subjective and it requires deeper understanding if there must be sound intervention. The social interaction that takes place between the physician and the patient provides an avenue for the physician to have objective and, more importantly, subjective knowledge of disease condition. It also provides an opportunity to gain knowledge of the patients' views of illness condition. Lay perspective or explanatory models are vital for effective evaluation and intervention. The interpretivists also explain that illness itself and accompanying responses are socially constructed. An illness is thus not a real condition but is defined by the society as such. This implies that illness categories are created; people are defined as ill through the process of social interaction. For instance, HIV/AIDS is defined as a dreadful disease with life-threatening consequences. In addition, mental illness is associated with stigma that affects social interaction in many societies. All of these definitions are not fixed but are relative from one society to another and are subject to change through gradual understanding and redefinition. For example, obesity is gradually assuming a disease status in many non-western societies (especially in many African countries) where it was not previously defined as such.

7.2.1 Criticisms of the Interpretive Perspective

Like other perspectives, social constructionism is also fraught with a number of criticisms. This shows that there is no perspective that is perfect. The adoption or adaptation of any perspective depends on the problem to be studied. For instance, for structural issues, any substantive theory from functionalism or the social production of health could provide a better explanation than the interpretive perspective. When it comes to micro-phenomena, a theory from the interpretive paradigm will be more appropriate. Some of the criticisms of interpretive perspective include, but are not limited to:

1. It is often difficult to apply interpretive perspective in the explanations of macro events. Macro events occur at the objective level, but the focus of constructionism is on the subjective level.
2. Research design based on interpretive perspective is often seen as less scientifically rigorous. This is due to its dependence on qualitative methodology, non-probability sampling, and relatively small sample sizes.
3. The perspective relies extensively on psychological reductionism, an idea which depicts that social phenomena are mental abstractions. They are constructed and can be reconstructed.
4. It underrates the pressure or influence of social factors and structures. This is because of its non-deterministic stance. The approach is based on the self-authorship of action without adequate consideration of modifying factors.
5. The perspective is the major source of conceptual disunity in observational endeavours. It often presents a problem of operational definition since, according to the perspective, the social process is not fixed and thus is relative with regard to time and space.

Having provided some background information on the interpretive perspective, some substantive theories derived from it in medical sociology will be discussed.

7.3 The Weberian Social Action Theory

Max Weber (1864–1920), a German sociologist, political economist, and philosopher, is often referred to as the father of interpretive sociology. In his classical works, especially *The Methodology of the Social Sciences* (first published in 1903 and later in 1949) and *Economy and Society: An Outline of Interpretive Sociology* (first published in 1921 and later in 1978), Weber devoted attention to the explanation of sociology as an interpretive social science. Weber (1978, p. 4) defined sociology as "a science concerning itself with the interpretive understanding of social action and thereby with a causal explanation of its course and consequences." Weber used the German word *verstehen*, meaning *understanding*, as the methodological approach in sociology. He claimed that sociologists should capitalise on and utilise the advantage they have over natural scientists; that advantage resides in the sociologists' ability to *understand* social phenomena—action, behaviour, and the actor (himself/herself), whereas the natural scientists could not gain a similar understanding of the behaviour of an atom or other inanimate objects (Ritzer 2011, p. 116). Weber observed that understanding involves the interpretive grasp of the meaning embedded in social realities. By implication, there is a need to understand how illness categories are constructed, as well as subsequent illness experiences and responses by the actors. This will then allow for interpretation of meaning and their implications for social existence and health interventions. Weber (1978, p. 5) clarified that all interpretation of meaning, like all scientific observations, "strives for clarity and verifiable accuracy of insight and comprehension." He observed that understanding could be direct observational or explanatory understanding.

The field of medical sociology provides an opportunity to apply this understanding, interpretive grasp of meaning based on observations and explanations as proposed by Weber. While Weber was not particularly interested in medical sociology, he was one of those who laid the foundation for the conceptualisation of sociology itself, methodology, and research directions in the field. Very often, Weber's social action theory has been adapted for the understanding of social capital in population health, and as the bureaucratic ideal type for the understanding of medical organisation.

Weber's theory of social action is sometimes referred to as the "Action Frame of Reference." Weber was preoccupied with the possibility of analysing human actions and relationships scientifically (Abraham and Morgan 2004). It is further observed that Weber's primary focus was on the subjective meanings that human actors attach to their actions in their mutual orientations within a specific sociohistorical context. Weber argued that the explanation of social affairs has to account for the way in which individuals attach subjective meanings to situations and direct their actions in accordance with their perception of those situations (Burrell and Morgan 1979). The individuals interpret and define the situation, and then act accordingly. This also signifies that behaviours are moulded within the socio-spatial setting. Human predisposition and cultural frame are exclusive functions of our mutual orientation. Hence perception of diseases or illness is a product of the sociocultural realm. This leads to the relativity of the sociocultural milieu that explains differentials in the local understanding of illness within and across cultures.

The major deduction from Weber's approach is that human action is social in nature because of the meaning attached to it—be it overt or covert and omission or acquiescence. Human action is *social* "insofar as, by virtue of the subjective meaning attached to it by the acting individual, it takes account of the behaviour of others and

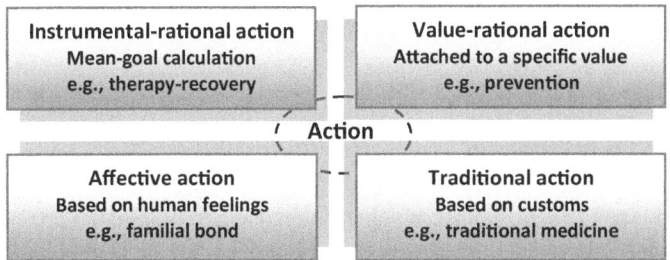

Fig. 7.1 Typology of social action

is thereby oriented in its course" (Weber 1978, p. 4). A *meaning* is the rationalised reason advanced by individuals as explanation for a specific action. Hence Weber asserted that the absence of assigned meaning by the individual makes the action meaningless. This contextual framework explains the intricacies in societal responses to disease and illness. The kind of actions taken by individuals in the management of ill-health depends on the sociocultural milieu. This refers to a sociohistorical context of health-seeking behaviour.

Practically, the foregoing discussion implies that human behaviour or action could be divergent in different social spaces. This behaviour or action is clearly relatable to health, first in terms of its local understanding which leads to a specific response from the individual and by extension the society at large. Weber (1978, p. 22) noted that "social action includes both failure to act and passive acquiescence, and is often oriented to the past, present, or expected future behaviour of others." "Others" in this sense could be given extended interpretation to include social institutions such as medical institutions. This explains that health and illness behaviours as well as non-participation in either of them can be explained within the limits of personal and relational understanding.

In this regard, Weber's typology of social action, as shown in Fig. 7.1, provides a reference point to understand both the basis and course of action. Weber identified that behavioural complex falls into four major categories: *zweckrationale*, *wertrationale*, affective, and traditional actions.

7.3.1 Instrumental Rational or Zweckrationale *Action*

It is that kind of action that defines a goal and chooses means purely in terms of the efficiency of attaining the end-in-view (Abraham and Morgan 2004). This is a goal-oriented rational action in which the actor deliberately acts to achieve a definite goal. Labinjoh (2002) also corroborated that in this case, the action is guided by consideration of ends, means, and secondary consequences. The end-in-view for the utilisation of a therapeutic regimen is to achieve recovery in the case of ill-health, and to avert occurrences of ill-health in the case of prevention. Individuals, based on their knowledge, act "logically" to avert or manage an illness condition. The actor assumes that the action will lead to the desired consequences.

7.3.2 Wertrationale *or Value-Rational Action*

The second type is *wertrationale* or value-rational action. Labinjoh (2002) observed that in this case, the agent consciously decides on the ultimate goal of his/her action and, as a result, systematically organises the action to achieve the goal. In this regard, action is based on individual beliefs, expectations, social imperatives, or honour. In other words, action is based on collective beliefs, values, and sanctions. It is, therefore, observed that culture creates illness labels, diagnostic categories, and health values. An actor who consistently uses traditional medicine no matter how severe the condition might be is motivated by the value of the efficacy of action based on sociocultural orientation.

7.3.3 *Affective Social Action*

In a case where emotion or impulse determines the means and ends of action, such action is called affective social action. Coser (2004) argues that affective action is anchored on the emotional state of the actor. Generally, care for a child is based on the emotion of the mother, but it could be guided by other kinds of motives as well. A major concern of the mothers in the domestic sphere is the provision of adequate care for the infants. This is why mothers are usually the first to perceive the health status of the child and act accordingly. This can be extended to other people in the society. *Care and support* for the sick is a major positive response towards recuperation and reintegration into the society.

7.3.4 *Traditional Action*

The last kind of action is called traditional action, which is guided by customary habits of thought and reliance on the external yesterday (Coser 2004). Every society has distinct traditional perspectives that are transferred from one generation to another. These traditions embed notions about health and illness. Cohen (1968) observed that Weber typically depicts the process of means-end motivation in social action. He observed that every actor has certain sentiments or affective dispositions which affect both his/her choice of goals. It is further averred that action is influenced not only by the situation but by the actors' knowledge of it. It is for this reason that both knowledge of available means and perceived efficacy of action play an important role in an individual's determination of what course of action to take in managing illness.

A traditional environment could explain the motive and means of social action. This last typology of action also signifies the relevance of culture on health.

The embedded notions about diagnosis, prevention and treatment, guide the actions of the ill and significant others. Heggenhougen et al. (2003) observed in this regard that disease control efforts need to pay attention to local realities (including cultural characteristics) that have a major influence in shaping ideas pertaining to health and illness. Each kind of action gives the basis for decisions or choices. The typologies can also be used to explain lifestyle choices, especially in relation to others. It is noticeable that Weber's typologies of social actions are individually distinctive, but they could be mutually inclusive: the health and illness behaviours/actions might combine the different kinds of motivations in a single action. Figure 7.1 shows that action, represented in the middle, could be a blend of the two or more kinds.

Weber's typologies of social action can be applied in the explanation of care and support or social capital. Action can also be motivated due to affection or good neighbourhood practices. This is because the social action theory emphasises social interdependence and interaction. Such interdependence can be examined within the personal control of health-endangering behaviour and care for others. The typology can be used to explain a household production of health and influence of what Weber (1978) called communistic solidarity of health. The framework of health intervention, especially in public health, has also promoted the use of "social action." There are usually calls for social action to help people who are in need of certain medical attention. This is often a call for community action to alleviate health-endangering behaviour for a safer social existence within the society. The action theory can be applied within this context to understand the purpose and orientation of action. Like the various dimensions of social action, it is important to set a goal and understand the values and traditions of the society.

7.4 Weber's Bureaucratic Rationality and Medical Institutions

Within the context of organisational studies or service delivery assessment, Weber's theory of bureaucracy is usually the starting point. Weber's ideal type, rationalisation, and bureaucracy have a wide range of applications including institutionalisation of medicine and health care, changing patterns in doctor-patient relationships, professional relationships (nurse-doctor, pharmacist-physician, etc.), organisational ethics/practices, power relations, professionalism, professionalisation and deprofessionalisation, organisational context of consumeristic attitude towards health, market relationships within health care, and global health phenomena. The genesis of Weber's discussion of bureaucracy started with his theoretical precept called the ideal type. Weber argued that one of the primary drives of sociology should be the construction of an ideal type, a kind of conceptual purity or perfection. This implies the provision of a utopian definition and attributes of sociological categories to serve as reference points in observational or explanatory analysis.

7.4 Weber's Bureaucratic Rationality and Medical Institutions

Ritzer (2011) noted that an ideal type is a heuristic device, which is useful and helpful in doing empirical research and in understanding a specific aspect of the social world. One major example of a (sociological) ideal type is bureaucracy. The first point is that bureaucracy or *officialdom* is based on formal rationality. Ritzer further observed that the domain of bureaucratic rationalisation involves universally applied rules, laws, and regulations. Allan (2010) explained that Weber used the word "rationalisation" in three different ways: first as means-ends calculation based on the most efficient means to achieve a given end; second, Weber relates it to bureaucracies which are structural methods of organising human behaviour across time and space; and, third, as the opposite of enchantment, free of mystery and magic. Modern medical practices are based on disenchantment that necessitates a scientific method of care and cure. It is also based on goal calculation, fulfilling the functional needs of the society, in this case, health care. Bureaucratic structures depict disenchantment and goal calculations.

The dominance of formal rationality leads to the proliferation of bureaucratic arrangements including the development of formal health care systems. The hospital is a domain of rational goal actions. Weber (1978, pp. 218–219) identified a number of characteristics of ideal bureaucracy such as medical institutions:

1. A continuous, rule-bound conduct of official functions (legalisation and legitimation of functions).
2. A specified sphere of competence (jurisdiction): This involves demarcation of obligations to perform functions, which have been marked off as part of a systematic division of labour. This is often referred to as specialisation.
3. The organisation of offices follows the principle of hierarchy (hierarchisation); that is, each lower office is under the control and supervision of a higher one.
4. The rules that regulate the conduct of an office are based on technical qualification, as are appointments.
5. A principle of separation of staff from owners or official from private: In principle, the modern organisation separates official activities from private activities or life.
6. A complete absence of appropriation of his/her official position by the incumbent: undue personal gains and interests should be eliminated.
7. Administrative acts, decisions, and rules are formulated and recorded in writing. This is called formalisation.
8. Organisational mobility or promotion is based on achievement. This helps the organisation to achieve efficiency and commitment to organisational goals. It also helps to nurse the aspirations of the members of staff.

Weber noted that official duties are bound by strict and systematic discipline and control in the conduct of the office. The profession of medicine is bound by definite rules and regulations. Some of these are defining functions or practices that are legal within a given society. Medical interventions or health care are carried out as official duties as specified within the organisation. Recruitment in the organisation is based on technical qualification. There is apparent regulation of entry and exit. Those who are recognised as professionals possess a number of qualifications or certificates. Such qualifications confer the competence to occupy a definite position and legitimise allocated functions. Moreover, there is also the compartmentalisation of activities. Medical institutions now have a high number of specialised practitioners. A medical institution is a complex organisation with various departments and specialisations. The division of labour is a critical aspect of bureaucracy.

Stratification of authority is a major feature of a bureaucratic organisation such as a hospital. The organisational chart often shows the hierarchies and flow of authority in a medical institution. This regulates professional relationships and could help to resolve conflict among professionals. Weber (1978, p. 223) noted that the primary source of the superiority of bureaucratic administration lies in the role of technical knowledge. Bureaucratic administration and hierarchies mean fundamental domination through knowledge. Arrangement is often based on technical qualifications and expertise. Those with higher qualification or competent knowledge are placed higher than others with low technical knowledge. Hierarchisation often generates conflict among various professionals (physicians, pharmacists, physiotherapists, senior nurses, etc.) involved in the healing process. Each of the professionals often claims expertise and superiority and often tries to oppose the "excesses" of the other professionals.

Rationality also reflects in official duties which should be regulated by what Parsons (1951) described as affective neutrality. Allan (2004, p. 152) noted that "the organizational, intellectual, and cultural movements towards rationality have emptied the world of emotion, mystery, tradition, and affective human ties," which are replaced with objective and scientific activities. The activities of medical professionals within the health sector should be based on legal conduct, which should be separated from affections or value judgments. Organisational property should not be mixed indiscriminately with personal property. Officialdom also extends to the explanation of some unethical practices, especially within the medical institution. The patient-physician should be guided by virtues and rules that would ensure that the interests of both parties are protected. The physician, who is more in the position of power relative to the patient, should ensure that exploitation in its entirety is avoided.

The critical link in the application of Weber's bureaucratic rationality is the conception that is very close to the modern perspective that integrates structures, process, and power (Ritzer 1975). Particularly, there are embedded power relations in a hospital. This power relation is very critical in the analysis of the rights of patients and the nature of service delivery. This perspective can also clarify the structures and processes and their implications in the delivery of health care. This perspective can also be used to assess the effects of bureaucratic structures on the functions of different specialties in medical professions. More so, Kleinman (2010) noted that Weber's bureaucratic rationality is directly pertinent to understanding how bureaucracies could create implementation bottlenecks for local and global health programmes.

On a final note, Weber's social action and bureaucratic rationality represent an adaptation of classical sociological theory in medical sociology. The adaptation of the two theoretical precepts depends on the study and the arguments the researcher wants to advance. The next chapter will dwell more on substantive theories in medical sociology.

7.5 Health and Illness Behaviour Models

A number of conceptual models have been developed over the years, especially to explain health and illness behaviours. The models are mostly microscopic-level-based theoretical models focusing on the individual in order to explain propensity to risk behaviours, use of preventive measures, health beliefs, and modifying factors (including social and normative factors) that could predict individual health-related behaviour. The models that will be explained in this section include the health belief model, the theory of planned behaviour, Suchman's stages of illness and medical care, and Andersen's model of health services utilisation.

7.5.1 The Health Belief Model (HBM)

The health belief model (HBM) is a well-known and widely applied social cognition model in medical sociology. It was developed by some social psychologists and has a link with the interpretive paradigm in sociology. The model presents a form of micro-analysis of behaviour, or phenomenological orientation relating to health. The model had its origin in the research of three psychologists, namely Godfrey M. Hochbaum, Irwin Rosenstock, and Stephen Kegels (Burns 1992). It was later developed and expanded by Godfrey M. Hochbaum (1958), Irwin Rosenstock (1960, 1966, 1974), Becker M. Howard (1974a), and Rosenstock et al. (1988). The model was developed due to serious concerns about the under-utilisation of various medical services, especially the tuberculosis (TB) screening program in the 1950s in the United States (Strecher and Rosenstock 1997). Hochbaum (1958) initiated the report of the model when he studied a large sample of those who participated in a TB screening exercise in the United States, stressing on the beliefs and related disease perceptions motivating acceptance of the screening exercise. The *Health Education Monograph*, edited by Becker (1974a), provided an extensive explanation and applicability of the model. The perspective has since assumed a substantive theoretical status because of its wide applicability and relevance in explaining various health concerns, including health and illness behaviours (see Kirscht 1974), drug adherence (see Becker and Maiman 1980), and sick role behaviour (see Becker 1974b). More so, Janz and Becker (1984) observed that the HBM has served as a conceptual framework for many researchers and has continued to be a major organising framework for explaining and predicting acceptance of health and medical care interventions.

In the beginning, the model was presented with only four key concepts: perceived susceptibility, perceived severity, perceived benefits, and perceived barriers (Rosenstock 1966). The concept of "cues for action" was added later to describe other factors that can trigger behaviour. Later in 1977, the concept of "self-efficacy or efficacy of expectation" was introduced by Bandura to explain how expectations can motivate behaviour (Bandura 1977). The concept of self-efficacy was added to the HBM by Rosenstock et al. (1988) to improve the applicability of the model. In addition, Stretcher and Rosenstock (1997, p. 115) provided a framework which

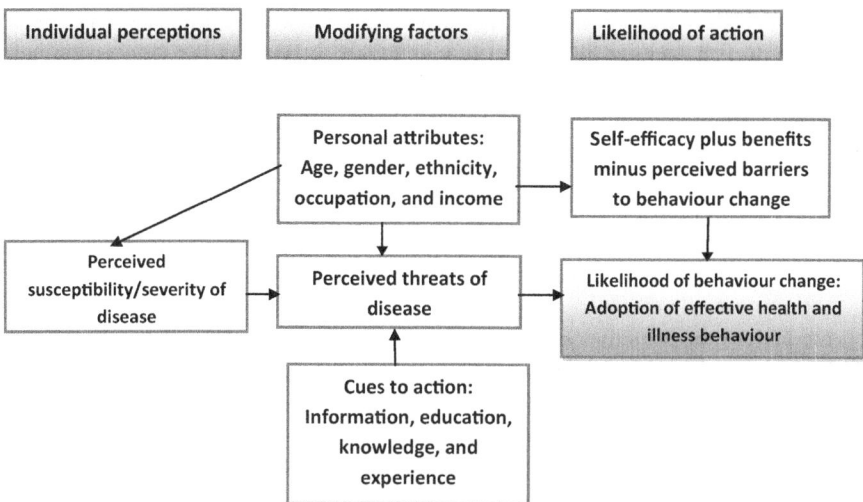

Fig. 7.2 The health belief model. (Source: Slightly updated from Strecher and Rosenstock (1997, p. 115))

includes "mediating factors," which was later added to highlight the influence of demographic variables (e.g., age, gender, ethnicity, occupation, education, and income). Now the major components of HBM include six key concepts and modifying factors (see Fig. 7.2 for the diagrammatic presentation of the model).

The HBM emphasises individual psychological processes in explaining individual behaviour towards health. It holds that health or illness behaviour is a function of the perception an individual has of his/her vulnerability to a disease and the perceived effectiveness of treatment, which affects the decision of whether to seek medical attention (Elder et al. 1999). Health behaviour and practices help to (a) prevent; (b) detect disease, defect, injury, and disability; (c) promote and enhance health; and (d) protect the individual and collectivity from risk of an actual disease, defect, injury, and disability (Alonzo 1993), while illness behaviour includes all activities undertaken by an individual considering himself to be ill, for the purpose of defining the state of his health and eventual actions towards recuperation. Some of the key elements of health and illness behaviours include prevention, detection, protection, and promotion (see Chap. 2 for more discussion on health and illness behaviour).

The HBM has various versions, but a comprehensive version was advanced by the proponents (by Rosenstock et al. 1988; Strecher and Rosenstock 1997), which provides an explicit account of the model by presenting the six major variables and the seventh modifying factors, which could influence course of action.

1. **Perceived susceptibility (to the disease)**: Each individual has his/her own perception of the possibility of experiencing an adverse effect on one's health. Knowledge of a disease may increase perceived susceptibility and the consequent use of preventive measures. The extent of the necessity to stay healthy following the perceived threat will go a long way to discourage or encourage

certain health-related behaviour. For instance, it may ensure drug adherence (i.e., taking of full doses at the correct time intervals to avert further complications). This variable is related to an individual's estimation of risk from a particular disease. More importantly, perceived susceptibility implies a belief in the reality of the disease and associated risk. Hence this could push an individual away from risk-related behaviour.

2. **Perceived severity**: If one contracts a disease, how serious will the effects be? The perceived experience of pain, discomfort, loss of work time, and financial burden may trigger a change in behaviour. This is sometimes referred to as "perceived seriousness of a disease." What is the emotional burden of a disease? These are the major questions that are asked when considering the perceived seriousness. The perceived effect of the complications (perceived threats) of a disease may influence a succession of change in behaviour of an individual to adopt preventive measures, seek appropriate treatment, or adhere to a therapeutic regimen. In sum, Janz and Becker (1984) observed that this variable involves evaluations of both medical/clinical consequences (e.g., death, disability, and pain) and possible social consequences (e.g., effects of the conditions on work, family life, and social relations).

3. **Perceived benefits**: How bearable or severe are the costs compared with the benefits of passivity or inaction? The answer to this determines health-seeking behaviour. In other words, what are the perceived benefits of taking action by using preventive measures or taking steps to avert complication for non-adherence to treatment or medical suggestions? This often depends on an adequate demonstration of the benefits of using a medical recommendation. It is assumed that if an individual understands and accepts that certain health actions will be beneficial in reducing threats from a disease, he/she might likely initiate such action.

4. **Perceived barriers**: The perceive benefits should be achievable at a subjectively acceptable cost. Cost herein refers to factors that may constitute constraints or impediments to a medically beneficial action. Such cost might be monetary, social, psychological, or even medical (e.g., adverse events). This is why the model suggests that the benefits minus the barriers may likely motivate action (especially when the benefits outweigh the costs [or barriers]). For instance, it is important to identify and understand the barriers to condom use in STD prevention, ITN use in malaria prevention, regular exercise to check weight, or medical checkups for the early detection of diseases.

5. **Self-efficacy**: Following the perceived susceptibility and seriousness of the outcomes of a disease, the beliefs regarding self-efficacy of action will influence the direction of action. This is the belief that a particular action can be implemented and will then lead to certain expected outcomes. This particular variable was acquired from the social cognitive theory formulated by Bandura. It is important not to confuse this with perceived benefits. Rosenstock et al. 1988 specifically defined self-efficacy as the conviction that one can successfully execute the behaviour required to produce the desired outcome. It goes beyond whether an action will be beneficial or not but extends to the capacity and ability to engage action necessary for the results.

Table 7.2 The health belief model and potential change strategies. (Source: Glanz et al. 2005, p. 14)

Concept	Definition	Potential change strategies
Perceived susceptibility	Beliefs about the chances of getting a condition	Define what populations(s) are at risk and their levels of risk
		Tailor risk information based on an individual's characteristics or behaviours
		Help the individual develop an accurate perception of his or her own risk
Perceived severity	Beliefs about the seriousness of a condition and its consequences	Specify the consequences of a condition and recommended action
Perceived benefits	Beliefs about the effectiveness of taking action to reduce risk or seriousness	Explain how, where, and when to take action and what the potential positive results will be
Perceived barriers	Beliefs about the material and psychological costs of taking action	Offer reassurance, incentives, and assistance; correct misinformation
Cues to action	Factors that activate "readiness to change"	Provide "how to" information, promote awareness, and employ reminder systems
Self-efficacy	Confidence in one's ability to take action	Provide training and guidance in performing action
		Use progressive goal setting
		Give verbal reinforcement
		Demonstrate desired behaviours

6. **Cues to action**: Cues to action could also be an important drive to action. Such could be a vicarious experience or verbal persuasion or conviction. Experience could come as a result of a direct observation of a disease condition or contact with sufferers. Cues could also be derived from information, education, and knowledge about a particular disease, its control measures, and access to health care. For instance, contact with a person living with a disease might convince those who do not believe in the reality of such a condition or trigger action to avoid falling into a similar condition.
7. **Modifying factors**: the factors include personal attributes or demographic characteristics. Apart from the level of susceptibility, other intervening factors such as level of education, occupation, proximity to health centres, income, age, sex, marital status, and so forth may influence the course of action taken.

The aforementioned variables propel individuals to act in response to health problems in certain ways. They could change individual behaviour regarding the use of preventive and treatment measures and adherence/non-adherence to a given health prescription/recommendation. It also goes further to affect the specific choice/measure in health maintenance. While the model explains both curative and preventive actions in line with the perception of diseases and other variables, it informs a number of practical applications in an attempt to (deliberately) change the behaviour of an individual. Table 7.2 shows some potential strategies that may be applied to change an individual's perception of a disease and encourage appropriate behaviour.

Basically, Glanz et al. (2005) presented how HBM can be used in the execution and promotion of health programmes. The model presents a form of the causal analysis of health-related behaviour, which is an important model for health care and planning. Davidhizar (1983) has since observed that a clear understanding of the cause of behaviour is necessary in order to predict change and determine methods to influence health behaviour. While the model continues to be utilised for a wide range of health programmes, it suffers a number of criticisms.

1. The model generally neglects the influence of social norms and other structural factors that may inform behaviour. The cultural context often modifies human behaviour.
2. The model over-relies on the assumption that every person is rational in thinking and acting and will therefore act (positively) in the case of perceived threats or severity of a disease. Some individuals might be indifferent to threats or deliberately take health risks. For instance, despite the evidence that smoking is risky, a lot of people continue to smoke.
3. The model is an individual-level theory of behaviour construed as a "victim-blaming" theory that lays the blame on individuals for not engaging in appropriate preventive health and illness behaviours (Tanner-Smith and Brown 2010).
4. The model often fails to adequately address certain contextual constraints that either directly or indirectly influence individuals' preventive health and illness behaviours (Tanner-Smith and Brown 2010). For instance, a limited supply of health services may be a major constraint.
5. It has been observed that most research utilising the model extensively relies on quantitative methods (Tanner-Smith and Brown 2010). Since the model stems from a phenomenological (micro) orientation, a qualitative method will add great value to uncover micro-phenomena.

7.5.2 *The Theory of Planned Behaviour (TPB)*

Icek Ajzen developed the TPB in 1985 and first published it in his article *From Intentions to Actions: A Theory of Planned Behaviour*. The theory was developed from the theory of reasoned action, which was developed by Martin Fishbein and Icek Ajzen in 1975 through their publication *Belief, Attitude, Intention, and Behaviour: An Introduction to Theory and Research*. In order to improve the applicability of the theory of reasoned action, Ajzen (1985, 1991) added new variables such as control beliefs and perceived behavioural control, then called the new framework a theory of planned behaviour. The TPB was developed from social psychology. It also has a link with interpretive sociology because it focuses on micro or subjective phenomena. This is why it is often adopted in medical sociology to explain health-related behaviour. The theory presents another approach in studying beliefs and health behaviour. Both the HBM and TPB are expectancy theory–based models, but there is a key difference. The TPB includes the consideration of social influence

Table 7.3 The theory of planned behaviour. (Source: Glanz et al. 2005)

Concept	Definition	Salient questions
Behavioural beliefs	Belief about consequences of particular behaviour	Do you think the behaviour will produce a good or bad outcome?
Attitude	Personal evaluation of the behaviour	Do you see the behaviour as good, neutral, or bad?
Normative beliefs	Perception about the particular behaviour, which is influenced by the judgment of significant others (social influence)	Do you think there are expectations from you regarding a particular behaviour?
Subjective norm	Beliefs about whether key people approve or disapprove of the behaviour; motivation to behave in a way that gains their approval	Do you agree or disagree that most people approve of/disapprove of the behaviour?
Control beliefs	Beliefs about the presence of factors that may facilitate or impede performance of the behaviour	Do you agree that you do not have any problem in carrying out a particular behaviour?
Perceived behavioural control	Perceived ease or difficulty of performing the particular behaviour (i.e., control over the behaviour)	Do you believe performing the behaviour is at your discretion or not?
Behavioural intention	Perceived likelihood of performing behaviour	Are you likely or unlikely to perform the behaviour?

(subjective and normative norms) but does not consider threats from a disease as shown in the HBM.

The TPB is based on the volitional control of behaviour and rationality of human beings. It is a self-responsibility approach in health behaviour—that individuals form their response based on personal evaluation of beliefs and responsive options. Actors then act as rational beings by selecting appropriate responses in terms of health and illness behaviour. Basically, the TPB was designed to predict behaviour from intention that is based on the correlation of beliefs, attitudes, intentions, behaviour and self-efficacy, or control beliefs. Table 7.3 presents the basic concepts and definitions in TPB. The basic argument is that people act based on intention, which requires adopting a positive attitude towards the behaviour, seeing it as a (approved) norm, and believing they have the ability to act. Ajzen and Manstead (2007, p. 45) observed that

> [i]n combination, attitude towards the behaviour, subjective norm, and perception of behavioural control lead to the formation of a behavioural intention. As a general rule, the more favourable the attitude and subjective norm, and the greater the perceived behavioural control, the stronger should be the person's intention to perform the behaviour in question.

The TPB examines causal antecedents of health-related behaviours, knowing why people perform, or fail to perform, recommended health practices (Ajzen and Manstead 2007). It is further explained that this model should generate a strong argument in studying lifestyle issues relating to health. The TPB, a framework to examine the determinants of particular behaviours, has been used to understand health-related behaviours such as exercising, donating blood, adhering to a low-fat diet, using condoms for AIDS prevention, avoiding illegal drugs, and wearing a safety helmet (Ajzen and Manstead 2007). It can generally be applied to predict varieties of health-related behaviours and can be the basis for implementation research.

There are three determinants in the TPB, namely attitudes towards the behaviour, subjective norms, and perceptions of behaviour. The three determinants are strongly connected to behavioural beliefs—the belief that an individual has about the consequences of a particular behaviour which helps to mould an attitude towards that behaviour. This implies that attitude reflects in the perception of the subjective outcome of a particular behaviour. Ajzen (2011) noted that beliefs about the likely consequences of the behaviour may be positive or negative. Such a belief might inform the expectations about the experience of pain, pleasure, regret, fear, elation, or other emotions. Both positive and negative expectations influence the nature of attitude. If there is a strong expectation that a particular behaviour is useful, positive, effective, and highly recommended, there is a greater possibility of developing a positive attitude.

Normative beliefs also influence the formation of a subjective norm. Normative beliefs are the aggregate of influence from significant others and social expectations, prescriptions, and proscriptions in the society. The subjective norm is then a personal evaluation and exhibition of the normative beliefs based on understanding and level of acceptability. An individual can form a subjective norm as perceived social pressure. Therefore, a subjective norm is determined by the total set of readily accessible beliefs concerning the expectation of important referents (Ajzen 2012, p. 443).

Furthermore, control beliefs also determine perceived behavioural control. Control beliefs are the aggregate of enabling or disabling factors relating to a particular behaviour. Such factors may impede or facilitate the performance of a particular behaviour. The resources and opportunities available to a person must (to some extent) inform the possibility of behavioural achievement (Ajzen 1991). If there are enabling factors, there is a greater chance to have confidence over a particular behaviour. Ajzen (2012) noted that perceived behavioural control is synonymous with self-efficacy (in HBM or social cognitive theory). It is the perception of the capacity to exercise control over the behaviour. As shown in Fig. 7.3, perceived behavioural control and behavioural intention can be used directly to predict behavioural achievement.

Therefore, behavioural intention, which could lead to actual behaviour, is based on three sets of determinants—behavioural beliefs and attitude; normative beliefs and a subjective norm; and control belief and perceived behavioural control (Ajzen 2011). These determinants are also influenced by demographic, environmental, and personal characteristics as shown in Fig. 7.3. Ajzen (2011) observed that a number of factors relating to personality and broad life values; demographic variables such as education, age, gender, and income; and exposure to media and other sources of information greatly influence the formation of beliefs.

In addition, intention may lead to actual behaviour. Behavioural intention is *trying* to perform a particular behaviour. The transition between intention and behaviour is simple because intention is a necessary condition for behaviour. On the other hand,

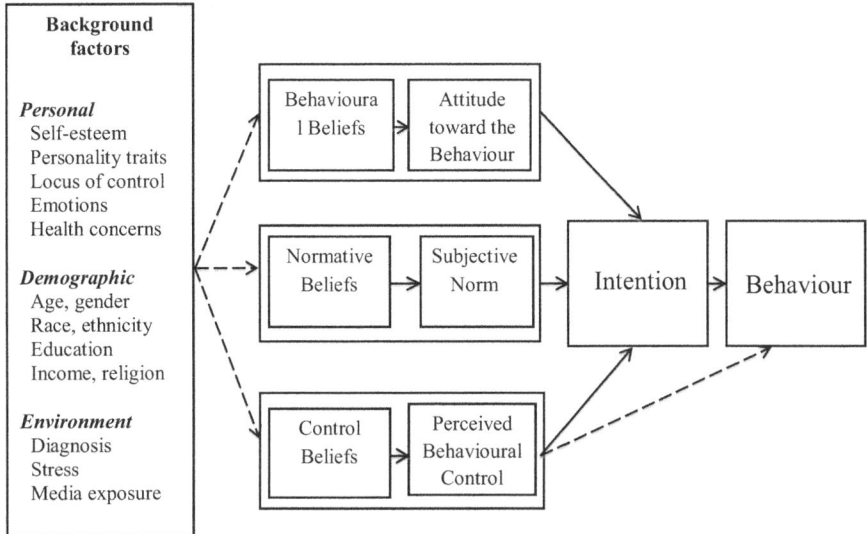

Fig. 7.3 The theory of planned behaviour. (Source: Ajzen and Manstead 2007, p. 46)

the transition is also complex because not all intentions lead to behaviour. Many people have the intention to quit smoking or lose weight without implementing the actual behaviour that will lead to such outcomes. Ajzen (2011, p. 1115) observed that whether intentions predict behaviour depends in part on factors beyond the individual's control; for example, the strength of the intention-behaviour relation is moderated by actual control over the behaviour. As a general rule, the stronger the intention to engage in the behaviour, the more likely its performance should be (Ajzen 1991). Moreover, Ajzen (2011) averred that beliefs can be formed based on the information or knowledge people have, and sometimes information could be inaccurate and incomplete. This signifies that beliefs formed based on inaccurate or a low level of knowledge may not produce positive behaviour. The preceding statement illustrates that the TPB does not show that behavioural, normative, and control beliefs are always formed based on rational and accurate premises.

In sum, the TPB distinguishes between three types of beliefs—behavioural, normative, and control—and three related constructs of attitude, subjective norm, and perceived behavioural control (Ajzen 2011, 2012). A meta-analysis found that the TPB is an appropriate framework as a predictor of intentions and behaviour (Armitage and Conner 2001). Despite the fact that the theory is a useful conceptual framework for dealing with the complexities of human social behaviour, it suffers a number of criticisms. Intentions are sometimes found to be poor predictors of behaviour (Kor and Mullan 2011). As Ajzen (1985) noted, intentions are predictors of behaviours but not all intentions are carried out. This shows that there is still a major element of probability in the intention-behaviour relation.

7.5.3 *Suchman's Stages of Illness and Medical Care*

In 1965 Edward Suchman proposed a model for the study of illness behaviour (cf. Sect. 3.5). The model has since become one of the major conceptual frameworks for many studies. The model is an advancement of the sick role model by Parsons. The primary concern of Suchman was to explain illness experience and medical care. Then, he described and analysed five major stages of illness that show critical transition and decision-making points in medical care and behaviour. Suchman (1965) grounded the stages of illness experience by distinguishing four principal elements: (a) the content, (b) the sequence, (c) the spacing, and (d) the variability of behaviour during different phases of medical care. Before describing the stages, Suchman introduced a number of terms to describe the content and variability of illness behaviour.

1. **Shopping**: this refers to seeking multiple sources of medical care, especially by combining traditional/folk medicine with modern medicine. Many patients engage in self-medication before seeking care from the official health sector.
2. **Fragmentation of care**: a situation where the patient is treated by a variety of medical practitioners at a single source of medical care. For instance, a patient with a fracture might need to be seen by a physician, radiologists, and physiotherapists.
3. **Procrastination**: this simply means a delay in seeking care following the recognition of symptoms. This is based on the observation that not all patients spontaneously or automatically seek care.
4. **Self-medication**: this is the use of self-treatment or home remedies. Some patients buy medication over-the-counter and administer it without a prescription.
5. **Discontinuity**: this means interruption of care. It is possible for a patient to miss a medical appointment or simply withdraw from treatment.

Suchman then divided the sequence of medical events into five stages (see Fig. 7.4), showing major transition and decision-making points. He, however, noted that all the stages might not be present in every case of illness.

A transition from one point to another requires the decision of the patient to situate the need for a transition and accept such a need. The stages are briefly explained in the following subsections.

7.5.3.1 The Symptom Experience Stage

Illness experience means the feeling of pain, discomfort, or any form of abnormality. This implies that there is a perception that something is definitely wrong. It is through this experience that the patient can define himself or herself as ill or unhealthy. This stage is critical because the experience depends on physical, emotional, or mental indications. It also depends on the ability to recognise the signs and symptoms of ill-health. The experience of illness may also reflect the severity of the illness. A patient may consider illness as serious or mild. This also considers the patient's knowledge of the symptoms of the disease or illness. It is important to note that

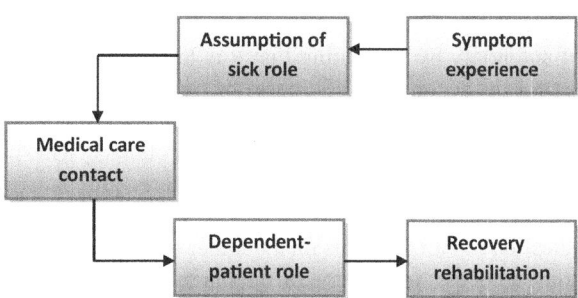

Fig. 7.4 Suchman's stages of illness and medical care

Suchman is particular here about symptomatic disease or illness. Apart from the physical dimension, Suchman (1965, p. 114) observed that the cognitive aspect is very important because it involves the interpretation and derived meaning for the individual experiencing the symptoms. It is further observed that this stage also involves an emotional response, or the fear or anxiety of perceived threats (in HBM), which may be attached to the physical experience and cognitive interpretation. The variability in the experience of symptoms often functions to initiate the patient into the medical care process and explains why some may not seek medical care. The variability also informs the selection of a care provider, whether in the traditional or modern care system. Suchman noted that three aspects of decision-making may be indicated at this stage: denial of illness, "flight to health," and procrastination. "Flight to health" will encourage the patient to proceed to another stage.

7.5.3.2 The Assumption of the Sick Role Stage

If the symptom experience is accepted as real and requiring medical attention, the patient may then assume the sick role. In this stage, the patient may be exempted from normal roles and depend on significant others. Here, there should be a wish to get well and seek assistance in the process. For instance, an individual seeks consent and confirmation to suspend normal roles in the society (Suchman 1965), and this exemption from duties must be sanctioned within an approved and acceptable standard. This is necessary to prevent undue excuses. It is also necessary to seek medical assistance to ensure a quick return to normal duties. Then, the individual needs to decide to move to the next stage (i.e., seek medical care).

7.5.3.3 The Medical Care Contact Stage

According to Suchman (1965, p. 115), "at this stage of illness, the sick individual seeks a medical diagnosis and a prescribed course of treatment from a *scientific* rather than *lay* source." The ill needs to seek competent help from those with technical qualifications. This helps the patient to legitimise the sick role process and confer sick role entitlements. It is at this stage that an actual medical diagnosis is reached and a course of treatment is recommended. Suchman recognises the notion of autonomy by stipulating that it is left to the patient to accept the diagnosis and accept the recommended course of treatment or continue to search for alternative explanations. He stressed that, in the case of a non-acceptance of the diagnosis and recommendations, this stage could be prolonged. This prolongation is due to repetition of activities—another diagnosis and recommendation probably by another care provider in another health facility or because of shopping. It is also noted that the selection of care depends on a number of factors, including access to care and other conveniences. Acceptance of the diagnosis and course of treatment will determine the future of the patient's medical behaviour and subsequent move to another stage.

7.5.3.4 The Dependent-Patient Role Stage

This stage indicates the acceptance of professional help and course of treatment. According to Suchman, the critical decision here is the transfer of control to the physician. It is at this stage that the individual actually becomes a patient (assumes patienthood). Acceptance of the course of treatment also means acceptance of the social and physical adjustments and perhaps pains involved in the treatment process. For instance, the treatment may involve some physical and dietary restrictions. In the case of hospitalisation, the patient is confined to the hospital where there may be a limit to visits by significant others. The patient has to accept medical instructions regarding medication and activities to ensure effectiveness of the therapeutic regimen. Suchman noted that the care process might lead to conflict between the patient and physician regarding the meaning and interpretation of symptoms.

7.5.3.5 The Recovery or Rehabilitation Stage

Patienthood often ends following a perceived wellness and confirmation of such by the professionals. This stage indicates the decision to relinquish the sick role and return to normal duties. An individual may fully regain his/her health and resume old roles or return as a chronic invalid or long-term rehabilitee (Suchman 1965, p. 116). Suchman noted that the return to a normal role is easy in cases of acute illness, but some difficulties may prevail in cases of chronic illness or physical impairment. In fact, in some cases, an individual may require a period of grace before returning to his/her normal role, while in some others an individual may never return to normal roles again.

Suchman also observed that some demographic characteristics such as age, sex, and income might determine an individual's response to illness. This implies that variation in the stages in terms of sequence and content may be due to some of these personal attributes. The model also has some practical applications: it is important for a care provider to understand the patient's complaints, point of view, and experience of illness; the physician needs to consider whether the patient has *shopped* before coming to a particular care facility; understand and prioritise the needs of the

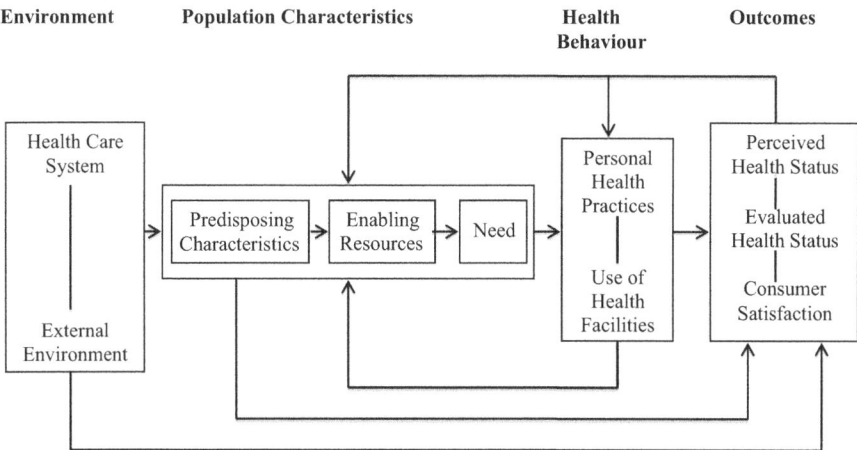

Fig. 7.5 Andersen's model of health services utilisation. (Source: Andersen 1995, p. 8)

patients; minimise inconveniences during patient-dependent role; and so on. As a microsociological model, it has been widely applied, but it also suffers some criticisms similar to those of its microanalytic counterparts previously examined.

7.5.4 Andersen's Model of Health Care Utilisation

Ronald Max Andersen (1968) presented another conceptual model to explain the utilisation of health services. The model was first developed to understand why families use health services and examine equitable access to such services (Andersen 1968). The model was first presented with three categories of determinants: predisposing characteristics, enabling characteristics, and need-based characteristics. Since then, the model has undergone a lot of modifications with the incorporation of more variables. Andersen (1995) identified the number of progressions in the modification of the model and finally arrived at the current model based on a number of modifications observed through a series of studies that have applied the initial model. Figure 7.5 presents the model.

Unlike the previous model, which was mainly based on microanalysis of health services utilisation, the new model incorporates some macro issues influencing health services utilisation.

According to Andersen (1995), an individual is more or less likely to utilise health services based on demographics, position within the social structure, and beliefs of health services benefits. Andersen claimed that the basic argument is that the utilisation of health services is based on people's disposition, or factors that enable or impede use of and need for health care. The key factors presented in Fig. 7.5 will be itemised and briefly explained.

1. **The predisposing characteristics**: these include demographics, social structure, and health beliefs. Like previous models discussed, this model also considers the importance of population characteristics that form part of the predisposing characteristics (age, gender, and attitudes). The social position of the individual in the social structure and social network also play a role. Andersen (1995) explained that the social position could be measured by level of education, income, and occupation. More so, the health beliefs (which include attitudes and values) of an individual determine the conception of illness symptoms and probable consequences.
2. **The enabling factors**: these are the factors that enable the individual to seek medical care. They constitute empowerment factors such as affordability of health services, possession of a health insurance policy, and adequate income. Low SES may be a disabling factor in a case in which the patients have to bear the direct cost of care. Those with a relatively high income may have better access to health services.
3. **The need factors**: these reflect the needs of the patient, especially based on the disease characteristics. A severe condition or accident may require urgent medical attention. Most times, in the case of an accident, the patient may not be able to make any decisions but will be rushed to a health facility for attention. The need factors also include the nature of the disease, whether acute or chronic, which could also determine the urgency of health services utilisation.
4. **Health system characteristics**: the type and nature of the health care system are major determining factors in health services utilisation. A socialised medical system may provide more opportunities in terms of access than a capitalist health care system. In addition, the availability and supply of services are part of the health system's characteristics. A health facility or services may not be available. The organisation of the health care system is also as important. It shows how health care resources are maximised and organised to meet the needs of the population.
5. **The external environmental factors**: these are structural factors that may determine the nature and organisation of the health system. These factors include political, geographic, environmental, and economic factors. For instance, the political environment plays a significant role in the allocation of resources. The role also extends to policy formulation and implementation.
6. **Personal health care practices**: these include lifestyle issues such as diet, exercise, and self-care, which might determine the outcome of care. The practices may include subjective norms towards health care utilisation. The central issue in health care practice is health behaviour, or the extent to which an individual adopts modalities that aid in the prevention of diseases or infirmities.

The other factors presented in the figure include "use of health services," which involve type, purpose, and place; perceived health status; and consumer satisfaction, which includes convenience, availability, proper financing provider characteristics, and quality of services received. All of these factors also contribute in determining the outcome of care.

In sum, Andersen's modified model indicates that the environment (health care system and external environment) determines the population characteristics (predisposing characteristics, enabling factors, and health needs), which invariably influence health behaviour (personal health resources and use of health services) and consequently leads to health outcomes.

References

Abraham, F., & Morgan, J. H. (2004). *Sociological thought*. New Delhi: Macmillan.
Ajzen, I. (1985). From intentions to actions: A theory of planned behaviour. In J. Kuhl & J. Beckman (Eds.), *Action-control: From cognition to behaviour* (pp. 11–39). Heidelberg: Springer.
Ajzen, I. (1991). The theory of planned behaviour. *Organizational Behaviour and Human Decision Processes, 50*, 179–211.
Ajzen, I. (2011). The theory of planned behaviours: Reactions and reflections. *Psychology & Health, 26*(9), 1113–1127.
Ajzen, I. (2012). The theory of planned behaviour. In P. A. M. Lange, A. W. Kruglanski, & E. T. Higgins (Eds.), *Handbook of theories of social psychology* (pp. 438–459). London: Sage.
Ajzen, I., & Manstead, A. S. R. (2007). Changing health-related behaviours: An approach based on the theory of planned behavior. In K. van den Bos, M. Hewstone, J. de Wit, H. Schut, & M. Stroebe (Eds.), *The scope of social psychology: Theory and applications—essays in honour of Wolfgang Stroebe* (pp. 43–63). New York: Psychology Press.
Allan, K. (2010). *Explorations in classical sociological theory: Seeing the social world*. California: Sage.
Alonzo, A. A. (1993). Health behaviour: Issues, contradictions and dilemmas. *Social Science & Medicine, 37*(8), 1019–1034.
Amzat, J., & Omololu, F. (2012). The basics of sociological paradigms. In I. S. Ogundiya & J. Amzat (Eds.), *Basics of the social sciences* (pp. 115–134). Lagos: Malthouse.
Andersen, R. M. (1968). *A behavioural model of families' use of health services*. Research Series No. 25. Chicago, IL: Centre for Health Administration Studies, University of Chicago.
Andersen, R. M. (1995). Revisiting the behavioural model and access to medical care: Does it matter? *Journal of Health and Social Behavior, 36*, 1–10.
Armitage, C. J., & Conner, M. (2001). Efficacy of the theory of planned behaviour: A meta-analytic review. *British Journal of Social Psychology, 40*, 471–499.
Bandura, A. (1977). Self-efficacy: Toward a unifying theory of behavioural change. *Psychological Review, 84*, 191–215.
Barbie, E. (2005). *The basics of social research*. Belmont: Thomas Wadsworth.
Becker, M. H. (Ed.). (1974a). The health belief Model and personal health behaviour. *Health Education Monographs, 2*, 324–508.
Becker, M. H. (1974b). The health belief model and sick role behaviour. *Health Education Monographs, 2*, 409–419.
Becker M. H., & Maiman, L. A. (1980). Strategies for enhancing patient compliance. *Journal of Community Health, 6*, 113–135.
Burns, A. C. (1992). The expanded health belief model as a basis for enlightened preventive health care practice and research. *Journal of Health Care Marketing, 12*(3), 32–45.
Burrell, G., & Morgan, G. (1979). *Sociological paradigm and organization analysis*. London: Heinemann.
Cohen, P. S. (1968). *Modern sociological theory*. London: Heinemann.
Coser, L. A. (2004). *Masters of sociological thought: Ideas in historical and social context* (2nd ed.). New Delhi: Rawat.

References

Davidhizar, R. (1983). Critique of the health belief model. *Journal of Advanced Nursing, 8*(6), 467–472.
Elder, J. P., Ayala, G. X., & Harris, S. (1999). Theories and intervention approaches to health behaviour change in primary care. *American Journal of Preventive Medicine, 17*(4), 275–284.
Fishbein, M., & Ajzen, I. (1975). *Belief, attitude, intention, and behaviour: An introduction to theory and research*. Reading: Addison-Wesley
Foucault, M. (1970). *The order of things: An archaeology of the human sciences*. London: Routledge.
Glanz, K., Rimer, B. K., & Su, S. M. (2005). *Theory at a glance: A guide for health promotion practice* (2nd ed.). United States: National Cancer Institute (A Monograph).
Glaser B. G., & Strauss, A. L. (1967). *The discovery of grounded theory: Strategies for qualitative research*. New York: Aldine de Gruyter.
Heggenhougen, H. K., Hackethal, V., & Vivek, P. (2003). *The behavioural and social aspects of malaria and its control: An introduction and annotated bibliography* (Vol. 03:1). Geneva: TDR/STR/SEB.
Hochbaum, G. M. (1958). *Public participation in medical screening programs: A sociopsychological study*. Washington DC: Public Health Service.
Janz, N. K., & Becker, M. H. (1984). The health belief model: A decade later. *Health Education & Behaviour, 11*(1), 1–47.
Kirscht J. P. (1974). The health belief model and illness behaviour. *Health Education Monographs, 2*, 387–408.
Kleinman, A. (2010). Four social theories for global health. *The Lancet, 375*, 1518–1519.
Kor, K., & Mullan, B.A. (2011). Sleep hygiene behaviours: An application of the theory of planned behaviour and the investigation of perceived autonomy support, past behaviour and response inhibition. *Psychology and Health, 26*, 1208–1224.
Labinjo, J. (2002). The sociological trio: An introduction to Marx, Weber and Durkheim. In U. C. Isiugo-Abanihe, A. N. Isamah, & J. O. Adesina (Eds.), *Currents and perspectives in sociology* (pp. 1–31). Ibadan: Malthouse.
Parsons, T. (1951). *The social system*. Glencoe, IL: The Free.
Ritzer, G. (1975). Professionalization, bureaucratization and rationalization: The views of Max Weber. *Social Forces, 53*(4), 627–634.
Ritzer, G. (2011). *Sociological theory* (8th ed.). New York: McGraw-Hill.
Rosenstock, I. M. (1960). What research in motivation suggests for public health. *American Journal of Pubic Health, 50*(3), 295–302.
Rosenstock, I. M. (1966). Why people use health services. *Milbank Memorial Fund Quarterly, 44*(3), 94–127.
Rosenstock, I. M. (1974). Historical origins of the health belief model. *Health Education Monographs, 2*, 328–335.
Rosenstock, I. M., Strecher, V. J., & Becker, M. H. (1988). Social Learning Theory and the Health Belief Model. *Health Education & Behavior, 15*(2), 175–183.
Strecher, V. J., & Rosenstock, I. M. (1997). The Health Belief Model. In A Baum, S. Newman, C. McManus, & K. Wallston (Eds.), *Cambridge handbook of psychology, health and medicine* (pp. 113–116). Cambridge: Cambridge University Press.
Suchman, E. (1965). Stages of illness and medical care. *Journal of Health and Human Behaviour, 6*, 114–128.
Tanner-Smith, E. E., & Brown, T. N. (2010). Evaluating the Health Belief Model: A critical review of studies predicting mammographic and pap screening. *Social Theory & Health, 8*, 95–125.
Weber, M. (1949). *The methodology of the social sciences* (translated and Edited by E. A. Shils & H. A. Finch). Glencoe: The Free.
Weber, M. (1978). *Economy and society: An outline of interpretive sociology*. Berkeley: University of California Press.
Young, J. T. (2004). Illness behaviour: A selective review and synthesis. *Sociology of Health & Illness, 26*(1), 1–31.

Chapter 8
The Interpretive Perspective in Medical Sociology: Part II

8.1 Introduction

As previously mentioned, the interpretive paradigm deals with microanalysis (see Sect. 7.2 for basic features of the interpretive paradigm). This chapter will further explain some of the interpretive substantive theories in medical sociology including social construction of illness, the chronic illness trajectory model, labelling theory, theory of social stigma, the total institution theory, and postmodernism. The general discussion focuses on the social conception of illness, the course of illness, reaction to illness and the sick, and the experience of patienthood. This focus forms the stronghold of the social understanding of human health.

8.2 The Social Construction of Illness

The social construction of illness focuses on how social forces or context shape human understanding of illness. The social constructionist polemics stem from interpretive paradigm in sociology (see basic views in Table 7.1). Particularly in medical sociology, the application of the perceptive has been traced to the works of Erving Goffman, Anselm Strauss, Eliot Freidson, Becker S. Howard, and Michel Foucault, among others. The perspective here stems from the traditional conception of social constructionist approach and not that of Brown (2008), which is a fusion of constructionism and structuralism. In sum, the perspective is based on microanalysis, subjectivity, idiographic approach, and voluntarism. The foundation of this microanalysis is the belief that realities are socially constructed. The meanings of any phenomena are not necessarily inherent to the phenomena themselves but develop through interaction in a particular social context (Conrad and Barker 2010). Patients often construct realities around the disease based on sociocultural milieu. As Singer (2004, p. 9) observed, this perspective is an alternative to the biomedical notion of disease "as a category in nature, a finite and objective reality discoverable through scientific endeavour..." It is also an alternative to the structuralist perspective of health. It focuses on the social origin of disease and how individuals construct certain responses to illness within a sociocultural context. The social construction of illness indicates that illness does not mean the same across cultures and that it depends on the perception of individuals. This perspective also unravels the nature of clinical interaction.

Kleinman et al. (2006) noted that the illness process begins with personal awareness of a change in the way the body feels and continues with the labelling of the sufferer by family or by self as "ill." This definition of being ill marks the beginning of the sick role process. It also marks the selection of a care provider and associated modalities channelled towards recovery. The starting point in the understanding of illness behaviour is to understand the perception of illness based on the social construction of illness or what could also be called lay perception or the explanatory model of illness. More often than not, the lay perception is different from the biomedical notion of disease (refer to the distinction between illness and disease in Chap. 2). In short, illness refers to the personal, interpersonal, and cultural manifestation or experience of disease or discomfort (Frankenberg 1980; Kleinman et al. 2006). The definition of illness requires personal and social interpretation and judgment. Such interpretation is based on cultural factors governing perception, labelling, explanation, and valuation of the discomforting experience (Fabrega 1972; Kleinman et al. 2006). The interpretation of illness also depends on many individual attributes such as knowledge, education, and class position. This is why illness is often experienced within a cultural milieu.

The construction of illness which forms the patient's explanatory model comprises five indices (Kleinman 1978; Kleinman et al. 2006). These indices include:

1. **Aetiology:** causal categories may include natural, supernatural, mystical, and genetic/hereditary causes. An individual may develop causal explanations that are "unthinkable" in biomedical terms. A supernatural explanation of disease is beyond scientific comprehension. It is a part of the cultural beliefs as it forms an important defining stance in the understanding of disease. This is similar to the first stage in the construction of disease, which Brown (1995) called *identification and diagnosis*. The beginning involves recognition of a medical problem through direct experience. According to Brown, there may be conflictual notions of the disease. AIDS was first associated with zoosexuality and homosexuality, and later with physical contact with infected persons and subsequently with the unsafe exchange of bodily fluid through various means, especially sexual intercourse. There may be a gradual shift in belief or lay conception as more facts are emerging.
2. **Onset of symptoms**: patients also experience illness through perceived symptoms. The cultural repertoire designates certain signs attributable to disease, from which disease could be categorised. If such symptoms are identified, then the individual can be categorised as ill. Most times, the extent to which a condition disrupts daily activities may indicate the signs and symptoms from a lay construction of illness. This is close to what Brown described as *experience of illness*. There may not be uniform experience from a particular disease. The experience of illness also shapes how the disease is defined and how rights and obligations are constructed. While obesity may be found in the medical classification as a disease, some obese people would actually be regarded as "big and beautiful."
3. **Pathophysiology**: experience of illness often manifests with the obstruction of normal roles in the society. In other words, illness may have disabling manifestations. Therefore, patients evaluate the extent of disturbances of bodily functions

caused by a disease. This shows the level of underlying and potential abnormalities or threats from the disease. The perceived threat is also socially defined. This is also part of the experience of illness. It should be noted that in social construction, the physical manifestation is not in itself a problem but the consequences of such manifestation. Such consequences may involve interpersonal crisis, alienation, and stigmatisation.
4. **Course of illness** : the construction of illness also involves determining of the duration of illness. This may involve consideration of the illness whether acute or chronic. The course of the illness may be defined by the visibility of the symptoms, or whether the symptoms can be concealed and managed. Previous experience of disease management would also give a clue about the prospect of the duration or course of the illness.
5. **Treatment**: treatment pattern is a form of response that is constructed, which may be based on some indicators. For instance, causal explanation may define which care provider (whether folk or modern medicinal practitioners) will be appropriate. Apart from which kind of treatment, the patients also decide when and where to seek treatment. In some instances, there may be procrastination in seeking treatment. This may be based on perceived threats and the course of illness. The professionals also *construct* what kind of treatment to give or whether to withhold or withdraw treatment. While some decisions are ethical, some may be based on biased social considerations such as race or SES. Brown (2008) noted that there are still a lot of politics involved in the allocation of medical resources.

There are two systems involved in the construction of the indices: the lay and professional systems (Freidson 1960). The professional system emanates from medical knowledge, dominant medical frameworks, education, and the socialisation of medical providers (Brown 1995). The lay or explanatory model develops mainly from cultural experiences and beliefs.

Kleinman (1980) defined the explanatory model as the notions about an episode of sickness and their treatment that are employed by all those engaged in the clinical process. There are often two major notions: the patient's and the physician's notions. In other words, an explanatory model reveals the meaning people attach to their illness and their experiences of it. The patient's model reveals how people view their illness in terms of how it happens, what causes it, how it affects them, and how it can be resolved. The major goal of most qualitative research is to understand the explanatory model of illness or disease held by individuals in the community by revealing the local understanding and knowledge of the health problem. There is often more focus on the patient's explanatory model because it is borne out of illness experience and cultural context.

The construction of illness unravels illness experience within the society—the trajectories that individuals go through—the suffering, pains and gains, consequences of illness on self, identity, autonomy, and the social imperatives and medical dispositions that shape such experiences. Relating to illness experience, there is a distinct model called the *biographical disruption model*. Bury (1982) conceived biographical disruption as the extent to which individual structures of everyday life are disorganised by illness—a form of disabling changes (both social and biological) as a result of illness (see also Reeve et al. 2010). Utilising this model involves the examination of varieties of social changes in one's personal life as a result of illness.

Furthermore, the focus is also on interpersonal interaction and other subjective forces that shape the evaluation of symptoms and treatment patterns. Brown (2008) noted that notwithstanding the scientific basis of the biomedical definition of disease and diagnosis, people based their conceptions on social-cultural indices. Illness experience depicts an insider's view, a kind of subjective experience (Conrad and Barker 2010). Apart from the personal experience of discomfort, there is the relational dimension. When people discriminate against other people living with a particular disease, it becomes part of the experience of the illness. A person living with a certain disease may find it difficult to socialise with others, engage in recreational activities, and adhere to certain diets. Activities that were previously conventional may become unconventional, and this accounts for a shrinking social world (Charmaz 1991). Moreover, the experience of a medical condition is mediated by its meaning both to the sufferer and the social network.

A study of asthmatic patients observed a transition phase which signified the need to integrate knowledge, experience, and self-awareness, which will lead to acceptance and self-control (Snadden and Brown 1992). As the patient progresses to accept and manage their condition, they experience diminishing fear of the disease and develop a sense of self-control or self-immunity. For some diseases, the initial reaction could be denial, an attempt to assume the condition is not real or the diagnosis could be wrong. With progression towards the experience of the symptoms of the condition, fear may arise; this could be fear of pain, incurability, financial burden, judgement of others, and other associated pressures. The social experience of illness is a critical part of what Timmermans and Haas (2008) described as the exploration of the dialectic between social life and disease, to examine how social life matters for morbidity and mortality and vice versa. It is in the same vein that Sontag (1978) noted that the negative subjective experience of disease condition (e.g., cancer) and the symbolic meaning of horror attached to it are detrimental to the patient and exact adverse effects on disease control. Such negative metaphors or myths of a disease kill faster than the disease itself (Sontag 1978) because it forces the patient to accept death as the last resort.

The response to illness or illness behaviour is also governed by cultural and normative beliefs. Choice of a care provider is made based on personal comprehension of the condition and other personal attributes such as income, education, and gender (Brown 1995). This explains why there are variations in illness behaviour across cultures. This is why local concepts of disease/illness are important in disease control. It is through the understanding of the local conception of illness that the physician can relate with the experience of the patient. Kleinman et al. (2006, p. 147) submitted that

> [e]liciting the patient model gives the physician knowledge of the beliefs the patient holds about his [/her] illness, the personal and social meaning he [/she] attaches to his [/her] disorder, his [/her] expectations about what will happen to him [or her] and what the doctor will do, and his [/her] own therapeutic goals. Comparison of patient model with the doctor's model enables the clinician to identify major discrepancies that may cause problems for clinical management.

Giving a voice to the patient and discussing the professional model will lead to a mutual understanding and possibly better treatment outcomes.

8.3 Chronic Illness Trajectory Theory

The meaning and characteristics of chronic illness have been discussed (see Sect. 2.6.2). Chronic illness is often incurable with a long lifespan, but manageable. The trajectory model is another constructionist substantive theory in medical sociology developed by Anselm L. Strauss, medical sociologist, and Juliet Corbin, a nurse theorist. The theory is sometimes referred to as the Corbin-Strauss trajectory model, and it was developed from qualitative studies of chronic illness (see Corbin and Strauss 1988). The trajectory presents a retrospective mapping of illness experiences, which now serves as an important framework to study those living with chronic illness.

The central concept of the framework is "trajectory," or a course of illness which accounts for the gradual development (in terms of phases) of the illness. The trajectory also accounts for the actions taken by the patients, significant others, and caregivers in managing the illness condition. In other words, the illness trajectory refers to the course of an illness, to all the related work, as well as the impact on both the workers and their relationships that further affect the management of the course of illness and the fate of the sick person (Corbin and Strauss 1985). Burton (2000) observed that the trajectory represents the cumulative effects of an illness, including the manifestation of symptoms and impacts of the illness on an individual's social world/roles. Sometimes, the illness might lead to a shifting of roles and activities, sometimes referred to as biographic disruption.

The pattern of health over time is called a health trajectory and, incidentally, chronic illness presents with a changing health status over a long period of time. Henly et al. (2011) noted that the understanding of the trajectories of chronic illness over time enable individuals to prepare for a changing health status and the (medical and personal) factors that could influence such changes. Consistently, the patients and family members struggle with the illness course vision which includes five dimensions: meaning of the illness, meaning of symptoms, meaning of disability, meaning for biography, and time (Cooley 1999).

In general, Fig. 8.1 shows the eight stages of the course of disease of the Corbin-Strauss model which have been identified in the literature (McCorkle and Pasacreta 2001):

1. **Initial or pre-trajectory phase:** The risk of a chronic illness can be embodied without the manifestation of symptoms. At this stage, the individual lives a normal life without any signs or symptoms. Additionally, at this point preventive activities are vital to delay the onset of the disease. Depending on the nature of the disease, in cases where the disease is controllable, the onset of symptoms could be delayed as much as possible through regular checkups and healthy behaviour.

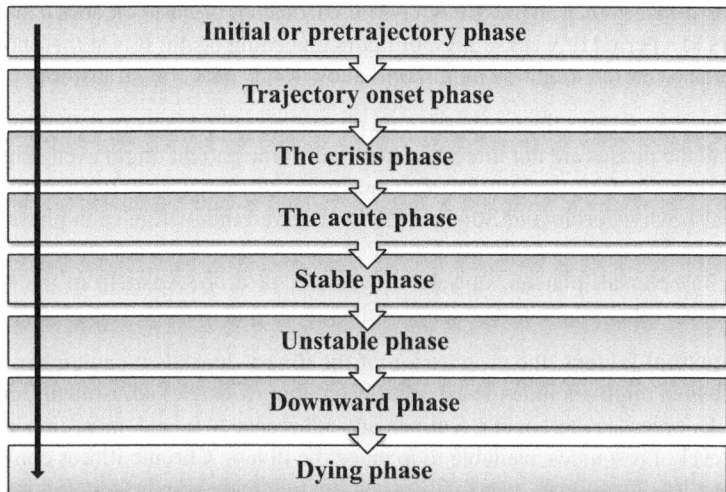

Fig. 8.1 Eight phases of the course of chronic illness

2. **Trajectory onset phase**: The actual illness experience begins upon the manifestation of symptoms and diagnostic confirmation of the disease. This could be mild if there have been some risk assessment and coordinated preventive activities. This also means that the disease is detected at an early stage. In most cases, this may involve a number of behavioural adjustments and forms of therapy.
3. **The crisis phase:** In most cases of chronic illness, there may be times of complications, and sometimes urgent attention might be needed to stabilise the patient. The complications could be life-threatening. At this stage, the patient is confronted (perhaps for the first time) with the sociomedical implications of the illness. This might serve as a strong cue to more behavioural adjustments, as well as the significance of therapies and drug adherence.
4. **The acute phase**: Following a complication or crisis, the patient may be stabilised and the symptoms may have subsided. This means that the symptoms can be controlled by a prescribed regimen or intervention.
5. **Stable phase:** The patient may stay for a long time without episodes of complication following appropriate management of symptoms (through therapeutic regimen). In this phase, the patient can live a normal life without transgressing medical recommendations. He/she would be conscious of risk factors that could trigger or aggravate the condition.
6. **Unstable phase:** This stage represents a cursor towards a more serious crisis. It is a situation in which a previous regimen fails to control the symptoms. This may necessitate a change in therapeutic measures for proper remediation of the health problem.
7. **Downward phase:** This phase is characterised by the progressive deterioration of a condition (in mental and physical status). The patient often presents with refractory symptoms that signal the imminent end of life.

8. **Dying phase:** When all measures have failed, death is the last outcome. This phase refers to a period of weeks, days, or hours preceding death. It is at this stage that terminal sedation might be required to allow for a "peaceful" transition.

While Fig. 8.1 presents the most elaborate phases, not all patients pass through all of them, and the phases are not directly sequential; some patient might even skip some phases. This is why the straight arrow on the figure indicates a very sloppy movement. This is also why Corbin and Strauss (1991) observed that within each phase exists fluctuations and periods of the illness called subphases, which are characterised as existing in reversal, plateau, upward movement, or drop. Apart from the phases, there are two other major components of the theory that must be considered.

1. **Contextual factors**: the progression of the illness depends on a number of factors which might include the extent of behaviour (lifestyle) adjustments, cultural beliefs, access to therapeutic regimen and adherence to it, and, more importantly, the level of resources available to manage the illness. Chronic illness could consume a lot of resources, especially when life treatment is indicated. For instance, constant dialysis might be too expensive for a poor household in which there is no functional health insurance system. Inadequate resources might speed up the progression towards the dying phase.
2. **Work related to chronic illness**: Corbin and Strauss (1985) identified three types of work—illness work, everyday life work, and biographical work— which interplay to produce consequences in terms of the illness outcomes. For instance, Corbin and Strauss recognised that families provide a great deal of caregiving for the chronically ill. While the sick person faces a number of challenges, he/she requires a lot of support (Conrad and Bury 1997). This is why Corbin and Strauss (1988) extensively described "unending work and care at home." They observed that the nature of chronic illness is social and that social context must proffer adequate aid and care for those with chronic illnesses (Conrad and Bury 1997). On the other hand, *illness-related work* "consists of regimen work, crisis prevention and management, symptom management, and diagnostic-related work" (Corbin and Strauss 1985, p. 226). *Everyday life work* refers to "the essentially daily round of tasks that keep the household going. It includes housekeeping and repairing, occupational work, marital work, child rearing, sentimental work and activities such as eating" (Corbin and Strauss 1985, p. 226). *Biographical work* refers to tasks that reflect one's self-identity. It could be the expression of professionalism or professional engagement. A writer who experiences a stroke that paralyses the hands will face a huge biographical challenge following the inability to write.

The essence of home care and cooperation among the spouses, children, and significant others are evident from the type of work involved in chronic illness (Corbin and Strauss 1984). For instance, living with muscular dystrophy or stroke might require support like food preparation, bathing, and bedding. Importantly, the level of support/work required depends on the phases of the illness whether in the crisis, stable, downward, or dying phase. These works must, however, be supported with professional input. The illness trajectory, patient's responsibilities, work required, and professional input are influenced by contextual factors, especially the socioeconomic characteristics of the patients and the household.

8.4 Social Reaction Theories of Illness

The two social reaction theories that will be discussed here, namely labelling theory and the theory of social stigma, are derived from the social constructionist perspective. These two theories have different intellectual trends and domains but are closely linked.

8.4.1 Labelling Theory

It is important to single out labelling theory as a distinct perspective from the social construction of illness. More importantly, labelling theory has some definite theoretical precepts and peculiar development. The theory has wide applications but has been specifically applied in illness definition and behaviour. The approach is unique because it is a social reaction perspective; it focuses on how people perceive, define, and react to illness condition. While Howard S. Becker is labelled as the founder of the labelling theory, the idea can generally be found in the works of previous interactionists such as Charles Cooley (1902), Herbert Mead (1934), Frank Tannenbaum (1938), and Edwin Lemert (1951). Mead is regarded as a classical proponent of symbolic interactionism who argued that interaction, the essence of life, is facilitated through symbols, meanings, and interpretation. In essence, actors subjectively create social realities. Tannenbaum (1938) introduced the idea of "tagging" behaviour among delinquent youth. His theoretical model is often referred to as the "dramatisation of evil," which denotes that individuals live according to a social tag attributed to them. Lemert (1951) was perhaps the first to describe social condemnation and how it could lead to a "career status" (what he described as secondary deviance).

Becker (1963) introduced the concept of labelling—and provided an explanation of labelling, attribution, and "acceptance" of status—and laid the foundation of a theoretical movement called labelling theory. What then are labels? Labels are constructed as working definitions of a condition within a sociocultural context. Theoretically, a label is not the same as stigma, although it is a part of the process that could produce stigma. A disease might be labelled as mild or serious; it might not elicit a negative reaction. A condition might be labelled as inevitable and normal. Nausea during pregnancy is generally labelled as normal and societies sometimes help pregnant women with supportive measures. More so, through the medicalisation of a problem, condition or behaviour is given a clinical name (label) in the process of scientific legitimation. In sum, labelling simply refers to the construction of social or technical understanding and designation of a condition.

Becker's arguments are first applied in the study of deviant behaviour. The central argument is that society creates labels and applies them in the definition of any pathology or condition. It is argued further that the label is not the quality of the act/behaviour but the subjective attribution of the audience. A similar act/behaviour may be defined differently by another audience or in another context. Becker (1963, p. 9) observed that

8.4 Social Reaction Theories of Illness

[s]ocial groups create deviance by making rules whose infraction constitutes deviance, and by applying those rules to particular people and labeling them as outsiders. From this point of view, deviance is *not* a quality of the act the person commits, but rather a consequence of the application by others of rules and sanctions to an "offender." The deviant is one to whom that label has been successfully applied; deviant behaviour is behaviour that people so label.

By creating social prohibitions and prescriptions, society delineates normality and abnormality. This delineation is therefore consequential for group interaction by generating social constraints whose infraction are labelled or disapproved. Society could also generate opportunities that are positively labelled or approved. The idea of labelling shows how a range of social forces moulds human behaviour that attempts to ensure compliance with societal goals and values (Winter 1996). The definition of an act or behaviour is not universal; it is highly relative across societies and groups. The contestation of behavioural labelling is a major source of conflict. Winter (1996) further noted that abnormalities or social problems in general are hard to explain as aberrations of individual behaviour because of the influence of social determinants; however, there are other critical issues in labelling theory.

Power relations involved in labelling facilitate the imposition of the definition of a condition. This indicates that the vulnerable are often at the receiving end. Generally, abnormal behaviour is a consequence of the responses of others to a person's behaviour. It is the reaction that shows how the behaviour is categorised. A similar behaviour may attract different reactions and categorisation. Here are other notable variations that may occur:

1. **Time:** there is variation over time; the definitions or labels are not static. They could change over a period of time. A condition previously considered as deviant or destructive may be relabelled.
2. **The actor/labelled:** labelling through the subjective definition rather than the object of the definition. The definition varies from person to person. The individual's characteristics affect how others react to the condition.
3. **The labellers:** labelling relates to how people define situations, persons, processes, or events as deviant or abnormal and examines the values, interests, and positions of those who define deviance. A professional may define a condition based on professional interest, while policy implementers will consider the allocation of resources.
4. **Outcome:** even when the action is similar, there may be variation in the labelling and consequences of the label. Some labels may have implications for social participation and self-concept.

The foregoing discussion provides a general explanation of labelling theory. Figure 8.1 shows a typical labelling framework. The characteristics of the individual, social networks, disease, and structural context play important roles in the definition of a condition and application of the label. The disease characteristics mediated by the form of social, behavioural, and physical manifestations as well as sociomedical consequences create subjective attributions which lead to the formulation of a definition and application of a label. Sociomedical consequences especially relate to the control of the disease (e.g., whether curable or not) and the extent of biographic disruption. While labelling theory has been applied to examine a number of medical conditions, it has gained a keen relevance in sociology of mental health. The following discussion will explain the relevance of labelling theory in mental illness.

In the application of labelling theory to mental illness, Thomas Scheff is a leading proponent with his publication *Being Mentally Ill: A Labelling Theory*. Actions that are often labelled are typically those that do not fit socially constructed norms. Such behaviours constitute social deviance in the society. Scheff (1966) argued that society generates mental illness by labelling social deviance as such. In other words, those behaviours that are not within societal norms are often regarded as indicators of mental illness. Those who are regarded as mentally derailed are subjectively defined as such, and all their behaviours are considered abnormal. The label situates them as defined, and over time they tend to fulfil the expectation of the label by exhibiting abnormal behaviours.

Scheff (2010) argued that labelling theory is a social model of mental illness that illustrate that the symptoms of mental illness are recast as violations of social norms. In line with Scheff's arguments, Kroska and Harkness (2008) observed that when an individual is diagnosed with a mental illness, cultural ideas associated with the mentally ill become personally relevant. The societal expectations (from the mentally ill) become a lens through which a patient's behaviour is evaluated. People are being labelled; they are seen as being mentally ill instead of having a mental illness (Pasman 2011). Therefore, according to labelling theory, the label of being mentally ill actually causes one to be mentally ill as a result of effects described as the Thomas theorem. The theorem (which is also in line with the notion of a self-fulfilling prophecy) stipulates that situations that men describe as real will be real in their consequences (Thomas and Thomas 1928). This means that perception and interpretation of a situation tend to fulfil the expectations.

Scheff (1974) noted that the social characteristics of patients help to determine the severity of the societal reaction irrespective of psychiatric condition. In most situations, the label outweighs self-concept and reduces self-esteem (Scheff 1966); however, a modified labelling theory of mental illness has been proposed (see Link et al. 1989). The modified version tries to underplay the causal indices in the theory by looking more at the consequences of the label. The modified version tends towards stigmatisation by indicating that the label often results in self-stigma. Whichever form, a labelling theory should be more concerned with the social negotiation of illness which produces lay understanding and a working definition of a condition.

The attempt at the modified version was a result of alternative explanation or criticism of Scheff (1966), especially by Gove (1970a, b, 1975). Gove (1970a, 1975) identified some theoretical faults in labelling theory. He claimed that Scheff simply reified the labels as if they actually cause mental illness without considering the psychiatric perspective which focuses more on actual (biomedical) diagnosis. Gove observed that Scheff neglected to take into account the influence of psychopathological variables in mental illness. To him, labelling theory should be integrated into the psychiatric perspective as an adjunctive theory which highlights potential problems in psychiatric practice. Therefore, the objective theoretical thinking should be at the mid-point between Scheff and Gove. This signifies a fusion of social and biomedical models. It upholds Gove's argument that labelling is not the full cause of mental illness but significantly contributes to the definition of mental illness. The fact still remains that most manifestations of mental illness have behavioural dimensions which usually create social reaction.

Labelling also has some positive aspects. Labelling suggests the adoption of the sick role, especially excusable behaviour and exemption from normal duties. It suggests the possibility of a discrepancy between an acceptable standard of behaviour and abnormality. This may stimulate the labelled to seek treatment. It helps the patient to seek competent help in order to normalise behaviour. Labelling is also a form of lay diagnosis. It creates awareness and understanding of illness condition. Unfortunately, the consequences of a negative label could be harmful. It leads to low self-esteem, impaired self-efficacy, and self-stigma. This is a situation in which labelling leads to stigmatisation. The next section presents the theory of social stigma.

8.4.2 Theory of Social Stigma

The theory of social stigma is a landmark contribution of medical sociology to the understanding of human health. It is one of the social reaction theories which has considerable practical applications in health, health care, and health policy. Erving Goffman (1922–1982) is the father of stigma theory as a result of his 1963 publication, *Stigma: Notes on the Management of Spoiled Identity*. Since then, the theory of social stigma has been a major theoretical stance in medical sociology and health care in general. While Goffman's classical ideas will form the starting point and background of the discussion, ideas from some recent contributors (especially Falk 2001; Jones et al. 1984; Link and Phelan 2001) will provide an appropriate intellectual blend of the theory of social stigma. Stigma (plural: stigmata) is a Greek word which means a sign, mark, tattoo, or label placed on criminals and other morally degrading persons as a blemish in order to identify them (see Goffman 1963; Falk 2001; Jones et al. 1984; Link and Phelan 2001). The first account of stigma as a symbolic mark on humans is documented in the Bible (later in the Quran) as the mark of Cain; the mark has its origin in the criminal act (murder of his brother, Abel) committed by Cain. Since then, various degrading stigmata have been used in human history.

Social stigma is a mark or attribution of shame, disgrace, or social devaluation. Goffman (1963) defined social stigma as a gap between virtual social identity and actual social identity; the gap shows a discrediting effect. A virtual social identity is one created by people through subjective evaluation of other people; it acts as an interaction interface that has the tendency to predominate the actual social identity. Stigma exists when there is a negative gap between the virtual identity and actual identity. Impliedly, stigma emanates from social interaction; this is why Goffman called it a language of relationship and not an attribute. It is a socially discrediting status ascribed to an individual that is indicative of a social difference from others. Simply, according to Goffman, stigmatisation is a process by which the reaction of others spoils a normal identity.

Goffman (1963) argued that there are three types of stigma. First, there are abominations of the body (i.e., various physical deformities). Physical characteristics could form a source of social degradation. Campbell and Deacon (2006) referred to these bodily abominations as overt or external deformities that are often visible, such as scars or physical manifestations of some medical conditions such as leprosy, obesity, dystrophy, dwarfism, and autism. Blemishes of individual character or deviations in personal traits constitute the second type. These are traits which are unusual, unnatural, or asocial. These forms of deviation present a discrepancy from the normative and collective norms of the society. Examples include treacherous and rigid beliefs, dishonesty, mental disorders, imprisonment, addiction, alcoholism, unemployment, suicide attempts, and radical political and religious behaviours. Falk (2001) described this deviation of personal traits as achieved stigma—where the role or behaviour of an individual is the source of stigma. The last type is tribal stigma of race, nation, class, and religion. Goffman noted that these types of stigma can be transmitted through lineages and can equally contaminate all members of a family. Falk (2001) described this as existential, a kind of stigma that is a result of ascription or natural attributes. The stigmatised have no control over the attributes. In this case, caste and class systems, especially where the social gap is wide, are accompanied with stigma. Atrocities committed by some members of a group may put others at the risk of stigma. For example, a long-bearded Muslim cleric may be branded as a fanatic and thus as a possible terrorist suspect, especially in the United States after the September 11th attack.

Goffman stopped at three types, but normative stigma should be the fourth category. Normative stigma is a discredited status based on the norms and values of society. The stigmatisation of women in a patriarchal society could fall into this category. Unmarried aged adults, infertile couples, widows, or a woman or family without a male child in most African and Asian communities can experience a form of normative stigma. It is neither existential nor achieved; it is generated based on the norms and values of the society.

Goffman (1963) included homosexuality as a personal trait that is stigmatised. During that time, homosexuality was not tolerated and was considered a medical abnormality and even a criminal act. While it has been normalised in many western nations, it is still a contested or stigmatised trait in many African societies. The implication is that stigma is a relative attribution. It varies by period, place, and person. There may be successions of alteration in attributes that are stigmatised over a period of time. Goffman (1963) observed that "an attribute that stigmatises one type of possessor can confirm the usualness of another, and therefore is neither creditable nor discreditable as a thing in itself." This also signifies that stigma is a social creation, not the attribute of the "mark" itself. A dwarf who belongs to the upper class may enjoy adequate social tolerance unlike one in the lower class.

Goffman discussed three categories of individuals in relation to stigma. The first are the stigmatised, or those who bear the stigma or label that is discreditable or discredited. They live with the burden of the stigma in everyday life. For them, the experience of stigma is a reality that creates a "battle" between them and others in the society. Most times, it limits their social participation and forces them to explore life opportunities only at the margins of the society. Stigma can be dehumanising and depersonalising. Second, the "normal" constitute the majority who do not bear any stigma. Most times they are those who place stigma on others by imposing discredited status on others. The last category is the wise, those who are tolerable of the stigmatised, those who hold unconditional love for the discredited persons. The wise are often empathetic and sympathetic; hence, they are highly tolerable of the stigmatised and do not allow the stigma to mediate social interaction.

One major criticism of this theory is the vagueness of the concept of stigma. Link and Phelan (2001) noted the criticism and conceptualised stigma with the use of four specific components. They observed that the conceptualisation proposed a fuller and more operational meaning of stigma. Stigma exists when the following four interrelated components converge. According to Link and Phelan (2001, p. 367), these include "elements of labelling, stereotyping, separation, status loss and discrimination [that] co-occur in a power situation that allows the components of stigma to unfold." The four components will be briefly explained later on.

8.4.2.1 Labelling Differences

Social differences are part of the realities of the social world. It only becomes a basis for discrimination when some differences are valued or reified and others are not. The value attached to social differences emanates through social construction and is relative across cultures. Link and Phelan (2001) concurred that there is a social selection of human differences when it comes to identifying differences that will matter socially. A label is like a tag that is affixed, beckoning to be seen or recognised, like the band with the captain in a football match. For stigma to exist there must be labels, such as addict, blind, gay, handicap, drunkard, and the like. Philips and Gates (2011) observed that labels become meaningful through language and in the context of human relations. Therefore, some labels are innately consequential for the possessors.

8.4.2.2 Differences Associated with Negative Attributes

Labels do not automatically lead to stigma unless they are associated with negative attributes. This component occurs when labelled differences are linked to stereotypes. Within a particular context, labelled differences are linked with undesirable attributes. Drinking alcohol in and of itself might not be a negative act, but among the groups that forbid such act it can generate a label (drunkard) and induce a negative attribute. Additionally, a label of "mentally ill" may link a person to a stereotype of being dangerous, unfit, unstable, unreliable, incompetent, and so forth. The visibility of a potential discreditable attribute contributes to stigmatisation. For instance, HIV status has the potential to be stigmatised if it is known within a social network. If a person is able to conceal such a status, he/she may be saved from stigmatisation. This is why most people with a "discreditable" attribute such as a HIV-positive status hide it. Philips and Gates (2011) also observed that negative attitudes about labelled differences are also influenced by the degree to which they are believed to pose a danger or threat to a particular group. If an individual living with mental illness is perceived to be dangerous, he/she may experience social distance, the same way many people will keep away from PLWHA because of the misunderstanding that it could be contagious through mere interaction. The perception that an illness may be the victim's fault (or responsibility) can also lead to stigmatisation. Stigmatisation occurs by apportioning blame to the individuals with labelled differences. The incorrect notion that only people who are sexually reckless or promiscuous contract HIV plays a role in the stigmatisation of PLWHA. This is a form of moral judgment (by apportioning blame), which has adverse effects on labelled differences.

8.4.2.3 Separation of "Us" from "Them"

The third component involves social separation of the normal and the stigmatised. This means the "outsiders" are separated from the "insiders." The labelled differences with negative attributes provide a "rationale for believing that negatively labelled persons are fundamentally different from those who do not share the label" (Link and Phelan 2001, p. 370). The labelled are perceived as a different kind of people that are below normal social or human standards. Such people could be called different names such as moron, imbecile, criminal, HIV patient, pauper, beggar, ex-convict, street children, and so forth (see Rose et al. 2007 for labels used for the mentally ill). The emphasis of the label is on the perceived difference and a clear demarcation of social boundaries. The social web is the domain of the expression of stigma. For instance, a child may be chastised for mingling with the stigmatised.

8.4.2.4 Status Loss and Discrimination

The negative attributions then lead to experience of status loss or devaluation. Link and Phelan (2001) observed that this fourth component is very central and fundamental. It is the aspect that often generates concern. Status loss means dehumanisation or depersonalisation. Stigmatised groups are usually disadvantaged because they have fewer opportunities in various aspects of life, including education, housing, employment, and medical treatment. Link and Phelan observed that the immediate consequence of stigma is a general downward placement of a person in a status hierarchy. This is part of what Harold Garfinkel (1956) described as moral indignation, which portrays shame and guilt. This leads to a number of adverse exposures such as violence, like lesbians facing "corrective" rape in South Africa. At the extreme end, some of them could be maimed and murdered similar to what happens to the persons with albinism in Tanzania and Burundi (Cruz-Inigo et al. 2011) and people with kyphosis (hunchback) in southern Nigeria. The people with albinism and kyphosis are believed to be spirits who can be murdered and used for various forms of rituals. In addition, the Yoruba of southwestern Nigeria and the Benin Republic have a proverb, *inu igbo ni adete gbe*, meaning that a person with leprosy should live in the forest, not among the people. Among the Hausas of northern Nigeria and the Niger Republic, people are often called by the kind of disability they suffer, like *makaho* (blind person), *musaki* (disabled person), and *kurma* (deaf person). Such name-calling adversely affects their status in the society.

Link and Phelan (2001) noted that power relations mediate the four components of stigma. It takes power to stigmatise. Social, political, and economic powers play defining roles in the social production of stigma. The power of the majority has a powerful voice in how a situation is defined. Such a voice is portrayed or convened through ideological apparatuses including the media. Gradually, a negative attribution becomes dominant and the stigmatised find themselves in the lower stratum of the society. This could lead to a struggle to challenge both the basis of their stigmatisation and the attendant consequences.

Another major landmark contribution to the theory of stigma was by Jones et al. (1984) who described six major dimensions of stigma, which include concealability, course, disruptiveness, aesthetics, origin, and peril.

1. **Concealability:** this implies how obvious, visible, or detectable a characteristic is to others. A stigma or character of a disease that could be stigmatised can be concealed while others cannot. For example, HIV status can be concealed while disability or severe burns cannot.
2. **Course:** a stigma or discreditable character of a disease could be temporary while others are permanent. The course of the stigma implies whether the labelled difference is lifelong or ephemeral. An irreversible stigmatised difference may lead to perpetual stigma stress. For instance, most labelled attributes emanating from chronic disease are irreversible.
3. **Disruptiveness:** this can be examined in two ways: how the stigma leads to biographical disruption and how it interferes with interpersonal relationships. Biographical disruption refers to interference with everyday life of the stigmatised. For instance, deafness (where stigmatised) limits the level of interpersonal involvement with divergent social networks.
4. **Aesthetics:** this refers to the content of the stigma, whether the labelled difference elicits a reaction of disgust, revulsion, or is perceived as unattractive or unsightly.
5. **Origin:** this has to do with causes of the difference, particularly whether the individual is perceived as responsible for the labelled difference. A labelled difference as a result of self-inflicted harm or indiscriminate behaviour is often more stigmatised than a natural occurrence.
6. **Peril:** the perceived threats to others from a labelled difference. A condition which is believed to be contagious may lead to social distance and grievous discrimination. Additionally, a labelled attribute that signifies dangerousness or volatility could be highly stigmatised.

Furthermore, Goffman's theory concludes that stigmatisation leads to a spoiled identity. The management of such an identity is a burden on the stigmatised. The theory can be applied to study societal reactions to a number of medical conditions, including deafness, albinism, disability, obesity, leprosy, HIV/AIDS, diabetes, severe

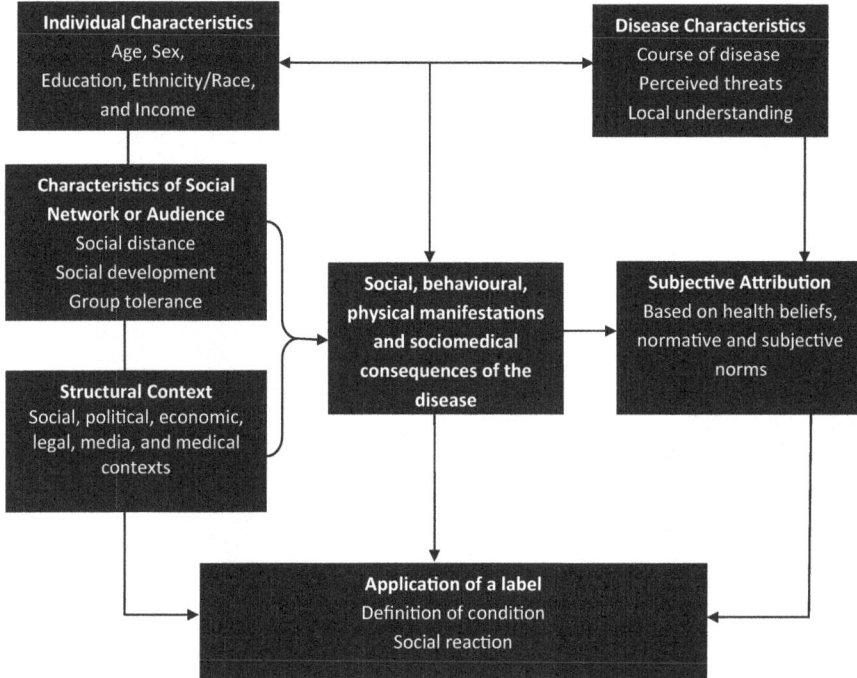

Fig. 8.2 Labelling framework

burns, mental illness, and countless others. The focus is often on the nature of the societal reaction and its consequences for health care and the individual living with the condition. Figure 8.2 presents a simple framework for the analysis of stigma related to health conditions. The figure was developed with some variables from an elaborate framework advanced by Pescosolido et al. (2008).

The first major consideration in stigmatisation is the characteristic of the disease or medical condition. The attributes of the disease and local understanding affects the formation of a response. Some diseases (e.g., mental illness) affect social relationships and could be difficult to conceal. Responses (including behavioural disposition, attitude, and cognitive reactions) are formed based on such disease characteristics. Stigmatisation is consequential for the stigmatised through experience of both internal and external stigma. External stigma could be measured by a number of indicators including avoidance, rejection, moral judgment, unwillingness to invest in the stigmatised, discrimination, and abuse. Internal stigma, on the other hand, could be measured by self-exclusion from services and opportunities, perception of self, social withdrawal, and fear of disclosure (Fig. 8.3).

It takes an enabling environment for stigmatisation to exist and be reinforced. The existence and persistence are influenced by structural context (the sociopolitical, economic, legal, media, and health care environments). The experience of stigma has adverse consequences for population health and health care. Stigmatisation has a negative impact on disease control efforts. It leads to denial, low level of social support, and impaired self-efficacy. For instance, stigma continues to be the most

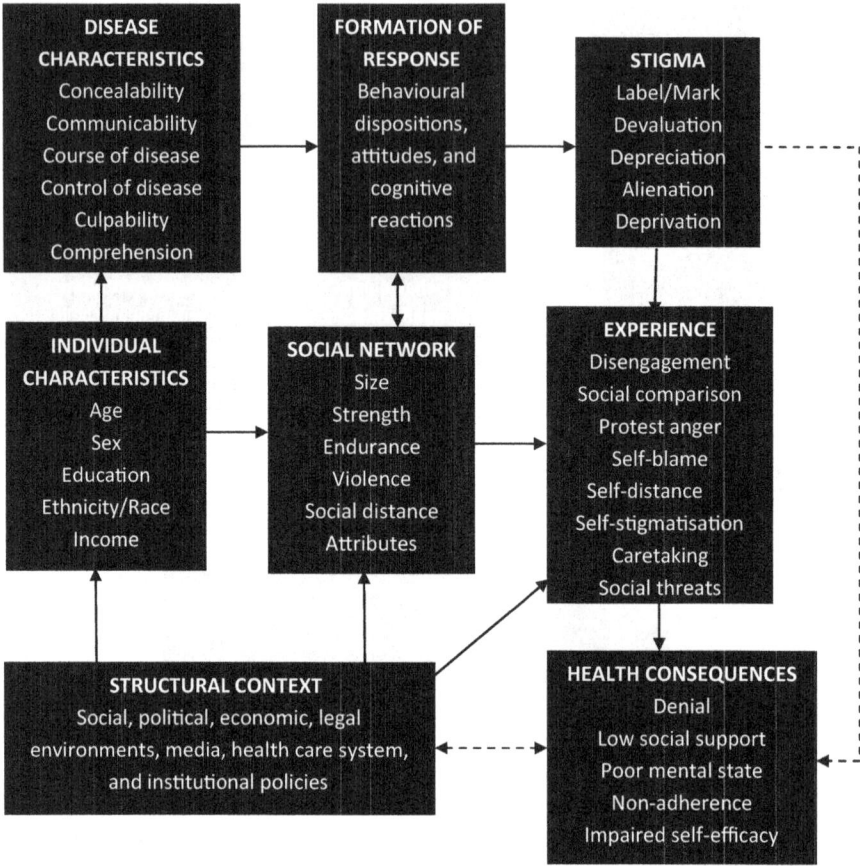

Fig. 8.3 Stigma and health. (Source: Adapted from Pescosolido et al. (2008))

detrimental challenge for PLWHA (see Herek 1999; Monger 2011). The PLWHA may isolate themselves from the community, be denied access to essential health care services, be rejected by significant others, and be unfairly treated in the workplace and in the society in general (Parameswari and Jayapoorani 2012).

The stigma theory will continue to be a major perspective in examining societal reactions to illness. Goffman conceived this long ago, and many researchers have continued to examine stigma in numerous human-related conditions. But stigma theory is not the only contribution of Goffman; the next section will examine his theory of total institution.

8.4.3 The Total Institution Theory

Whether the notion of "total institution" is viewed as a theory or critical perspective, the fact remains that it has a tremendous effect on the organisation of health service delivery the world over. It represents one of Goffman's significant intellectual contributions and a landmark input from medical sociology to health care (especially mental health). In 1961 Erving Goffman published *Asylums : Essays on the Social Situation of Mental Patients and Other Inmates* to explain the handling of patients, or the experience of patienthood in a mental health facility. The publication has been regarded as one of the top three books that revolutionised the organisation and delivery of health care, along with two others by Florence Nightingale: *Notes on Hospital* and *Notes on Nursing* (Black and Neuhauser 2006). This intellectual work observed the detrimental consequences of institutionalising people and fuelled a debate that led to radical changes in policy as to how services for those with mental illnesses and learning difficulties should be organised (Black and Neuhauser 2006).

Asylum is a work that facilitated the development of contemporary, community-orientated mental health practices or the process of deinstitutionalisation (Adlam et al. 2012; Suibhne 2011). Goffman's polemics favour the humanisation of a dehumanised group of people. The previously dominant practice in psychiatry was considered by critics to be close to brutality, horror, hell, misery, or terror. The mental hospital is a place of confinement, depersonalisation, and desocialisation. The *total institution* is a product of a three-year qualitative study, with the use of participant observation, of inmates in St. Elizabeth's Hospital in Washington, DC, to unravel the meaning of hospitalisation for mental patients. It is a sociological examination of the social situation of mental patients, the hospital, and life as subjectively experienced by the patients (Weinstein 1982). *Asylums* generally pictured the hospital as an "authoritarian system that forces patients to define themselves as mentally ill, change their thinking and behaviour, suffer humiliations, accept restrictions, and adjust to institutional life" (Weinstein 1982, p. 268).

Goffman, using the total institution model, placed mental hospitals in the same category as prisons, concentration camps, monasteries, orphanages, and military organisations. "A total institution is defined as a place of residence or work where a large number of like-situated individuals, cut off from the wider society for an appreciable period of time, together lead an enclosed, formally administered round of life" (Goffman 1961, p. xiii). In other words, a total institution is any place of confinement with regimented life under bureaucratic control. In this sense, life or daily activities are organised with little or no control by the participants. Goffman (1961, p. 4–5) identified a number of categories of total institutions, including:

1. Institutions established to care for people felt to be both harmless and incapable: homes for the aged, persons living with disability, orphans, and the poor or homeless.
2. Places established to care for people felt to be incapable of looking after themselves and a threat to the community, albeit an unintended one: TB sanatoriums, Leprosariums, and mental health hospitals.
3. Institutions organised to protect the community against what are felt to be intentional dangers to it, with the welfare of the people thus sequestered not the immediate issue: prisons, delinquent homes, concentration camps, prisoners of war (POW) camps, and penitentiaries.

8.4 Social Reaction Theories of Illness 173

4. Institutions established to congregate people who engage in work-like tasks for the instrumental facilitation of such activities: work camps, boarding schools, military barracks, and servants' quarters.
5. Establishments designed as retreats from the world, even while often serving also as training stations for the religious: convents, mission houses, abbeys, monasteries, and other cloisters.

Of particular interest here are those institutions established to cater for those with various medical conditions. Goffman's focus was on mental hospitals; the study leading to the publication was conducted in a mental health hospital. Other categories of persons with medical conditions who could be confined (for care) include persons living with disability (e.g., blindness, deafness, autism, Down syndrome, VVF). Goffman noted that the character of the confinement for the purpose of care has subjected them to a regimented condition which may be dehumanising.

Goffman identified major life activities—sleep, play, eat, and work—as basic social arrangements or necessities in modern society with which individuals are involved with numerous and divergent co-participants. Such involvements are sometimes unpredictable without an overall rational plan. The nature of total institution confines these four life activities within a limited circle of participants and place coupled with a rationalised plan.

Goffman (1961) identified basic characteristics of total institutions, stressing that every total institution might not necessarily have all the characteristics. First, all aspects of life are conducted under one roof and authority. A total institution is an establishment with definite structure or housing. Persons are formally accommodated based on certain criteria; everyone is under the authority of the establishment. Second, patterned activities are carried out with like-situated others with similar treatment. Daily activities are often specified for all members and are carried out with other persons with similar characteristics (e.g., a mental health facility is differentiated from a home for the blind). Third, activities are tightly scheduled and prearranged. Daily activities are structured using a daily time-table, with one activity leading to another at a prearranged time. Fourth, formal rules and officials guide daily life of the inmates. The organisation of daily activities is not a matter of choice but is imposed by the authority and implemented by officials. Fifth, activities are bureaucratically structured to fulfil an organisational goal: every total institution has a goal; for instance, a total institution may be organised to rehabilitate inmates. Sixth, restriction from wider social contacts is enforced. Social distance is prescribed in a total institution. This is a major defining characteristic of the institution; it controls the movement of individuals and tightly regulates contact with the wider society. There is even limited contact with the staff of the institution; the members of the staff are positioned to administer organisation materials and ensure strict compliance with the organisational rules.

In a total institution, daily needs are met as deemed necessary by the authorities. The inmates have little to no control over what material is provided. Some materials are intentionally banned and cannot be used. The inmate has no control over the decision of his/her fate (Goffman 1961, p. 9). All daily decisions are "dropped down" and compliance is required. In the case of movement, destination, travel distance, and time may not be disclosed. The diagnosis or treatment might not be disclosed. An attempt to withdraw from daily activities or prescriptions is a major infraction. When inmates work, they do not receive any benefits for their labour.

Goffman (1961) stressed on the major consequence of livelihood in a total institution, which is *mortification of self*. Admission into a social institution signifies a new life experience of abasement, humiliations, and profanations of the self. At the beginning of mortification of self, individuals are stripped of contact with the outside world. Specifically, Branaman (1997, p. liv–lv) reduced Goffman's process of mortification of self in a total institution to seven major aspects: role dispossession; programming and identity trimming; dispossession of property, name, and identity kit; imposition of degrading postures, stances, and deference patterns; contaminative exposure; disruption of usual relations of an individual actor and his/her acts; and restrictions on self-determination, autonomy, and freedom of action; and, in addition, the use of violence. Therefore, eight aspects of mortification of self will be examined:

1. **Role dispossession**: in a normal life, an individual has the opportunity to plan daily activities. There is a general choice in schedules and variety of contacts. There are no strict rules governing the sequence of roles. Branaman (1997, p. liv) observed that in a total institution, "membership disturbs role-planning because the separation of the inmate from the wider world can continue indefinitely." In essence, individuals are permanently withdrawn from conventional activities and have to live within the four walls of the institution. Goffman noted that an individual is automatically stripped of activities in the home world. This is a radical personal change in the life of an individual.
2. **Programming and identity trimming:** In Goffman's words, when processing inmates' admission, staff employ what are called admission procedures, such as the recording of life history, photographing, weighing, fingerprinting, assigning numbers, undressing, disinfecting, haircutting, issuing institutional clothing/uniform, giving specific instructions, and assigning to living quarters (Goffman 1961, p. 16). This is called identity trimming or programming, which allows the inmate to be coded into an official record. The trimming often changes previous bases of self-identification and imposes a new form of identification.
3. **Dispossession of property, name, and "identity kit":** inmates are stripped of their possessions and some are replaced with official provisions. The new possessions indicate institutional identification. Status material such as a wristwatch, comb, shaving set, cosmetics, and other beautification materials are dispossessed from the inmates. In most cases, the institutional number or medical case (e.g., patient with syphilis) predominates normal identity. Branaman (1997) observed that the absence of an individual's previous status or "identity kit" accounts for the loss of capacity to present one's usual image to others. All of the inmates look alike with a similar uniform, a number, or badge with other similar conditions. Goffman (1961) also refers to this as personal defacement.
4. **Imposition of degrading postures, stances, and deference patterns:** an individual may be forced to engage in activities in which symbolic implications

mortify the self. For example, hair may be shaved, individuals forced to change dress, to stand upright to take a photograph, and the likes. An inmate may be subjected to performing menial tasks or *disidentifying* roles, like a servant. The inmate is required to beg for cigarettes or for permission to use the telephone and to submit to staff expectations of verbal deference. Communication with significant others (where and when allowed) may be monitored and limited.
5. **Contaminative exposure:** inmates are open to undue exposures that are mostly detrimental to the notion of self. The companionship and interpersonal relationships of inmates are imposed. The blind mingle with other blind; so also the criminal with other criminals, or those that are more criminal; and persons with autism are grouped together. More so, the preservation of personal information is violated. Staff and occasional guests (including so-called charity-givers or religious preachers) may be provided with certain information about the inmates and permitted to move around. Branaman (1997) noted that the total institution offers no private spaces to conceal usual private activities; the person is compelled to expose himself/herself in humiliating circumstances. Within a total institution, the territories and embodiments of self are violated with impunity.
6. **Disruption of usual relations of an individual actor and his acts**: Goffman regarded the first aspect of disruption as *looping*, described as a lack of a self-protective expressive response to humiliating situations. Any form of response to assault on the self will be looped as the basis of the next assault or punishment in order to prevent further occurrence of defence. An inmate's margin of behaviour is used as evidence to justify further retention in a psychiatric facility. It is a deliberate act of *tyrannisation* or repression, forcing inmates into an internal world of their own. Another aspect is regimentation; inmates are expected to perform regulated activities in unison with blocks of fellow inmates. Any member of staff has the right to discipline any inmate and ensure compliance with laid procedures.
7. **Restrictions on self-determination, autonomy, and freedom of action**: particularly in a mental health facility, patients are treated as incompetent. Automatically, an incompetent person is devoid of autonomy. The inmate's "competent" wish is not regarded as one; it is subject to examination and the decision of officials prevails in every circumstance. Imposition of medication is thus a common occurrence. The denial of the right to self-determination, Goffman observed, produces a terrifying feeling. In a total institution, there is no freedom of choice or action as the inmates have a duty to surrender to the constitutive authority and, most importantly, to surrender his/her self and body. The inmate's body provides a means through which a number of "corrective or therapeutic" interventions are carried out.
8. **Use of violence**: probably one of the central points that Goffman made, while not precisely accorded a point of its own, is the use of violence on inmates. At the extreme end, as is the case in concentration camps, a deviant inmate may be killed. In the case of a mental home, inmates may be physically restrained, perceived as dangerous and a threat to others. An inmate may be repeatedly doped, sanctioned, and restricted from moving beyond certain circles. Apart from physical violence, the process of mortification of self or disfiguration itself is a form of violence.

That an individual is forced to shave or to wear a particular uniform constitutes psychological trauma. Admission in a total institution is a total declaration of violence on the self of any inmate.

Goffman (1961) described the career of a mental patient. Career, in this context, is meant to refer to any social strand of a person's course of life. He submitted that the career of the mentally ill is two-sided: first are internal matters such as image of self and felt identity and, second, on the other side includes official position and style of life. The idea of moral career is to examine the changes in the course of patienthood, the process of hospitalisation, which meddles with the social fate of the individual. The career of the mental health patient is then divided into three phases: pre-patient phase, the period prior to entry into the hospital; in-patient phase, the period in the hospital; and ex-patient phase, the period after recovery or rehabilitation.

In sum, the theoretical precepts of total institution have a wide range of applications. It can be applied to any institution (both medical and non-medical) with *totalistic* features or to examine how *totalistic* an institution is. The moral career of any would-be patient has three phases, but the "ex-patient phase" is vital for a discreditable condition (that can be stigmatised). There is no doubt that there has been a lot of reform in the organisation of medical care (especially in the mental health facilities) because of Goffman's intellectual contribution; however, there are still *totalistic* hospital practices. The use of violence, such as physical restraining and psychotropic medication for containment, is still prevalent in mental health hospitals and in homes for the elderly (Duxbury and Wright 2011). More specifically, *total institution* is still relevant in examining the experience of the patients (especially hospitalised patients). While an institution might not exhibit all the features of a total institution and mortification of self, it might be rewarding to continue to study various related and observable features in hospital settings and other institutions.

8.5 A Note on Postmodernism

The perspectives or paradigms including functionalism (see Chap. 5), Marxism (see Sects. 6.2 and 6.3), feminism (see Sect. 6.5), and interactionism or interpretivism (see Chaps. 7 and this chapter) previously discussed are generally termed as modern sociological theories (MSTs). The postmodern theorists assume that modernity signifies a historical period which has passed. Invariably, the postmodernists believe that the society is now in the postmodern era; in the last few decades, there have been some sociocultural, political, and economic advances that some scholars now think of as postmodern. For the purpose of understanding, some related terms to postmodernism, such as *postmodernity*, *postmodernism*, and *postmodern social theory*, will be defined. In specific terms, *postmodernity* refers to a period in history which comes after modernity; *postmodernism* refers to the cultural products of the new period, while *postmodern social theory* refers to a way of questioning the world differently from modern social theory (Ritzer 2011). Since the nature or character of the cultural products influence the epistemological approach in sociology, the

8.5 A Note on Postmodernism

term *postmodernism* will be used to refer to the sociological perspective sourcing from postmodern thinking. The postmodernist perspective is transdisciplinary, found in media, fashion, music, philosophy, theology, arts and humanities, architecture, technology, literature, communications, and the social sciences.

While the term "postmodern" has a long history in literature, its place in sociology can be dated back to the 1970s. Postmodernism represents an attempt at a paradigm shift following arguments that most modern theory cannot accommodate the new developments in human society and explain them appropriately. The first major criticism of the MSTs is that they are too ambitious through grand narratives and universalistic principles. Most MSTs proffer general rules governing the social worlds by focusing on the social aggregate and using a nomothetic approach. It is difficult to apply a single natural social law across social contexts (Keith 2005). Such difficulty questions the scientific (methodological) foundation of sociology—this is in line with postmodernist strictures of MSTs. The major proponents of postmodernism, including Jean-François Lyotard (1924–1998), Frederic Jameson, Jean Baudrillard (1929–2007), Jacques Derrida (1930–2004), Michel Foucault (1926–1984), Martin Heidegger, Gilles Deleuze, Felix Guattari, Nancy Fraser, and Linda Nicholson, question the rational foundation of MSTs.

Elaborating the features of the postmodern epoch, Frederic Jameson described postmodernism as a new cultural logic with five major elements: (1) heterogeneous cultural dominance and fragmentation, (2) superficiality and lack of depth, (3) the waning of emotion or affect (amplification of impersonal relations), (4) a loss of historicity (discontinuity or replacement of "real" history), and (5) new technologies (re-productive instead of productive technology) (Jameson 1991; Ritzer 2011). The society is becoming increasingly complex beyond what MSTs could describe and, consequently, postmodernism accounts for the basis of comprehending the new realities. It should be noted that postmodernism, like the MSTs, involves a range of different theoretical perspectives. This is why there are also a number of contentions within the postmodern perspective. There are also contentions in classifying some theorists such as Michel Foucault and Pierre Bourdieu as postmodernists. Despite the lack of total agreement within the perspective, there are still a number of general features that can provide a guideline in the understanding of postmodernism.

8.5.1 Some Features of a Postmodern Social Theory

Postmodernism presents a departure from some of the classical features of the MSTs. As previously mentioned, most postmodernists start with what they describe as the failures of modern theories, which inform paradigmatic crisis and the need for a shift to more encompassing theoretical ideas that will explain the drastic developments of the new era. Postmodernism materialised out of poststructuralism as a critique of MSTs (Cockerham 2011). The first major assumption is that there are new advances beyond modernism. There are two ways postmodernists have explained these advances: some (like Jean Baudrillard, Gilles Deleuze, and Felix Guattari) observed a drastic replacement of modernism, while others (like Fredric Jameson and Nancy Fraser) viewed it as an extension of modernism (Ritzer 2011). Despite having these two different ways, placing Africa within the postmodern context is difficult. Africa still consists of a majority of rural communities, some without the touch of modernity. Although globalisation is dragging Africa and other developing societies along, there are still unanswered questions regarding the application of the term "postmodernity" in African context.

Postmodernism proposes both theoretical and discursive engagement of mini-narratives as opposed to grand narratives. Ritzer (2011) noted that Fredric Emerson described postmodernism as incredulity to meta- or grand narratives of MSTs. The idea of a "unified" human society that can be explained with general principles is questionable and should be abandoned for more specific explanations that will recognise "differentiated" human societies. The mini-narrative approach is close to the idiographic approach of the interactionist approach (see Sect. 7.2). Since modernism is a result of social change that produced a new epistemological approach, it is logical that the postmodern era should also be treated with a new approach.

Postmodernism is also based on a relativistic view of reality. Relativism flows from the belief in cultural divergence, or cultural differentialism. To the postmodernists, a decentering tendency due to differences across "global" localities will promote an in-depth understanding of human societies. In essence, there is a need to activate the cultural differences to allow for more theoretical and empirical probing. To the postmodernists, there is no single universal truth or reality but truths or realities constructed by the participants based on their worldview. Therefore, it is important to situate facts within these worldviews. This is why postmodernism advocates for glocalisation in relation to culture and implementation projects (Scambler 2002).

Postmodernism is based on critical discourse involving deconstruction and reconstruction of realities. Deconstruction implies a discursive and critical questioning of traditional assumptions about realities to expose the underlying differences, especially their determinants and subjective foundation. For instance, Derrida deconstructed social structures and found only normative writings used in constraining people rather than actual "structures" (Ritzer 2011). As previously implied, the search for the meaning of social realities is often influenced not only by the subject but also by the contextual dynamics and space.

In addition, another postmodernist, Jean Baudrillard, insisted that the truth is what individuals project, since it can be created and controlled. The major implication is that, beyond subjective thinking, social dynamisms (e.g., power, hegemony, and hierarchy) affect human conceptualisation of realities and knowledge itself. This questions the objective foundation of knowledge and realities. Therefore, interpretation is the bedrock of reality, since interpretation is the act of making meaning of concrete and subjective experiences and writings. The process of interpretation is ever continuous. The continuity explains the fluidity of realities; it is unstable. The "truth" continues to emerge through the process of deconstruction and as more meanings are reconstructed. Invariably, the postmodernist implication for sociological theorising and empiricism is that a single coherent rationality should be avoided to pave the way for a kind of conceptual and observational multiplicity that will cater for cultural differentialism, or what Cockerham (2011) described as the fragmentation, diversification, and decentralisation of social life. Having provided some general foundations of postmodernism, it is pertinent to reflect on its relevance and central discourse in medical sociology.

8.5.2 Postmodernism in Medical Sociology

From the 1970s, postmodernism becomes an epistemological trend which has to be considered in most aspects of sociological investigation. Michel Foucault and Pierre Bourdieu are major postmodernist references in medical sociology. Bourdieu's work originated from poststructuralism. He is more interested in social inequality in relation to power and agency in human society. His assertion is that inequality still persists and accounts for various differences which are detrimental to living conditions. To Bourdieu, behavioural choices are typically a reflection of class position (Cockerham 2007). Bourdieu (1984) questioned consumption patterns and submitted that class-oriented consumption habits account for health inequality. There are various disparities based on class division relation to smoking, drinking, and eating (see Sect. 3.3.1). The health deterioration observed with the increasing chronic illness and overall downturn in life expectancy support Bourdieu's assertion (Cockerham 2007). While the idea of lifestyle in relation to health is not new, it buttresses the postmodernist claim of the new trend of consumption.

A major discourse that is prominent in postmodern thinking is the focus on the human body as a domain of power and desire. Deleuze and Guattari (1988) advanced a prominent perspective of body-without-organs (BwO). The "conservative" consideration of body-with-organs is associated with modernity. Such a conservative idea implies a human body that is restricted by time and space (Fox 1993). The postmodern idea of body-without-organs signifies the freedom of the body and its openness to contestations. It represents a literal body that is inscribed with power and desire (Fox 1993). For instance, in the postmodern era, there is more exercise of human desire through body modification or enhancement (see Sect. 9.1.5); the body is considered an entity which is flexible and not absolutely defined by its objects (the organs). It is still a living body, not stripped (physically) of its organs, but the BwO describes the virtual dimension of the body with unlimited potentials (Deleuze and Guattari 1988). The potentials signify an endless process of becoming, or, simply put, transforming the body. Therefore, the concept of BwO signifies a subjective and autonomous conception of self-identity, a drive towards pushing the body to achieve desired capacities without limitations. The idea of transhumanism in medicine typically fits into the notion of BwO.

Foucault's contribution to the development of sociology of the body is also in line with postmodern thinking. Foucault also described the body as a site of power (Petersen and Bunton 1997). The body is often regulated by medical knowledge and power of the professionals; such regulations are also sourced from religion and cultural norms. The medical knowledge and power inform Foucault's conception of clinical gaze, a perspective of the body defined by its biomedical essence and thus controlled by medical experts (Foucault 2003). The body is socially constructed and is a discursive entity (Petersen and Bunton 1997).

Fox (1993) discusses the postmodern discourse in health care organisation. He observed that the "organisation" is viewed as a process not as a "structure" which is constituted to serve particular interests of power. Organisation texts are like discourse, which may be produced and adjusted with time based on the interests at play (Fox 1993). Invariably, the organisation of health care needs to be deconstructed and reorganised to cater for postmodern developments.

8.5.3 *Some Criticisms of Postmodernism in Medical Sociology*

Following the previous arguments on the applicability of the term "postmodernity" in African context, there is a tendency to ask whether postmodernism is a perspective only for the advanced society. Africa is still very traditional in many respects, and the efforts to modernise are ongoing. If the wave of postmodernism has some effect on Africa, it is still considerably marginal in many parts. Perhaps the ideas of glocalisation and relativism, which consider cultural divergence and peculiarities, have a deeper essence in health considerations in Africa. As has been previously mentioned, the cultural frame of reference in an African setting is somehow different from what is obtainable in western societies. Such a cultural milieu must be considered for effective disease control.

Sociology considers both micro (nominalist) and macro (realist) approaches, but the postmodernist micro-conceptual stance is too "abstractual." Cockerham (2007) argued that the highly abstract orientation of postmodernism makes it difficult to be utilised for empirical research, especially in medical sociology. The highly abstractive stance is responsible for a lack of clear conceptualisations and an inability to account for social causation (Cockerham 2011, p. 242). Hence, postmodernism is vague and seems more meaningless as an analytical framework.

Furthermore, most arguments in postmodernism are not based on empirical confirmations (Cockerham 2011). The theory tends to downplay the observational-empirical approach in sociology for a discursive approach, or what Derrida calls the deconstruction of realities. It is difficult to use "deconstruction" as an approach in gaining practical knowledge about human societies. Therefore, postmodernism is not empirically oriented as there have not been empirical contributions from postmodernism.

Some postmodernists promote a propensity towards nihilism, anarchy of belief, and meaninglessness of realities. This undermines the interpretive power and use of symbols in human societies. The tendency to undermine the implication of meanings of (health-related) social facts may be a setback in the explanation of health-related behaviours.

8.6 Theoretical Triangulation in Medical Sociology

In Chaps. 5–7, and this chapter, a number of perspectives in sociology have been discussed with numerous substantive theories/models from each of the perspectives. Some of the theories could serve as alternatives to each other. While common ground could be observed in some theories, others present divergent views. The selection of a theory or theories could be a challenge at times. To resolve such a challenge, first, one needs to have general knowledge of theoretical perspectives and their methodological implications. Second, it is important to fully understand the problem to be studied in terms of issues to be investigated, especially whether it is micro, macro, or a combination of both. The two aforementioned issues will help to select a theory, or theories.

Each of the perspectives and substantive theories has both strong and weak points. It is necessary to counterbalance the weakness of one theory with the strength of the other. This is why it is possible to combine two or more perspectives or theories. The use of a combination of theories or perspectives is referred to as theoretical triangulation. Simply put, triangulation (also called multiple operationalism or mixed methods) is "the combination of methodologies in the study of the same phenomenon" (Denzin 1978, p. 291). Denzin asserted that triangulation involves the major aspects of the research process, especially theoretical frameworks (theoretical triangulation or pluralism), methods of data collection (methodological triangulation), and forms of data (data triangulation). Research in medical sociology will benefit from triangulation; of particular importance here is theoretical triangulation. Triangulation should generate more issues that might otherwise not available if a single theory is used. It also generates broad details by accounting for alternative explanations. For instance, while perception of disease is important in determining health and illness behaviours, so is fundamental social inequality. In sum, any research in medical sociology will benefit immensely from theoretical triangulation.

References

Adlam, J., Gill, I., Glackin, S. N., Kelly, B. D., Scanlon, C., & Suibhne, S. M. (2012). Perspectives on Erving Goffman's "Asylums" fifty years on. *Medicine, Health Care and Philosophy.* doi:10.1007/s11019-012-9410-z.
Becker, H. (1963). *Outsiders*. New York: Free Press.
Black, N., & Neuhauser, D. (2006). Worth a second look: Books that have changed health services and health care policy. *Journal of Health Services Research & Policy, 11*(3), 180–183.
Bourdieu, P. (1984). *Distinction: A social critique of the judgment of taste*. London: Routledge.
Branaman, A. (1997). Goffman's social theory. In C. Lemert & A. Branaman (Eds.), *The Goffman reader*. Oxford: Blackwell Publishers.
Brown, P. (1995). Naming and framing: the social construction of illness and diagnosis. *Journal of Health and Social Behavior,* Extra Issue, 34–52.
Brown, P. (2008). Naming and framing: The social construction of illness and diagnosis. In P. Brown (Ed.), *Perspectives in medical sociology* (pp. 82–103). Long Grove: Waveland Press.
Burton, C. R. (2000). Re-thinking stroke rehabilitation: The Corbin and Strauss chronic illness trajectory framework. *Journal of Advanced Nursing, 32*(3), 595–602.

Bury, M. (1982). Chronic illness as biographical disruption. *Sociology of Health and Illness, 4*(2), 167–182.

Campbell, C., & Deacon, H. (2006). Unravelling the contexts of stigma: From internalisation to resistance to change. *Journal of Community and Applied Social Psychology: Understanding and Challenging Stigma, 16*(Special Issue: 6), 411–417.

Charmaz, K. (1991). *Good days, bad days: The self in chronic illness and time.* New Brunswick: Rutgers University Press.

Cockerham, W. C. (2007). A note on the fate of postmodern theory and its failure to meet the basic requirements for success in medical sociology. *Social Theory and Health, 5,* 285–296.

Cockerham, W. C. (2011). Health sociology in a globalizing world. *Política y Sociedad, 48*(2), 235–248.

Conrad, P., & Barker, K. K. (2010). The social construction of illness: key insights and policy implications. *Journal of Health and Social Behavior, 51 Suppl,* S67–S79.

Conrad, P., & Bury, M. (1997). Anselm Strauss and the sociological study of chronic illness: A reflection and appreciation. *Sociology of Health & Illness, 19*(3), 373–376.

Cooley, C. H. (1902). *Human nature and the social order.* New York: Scribner.

Cooley, M. E. (1999). Analysis and evaluation of the trajectory theory of chronic illness management. *Scholarly Inquiry for Nursing Practice, 13*(2), 75–95.

Corbin, J. M., & Strauss, A. L. (1984). Collaboration: Couples working together to manage chronic illness. *Image—The Journal of Nursing Scholarship,16,*109–115.

Corbin, J., & Strauss, A. L. (1985). Managing chronic illness at home: Three lines of work. *Qualitative Sociology, 8,* 224–47.

Corbin, J., & Strauss, A. (1988). *Unending work and care: Managing chronic illness at home.* San Francisco: Jossey-Bass.

Corbin, J. M., & Strauss A. L. (1991). A nursing model for chronic illness management based upon the Trajectory Framework. *Scholarly Inquiry for Nursing Practice, 5,*155–174.

Cruz-Inigo, A. E., Ladizinski, B., & Sethi, A. (2011). Albinism in Africa: Stigma, slaughter and awareness campaigns. *Dermatologic Clinics, 29*(1), 79–87.

Denzin, N. K. (1978). *The research act* (2nd ed.) NY: McGraw-Hill.

Deleuze, G., & Guattari, F. (1988). *A thousand plateaus.* London: Athlone.

Duxbury, J., & Wright, K. (2011). Should nurses restrain violent and aggressive patients? *Nursing Times, 107,* 9.

Fabrega, H. (1972). The study of disease in relation to culture. *Behavioral Science, 17,* 183–203.

Falk, G. (2001). *Stigma: How we treat outsiders.* NY: Prometheus Books.

Foucault, M. (2003). *The birth of the clinic.* London: Routledge.

Fox, J. N. (1993). *Postmodernism, sociology and health.* Buckingham: Open University Press.

Frankenberg, R. (1980). Medical anthropology and development: A theoretical perspective. *Social Science & Medicine. Medical Anthropology, 14B,* 197–207.

Freidson, E. (1960). Client control and medical practice. *American Journal of Sociology, 65*(4), 374–382.

Garfinkel, H. (1956). Conditions of successful degradation ceremonies. *American Journal of Sociology, 61*(5), 420–424.

Goffman, E. (1961). *Asylum: Essays on the social situation of mental patients and other inmates.* NY: Anchor Books.

Goffman, E. (1963). *Stigma: Notes on the management of spoiled identity.* London: Penguin Books.

Gove, W. (1970a). Societal reaction as an explanation of mental illness: An evaluation. *American Sociological Review, 35,* 873–84.

Gove, W. (1970b). Who is hospitalized: A critical review of some sociological studies of mental illness. *Journal of Health and Human Behavior, 11,* 294–304.

Gove, W. (1975). The labelling theory of mental illness: A reply to Scheff. *American Sociological Review, 40*(2), 242–248

Henly, S. J., Wyman, J. F., & Findorff, M. J. (2011). Health and illness over time: The trajectory perspective in nursing science. *Nursing Research, 60*(3 Suppl), S5–14.

References

Herek, G. M. (1999). AIDS and Stigma. *American Behavioral Scientist, 42*(7), 1106–1116.
Jameson, F. (1991). *Postmodernism, or, the cultural logic of late capitalism.* Durham: Duke University Press.
Jones, E., Farina, A., Hastorf, A., Markus, H., Miller, D., & Scott, R. (1984). *Social stigma: The psychology of marked relationships.* New York: Freeman.
Keith, B. (2005). A century of motion: Disciplinary culture and organization drift in American sociology. *Footnotes, 33*(9), 6.
Kleinman, A. (1978). Concepts and a model for the comparison of medical systems as cultural systems. *Social Science & Medicine, 12,* 85–93.
Kleinman, A. (1980). *Patients and healers in the context of culture.* Berkeley: University of California Press.
Kleinman, A., Eisenberg, L., & Good, B. (2006). Culture, illness, and care: Clinical lessons from anthropologic and cross-cultural research. *The Journal of Lifelong Learning in Psychiatry, IV*(1), 140–149.
Kroska, A., & Harkness, S. K. (2008). Exploring the role of diagnosis in the modified labelling theory of mental illness. *Social Psychology Quarterly, 71*(2), 193–208.
Lemert, E. M. (1951). *Social pathology.* New York: McGraw-Hill.
Link, B. G., & Phelan, J. C. (2001). Conceptualizing stigma. *Annual Review of Sociology, 27,* 363–385.
Link, B. G., Struening, E., Cullen, F. T., Shrout, P. E., & Dohrenwend, B. P. (1989). A modified labelling theory perspective to mental disorders: An empirical assessment. *American Sociological Review, 54,* 400–423.
McCorkle, R., & Pasacreta, J. V. (2001). Enhancing caregiver outcomes in palliative care. *Cancer Control, 8*(1), 36–45.
Mead, G. H. (1934). *Mind, self, and society.* Chicago: University of Chicago Press.
Monger, M. (2011). Stigma: Barrier to quality of life and health care. *HIV Clinician, 23*(2), 1, 4–5.
Parameswari, S. J., & Jayapoorani, N. (2012). Effects of HIV related stigma on the lives of persons living with HIV. *BMC Infectious Diseases, 12*(Suppl 1), P52. doi:10.1186/1471-2334-12-S1-P52.
Pasman, J. (2011). The consequences of labelling mental illnesses on the self-concept: a review of the literature and future directions. *Social Cosmos*—URN:NBN:NL:UI:10-1-101264: (122–127).
Pescosolido, B. A., Martin, J. K., Lang, A., & Olafsdottir, A. (2008). Rethinking theoretical approaches to stigma: A framework integrating normative influences on stigma (FINIS). *Social Science & Medicine, 67,* 431–440.
Petersen, A., & Bunton, R. (1997). *Foucault: Health and medicine.* NY: Routledge.
Philips, S. D., & Gates, T. (2011). A conceptual framework for understanding the stigmatization of children of incarcerated parents. *Journal of Child and Family Studies, 20,* 286–294.
Reeve, J., Lloyd-Williams, M., Payne, S., & Dowrick, C. (2010). Revisiting biographical disruption: Exploring individual embodied illness experience in people with terminal cancer. *Health, 14,* 178–195.
Ritzer, G. (2011). *Sociological theory.* 8th ed. NY: McGraw-Hill.
Rose, D., Thornicroft, G., Pinfold, V., & Kassam, A. (2007). 250 labels used to stigmatise people with mental illness. *BMC Health Services Research, 7,* 97 doi:10.1186/1472-6963-7-97.
Scambler, G. (2002). *Health and social change: A critical theory.* Buckingham: Open University Press.
Scheff, T. J. (1966). Being mentally ill: A sociological theory. Chicago: Aldine.
Scheff, T. J. (1974). The labelling theory of mental illness. *American Sociological Review, 39*(3), 444–452.
Scheff, T. J. (2010). Updating labelling theory: Normalizing but not enabling. *Nordic Journal of Social Research, 1,* 1–7.
Singer, M. (2004). The social origins and expressions of illness. *British Medical Bulletin, 69,* 9–19.
Snadden, D., & Brown, J. B. (1992). The experience of asthma. *Social Science & Medicine, 12,* 1352–61.

Sontag, S. (1978). *Illness as metaphor*. NY: Farrar, Straus and Giroux.
Suibhne, S. M. (2011). Erving Goffman's *Asylums* 50 years on. *British Journal of Psychiatry, 198,* 1–2.
Tannenbaum, F. (1938). *Crime and community*. London: Columbia University Press.
Thomas, W. I., & Thomas, D. S. (1928). *The child in America: Behaviour problems and programs*. New York: Knopf.
Timmermans, S., & Haas, S. (2008). Towards a sociology of disease. *Sociology of Health and Illness, 30,* 659–76.
Weinstein, R. M. (1982). Goffman's asylums and the social situation of mental patients *Orthomolecular Psychiatry, 11*(4), 267–274.
Winter, M. F. (1996). Societal reaction, labelling and social control: The contribution of Edwin M. Lemert. *History of the Human Sciences, 9*(2), 53–77.

Chapter 9
Medicalisation and Client-Practitioner Relations

9.1 Introduction

The concept of medicalisation is another major contributions of medical sociology to medical practice and the understanding of human health. It depicts a cautionary note in the expansion of the medical domain. The notion of medicalisation is closely linked with the social construction of realities. Participants in medical practice construct issues that are termed as medical in order to expand the scope of medicine. Medicalisation describes how ordinary issues (usually non-medical) are defined as medical problems, thus requiring medical attention in terms of diagnosis, prevention, and treatment. In other words, medicalisation involves defining a problem in medical terms, usually as an illness or disorder, or using a medical intervention to treat it (Conrad 2005, p. 3, 2007, 2013). There is a growing tendency to define all social abnormalities or deviance as medical problems. The view stems from the notion that those who are healthy in a medical sense should not behave abnormally. In the same vein, Bell and Figert (2012, p. 776) observed that wider social processes such as rationalisation, systematisation of the medical domain, and rational application of science to everyday life foster the process of medicalisation. This implies that medicalising a situation gradually becomes a way to explain it, a form of medical explanatory model. Medicalisation also provides a way to eliminate mystical explanations of social events and gives room for the application of biomedical science to objectively explain such social events.

Medicalisation postulates that medicine has increased its relevance and domains in the management of human society. This reflects in all stages of human existence: pre-conception, conception, childhood, adulthood, old age, death, and posthumous condition. Invariably, medicalisation means increasing human dependence on medicine throughout the course of life, generated through professional expansions. At any point, anyone may be referred to the medical institution for certification. More importantly, the medical expansion of the domain of relevance involves the conversion of a social or moral problem to a disease (Filc 2004). Medicalisation is perpetuated through medical hegemony on social formation, especially in practitioner-patient relationships. It is further observed that physicians play a hegemonic role in the health care system. Filc (2004, p. 1277) specifically noted that apart from the professional expansion, medicalisation is also perpetuated through the "desocialisation of illness and disease so as to obscure the social processes working in their production." Desocialisation in this regard refers to the conversion of normal behaviour to abnormality (or deviance) or the labelling of more social traits as (medical) pathologies (see Sect. 8.4.1 for labelling theory). Desocialisation thus generates more interests for medical practitioners by underplaying the social context. Sociologists are interested in medicalisation because of its emerging consequences. These consequences are also part of the process through which medicalisation itself occurs. The consequences include, among others:

1. There is increasing hegemonic (professional) domination of practitioner-patient relationships, which is also referred to as medical paternalism (see sect. 9.2.1.1).
2. Professional expansion by converting or appropriating more social discourse into medical discourse. This implies the use of a medical model or gaze instead of a social model. This involves downplaying the sociogenic basis of events in order to reify the medical basis. This is synonymous to what Conrad (1992) described as *decontextualisation of social problems*.
3. There is increasing human dependence on medicine throughout the course of life. Every stage of life is medicalised, and so requires medical interventions. This is close to what Conrad (2013) portrayed as *pathologicalisation of everything*.
4. Another consequence is mass escalation of medical technology, products, and information. This is done through promotion of medical ideology, marketing of products, and unlimited access to lifestyle medications. Conrad (2013) called this *consumerisation of medicine*—a situation where medical procedures and care are becoming consumer items (see for instance, how beauty is increasingly commoditised through medicalisation [sect. 9.1.62]).
5. Dislocation of responsibility: this involves the shifting of responsibility for issues defined in medical terms from the individual to the experts (Conrad 1992). This is what Conrad (2013, p. 207) described as *the expansion of medical social control*. For all medicalised issues, the individual needs to seek medical attention.

9.1.1 The Rise of Medicalisation

The concept of medicalisation, sometimes called pathologisation, earned a place in medical sociology starting in the 1970s. This early application of medicalisation stems from psychiatry and deviance. The term is credited to the works of a number of scholars including Thomas Szasz, Ivan Illich, Eliot Freidson, Michel Foucault, Irving K. Zola, and Peter Conrad, among others. The scholars noticed increasing penetration and domination of medical ideology in all facets of life.

Thomas Szasz was part of the anti-psychiatry movement, a critical movement against the ways in which mental disorders are (sociomedically) constructed. The fundamental argument is that madness is manufactured through medicalisation, by describing more categories of social deviance as mental problems (Szasz 1970). Medical professionals continue to make attributions that define more individuals as mad, and, therefore, as requiring medical attention. The pathologisation of deviance

9.1 Introduction

is a critical way of ensuring social control, as more individuals try to "escape" medicalised situations to avoid being subjected to psychiatric testing and diagnosis. For instance, if a traffic offence (like speeding) is linked to a mental disorder, more individuals may try to avoid being subjected to psychiatric tests by avoiding such an offence. The discussion of medicalisation also relates to labelling (see Sects. 8.4.1 and 8.4.2.1). Labelling human conditions and attaching medical relevance create more medical categories.

Eliot Freidson (1970) used the term "professional dominance" to depict the process of medicalisation, arguing that the medical model predominates in health-related encounters. Such dominance involves not only the exercise of authority but also the expansion of (professional) relevance. In the classical book *The Profession of Medicine*, Freidson devoted a part to the social construction of illness (see Sect. 8.2). The definition of illness is beyond the control of the person or patient, but can be defined through the rational knowledge of the professionals, and thus can be managed by such professionals. Therefore, within the general realm of viewing illness as social deviance (like Parsons (1951) explained), the "deviants" need professional help. Freidson argued that there is often diagnostic bias and moral judgment of the patients by the physicians.

Another contribution to the concept of medicalisation is by Zola (1972), who viewed medicine as an institution of social control. Zola (1972, p. 487) argued that moral judgment in the name of health is "occurring through the political power physicians hold or can influence, but is largely an insidious and often undramatic phenomenon accomplished by 'medicalizing' much of daily living, by making medicine and the labels 'healthy' and 'ill' *relevant* to an ever increasing part of human existence." According to Zola, medicalisation is manifested in medical expansionism through which more aspects of social status are pathologised. Invariably, it is not uncommon to regard *social deviance*—any behaviour that negates normal pattern—as a medical issue. Many *excusable* behaviours require medical legitimation or sanction (e.g., absenteeism from work, international travel, employment, and study). Illich (1976, p. 76) described the application of a medical diagnosis on the general population as diagnostic imperialism, a limitless expansion of medicine in the legitimation of roles in the society.

Michel Foucault also contributed to the discourse of medicalisation through his concept of clinical or medical gaze. Foucault coined the concept in his book *The Birth of the Clinic* (first published in 1973) to describe the objectification of the body in clinical practice and how the human body is constantly under medical scrutiny. He described medical gaze as a dehumanising medical separation of the body from the person. The body thus becomes a medical domain with various ramifications. Foucault (2003, p. xiii) asserted that "at the beginning of the nineteenth century, doctors described what for centuries had remained below the threshold of the visible and the expressible ... revealing through gaze and language what had previously been below and beyond their domain."

From the foregoing discussion, it is evident that medicalisation as a notion of medical gaze is a useful device to shift the focus of medicine from the patients to the general population, or from ill-health to life itself (Illich 1975, 1976). This is why

Illich (1975) claimed that the world is suffering from too much medical interference, and, as expected, the extent of medical interference is growing unabated due to new medical possibilities. An entire human life and normal body are medicalised through the application of the medical model, a pathological view of the individual body or a form of medical reductionism. He observed that people are turned into patients without being sick. Counseling services are offered to apparently healthy individuals with checkups to *hunt* for diseases. Despite a lack of success in the cure of many diseases, medicine turns to the business of prevention care for prognosticated risks (Illich 1976, p. 89). Like Conrad (1992, p. 213) observed, both natural life processes (e.g., menopause, sexuality, childbirth, aging, and death) and deviant behaviours (e.g., madness, alcoholism, anorexia, gambling, and infertility) have been medicalised. Conrad (2007, 2013) has extensively discused various characters and characteristics of medicalisation. The next few subsections will examine some major aspects of medicalisation including pharmaceuticalisation, geneticisation, remedicalisation and demedicalisation, and medical enhancement.

9.1.2 *Pharmaceuticalisation*

Pharmaceuticalisation is the incorporation of more human conditions into the domain of pharmaceutical intervention (i.e., requiring medication). Prescription drug sales are growing worldwide. One of the reasons for pharmaceutical expansionism is business motive. Like other market products are expanding, so are pharmaceuticals in human care for enhancement, prevention, and treatment. The critical aspect of coverage is in the area of non-disease condition, or as a preventive measure. Vaccination is everybody's business because of probable exposure. There is growing pressure to improve human immunity in order to ward off predictable medical conditions. New drugs are being tested with attendant opportunities, but also ethical risks. More specifically, pharmaceuticalisation has been variously defined as "the transformation of human conditions, capacities or capabilities into pharmaceutical matters of treatment or enhancement" (Williams et al. 2011, p. 711). Enhancement involves non-disease treatment, especially to improve specific performances (see Sect. 9.1.5). On the other hand, pharmaceuticalisation is also "the process by which social, behavioural or bodily conditions are treated or deemed to be in need of treatment, with medical drugs by doctors or patients" (Abraham 2009, p. 100). It has been observed that there is more concentration on psychoactive and lifestyle drugs. For instance, the modern era has witnessed the rise of aphrodisiac drugs (Viagra and other related products) for sexual enhancement. In short, the bedroom has been pharmaceuticalised!

Pharmaceuticalisation is closely linked to medicalisation; it is one of the driving forces of medicalisation. Abraham (2010) differentiated between the two concepts. He argued that pharmaceuticalisation may occur without medicalisation, as the medical profession may be bypassed in pharmaceutical choice, purchase, and use. Direct consumer purchase of various forms of drugs is growing. In Africa, buying drugs over-the-counter (OTC) is common. With weak pharmaceutical regulations in developing countries, drugs can be purchased from street hawkers and in public places like bus stops. In essence, there is a growing demand for drugs by consumers rather than patients; a consumer's desire to use drugs recreationally is more likely the cause for the purchase (as opposed to purchasing to treat a medical condition).

Abraham (2010, pp. 606–607) identified five interwoven factors that have contributed to the growth of pharmaceuticalisation:

1. **The ideology or policy of the regulatory state**: there is ideological appropriation of pharmaceuticalisation through deregulation which promotes drug innovation and marketing. Deregulation also promotes commercial interest rather than health promotion interest. More relaxed regulations are created to generate access and meet consumer demand.
2. **Biomedicalism**: growing human health needs which are defined as pathologies require biomedical intervention. This aspect involves drug research and innovation which present with unending challenges because of the growing burden of chronic diseases. In essence, there is growing biomedical research aimed at providing solutions to many so-far incurable conditions, management of chronic diseases, and new improved treatment for old diseases (e.g., ACT for malaria).
3. **Consumerism**: this generally involves consumer movements. Abraham (2010) identified two aspects of consumerism. The first aspect is adversarial consumerism, which is consumer-based objection to drugs (due to drug-related adverse events) and drug marketing in the politico-legal sphere. The second aspect involves access-oriented collaborative consumerism, a movement to create access to new drugs and faster approval by regulatory agencies (e.g., call for mass production of HIV prevention drugs). It is this second aspect that actually produces pharmaceuticalisation, while the first aspect may lead to de-pharmaceuticalisation.
4. **Industry drug promotion and marketing**: the pharmaceutical companies are now aggressive in attracting sales. The internet is flooded with drug advertisements for drugs that are available for purchase without a prescription in many countries with low-level of regulations. Pharmaceutical companies often promote the positive side of drugs and fail to mention the long-term effects to enhance sales.
5. **Medicalisation**: increasing medical expansion in the diagnosis and treatment of life situations. Medicalisation promotes pharmaceuticalisation and vice versa. Medicalisation invariably increases drug preventive measures and treatment.

From the foregoing discussion, it is evident that five key actors with different values play complementary roles in enhancing pharmaceuticalisation (see Table 9.1). As Busfield (2010) explained, the actors include the pharmaceutical companies, government regulatory agencies and insurance companies, doctors, and the public. The fifth actor, pharmacists and chemist shop owners, is added to cater to the African context where they proliferate and play a substantial role in medicine sale, use, and primary care. All of these actors operate under the influence of external pressures/factors listed in Table 9.1.

Table 9.1 Key actors and influences on medicine use/pharmaceuticalisation. (Source: Busfield 2010, p. 940)

Actors	Role in medicine	Actor's own expansionary ideas and action	External pressures
Pharmaceutical industry	Developers, producers, promoters and sellers of drugs	Desire to increase profits Mechanisms:	(a) Cost controls of gov't and insurance cos[d]
		(a) Marketing/promotion to doctors and public	(b) Drug licensing and safety regulations[d]
		(b) Control over science	(c) Drug research and Innovations[a]
		(c) Disease mongering	(d) Drug needs for old and new illness conditions[a]
Doctors	Prescribers and gatekeepers; sometimes researchers	(a) Interventionism	(a) Industry's promotion of medicines[a]
		(b) Imbalances in risk assessment	(b) Patients' requests[b]
		(c) Limited knowledge	(c) Greater risk consciousness[b]
		(d) Medicalisation	(d) Cost controls of gov't and insurance cos[c]
The public	Potential users	(a) Desire to get better	(a) Industry's promotion of medicines[a]
		(b) Belief in the value of medicine	(b) Growth of consumer-oriented culture[b]
		(c) Active consumers/expert patients	(c) Gov't focus on choice and the expert patient[b]
Pharmacists and chemist shop owners	Dispenser, gatekeepers, retail sellers, prescribers	(a) Desire to increase sales and make more profit	(a) Users' demand[a]
		(b) Promotion of access to drugs	(b) Primary care role[a]
		(c) Promotion of medicine use	(c) Legal control[d]
Governments and insurance companies	Set framework of health care, including access to medicines, funders of health care, responsibilities in safety	(a) Improving access to health care	(a) Industry's promotion of medicines[a]
		(b) Supporting choice	(b) Growing cost of health care provision[c]
		(c) Value of industry to the economy	

[a] Strong expansionary pressure
[b] Weaker expansionary pressure
[c] Strong constraint on expansion
[d] Weaker constraint

9.1 Introduction

Invariably, the understanding of pharmaceuticalisation should revolve around the expansionist interest of the key actors (see Table 9.1). The roles of these actors often promote the expansionist idea that there are pharmaceutical solutions to most life and health problems. The major danger of pharmaceuticalisation, however, is that therapeutic interest is gradually undermined for nontherapeutic issues (see Sects. 9.1.5 and 9.1.6.2). There is also the tendency to undermine the interests of patients and public health. This implies that there is a shifting focus on the general consumers rather than patients. More so, a business motive (especially profit maximisation) that gives room for exploitation of consumers is being promoted. No wonder, Abraham (2007) observed that the pharmaceutical industry has been a major source of economic power. Additionally, the more the human society is pharmaceuticalised, the higher the number of drug-related adverse events. Busfield (2006) observed that the power of the pharmaceutical industry is encouraging the uncritical and extensive use of pills. Overuse may cause a gradual reduction in clinical benefits and development of drug resistance. The demise of Chloroquine in malaria treatment in malaria-endemic regions is a critical example of drug resistance as a result of overuse.

9.1.3 Geneticisation

Little did the world know when the term "geneticisation" was coined by Abby Lippman (a sociologist) in 1991 (see Lippman 1991, 1992) that the dawn of genetic revolution was very near. It is an aspect of medicalisation which is of increasing importance. Sociologists now use the concept of geneticisation to describe the increasing institutionalisation and globalisation of findings of the Human Genome Projects (HGP). The term is also used to critique the social impact of genetic testing (Hedgecoe 2009). Hedgecoe further noted that the social sciences' use of geneticisation serves to complement most bioethics commentaries on genetics, which tend to be structured around the ELSI (ethical, legal, and social implications) approach. The main thrust of sociological investigation is to apply sociological perspectives to unravel the social trends, dynamics, and implications of genetic testing and research. For instance, Lippman (1991) observed that the use of genetic testing is clearly more of a social use of genetic technology than a medical use.

The HGP completely mapped and sequenced all the genetic material of man in order to unravel how the human body functions. Genes string together to form chromosomes. They constitute units of hereditary traits, which can be passed from one generation to the next. Genomic sequencing is the process of decoding the human genome by examining the deoxyribonucleic acid (DNA) pattern composition. Geneticisation stems from biomedical domain but presents with enormous social impacts. Hence "geneticisation" is defined as the "socio-cultural process of interpreting and explaining human beings using the terminology and concepts of genetics, so that not only health and disease but also aspects of human behaviour and social interactions are viewed through the prism of biomolecular technology" (Ten Have 2012, p. 1). Geneticisation is a general term for genetic reductionism, gaze, or determinism, a process in which individuals are reduced to their DNA codes. This is why Lippman (1991, p. 19) described it as "an ongoing process by which differences in individuals and groups are reduced to their DNA codes, with most disorders, behaviour, psychological variations defined" by genetics. "It refers as well to the process by which interventions employing genetic technologies are adopted to manage problems of health."

Geneticisation leads to a belief in genetic essentialism by implying that human life is programmed by DNA or its genetic compositions. In this vein, genetics gives essence and direction to human existence, and social processes can be redefined in terms of genetic makeup. There is an interwoven, two-way focus in the understanding of geneticisation:

1. **The social construction of biological phenomenon**: an attempt is made to socially influence biological conditions to avoid random *allocation* of traits, to manipulate the genome to produce certain social outcomes. This is possible because of the understanding of genetic basis of human behaviour and personality.
2. **Biological construction of social realities**: this is the form of genetic gaze mentioned earlier; social realities, especially behaviours, are reduced to human genetics, a pre-programmed background. Inheritability of traits is reified and used in the explanation of social processes.

Sociology still needs to examine the genetic explanation of behaviour and scrutinise its basic assumptions, which sociologically are perceived as weak in the explanation of human behaviour (Freese and Shostak 2009). From sociological understanding of behaviour, what is perceived as genetic may be influenced by cultural variables. For instance, scientists have discovered a gene (dopamine D4 receptor gene variation) related to marital infidelity and sexual promiscuity (see Garcia et al. 2010). The gene is said to promote involvement in uncommitted sex (one-night stands). The question is: does this genetic discovery of an *adultery gene* mean that sociocultural and legal environments do not influence the prevalence of sexual infidelity in a community? The geneticisation of marital infidelity then holds a lot of sociocultural implications. Since most human beings value marital fidelity, is genetic testing required before marriage to determine whether a partner has the gene variant or not? What happens to groups in which the adultery gene is more common? One other implicit lesson from the scientific finding would be a desocialisation of sexual promiscuity: that racial/ethnic ancestry, age, and gender do not relate to sexual infidelity. This is a drive towards genetic determinism, which undermines the evidence that genetic traits and the environment (social as well as physical) account for human behaviour. Genes alone do not determine how people behave or succumb to a certain disease, but affect the risk.

The HGP is considered as social action on a large scale, and extends beyond the mere understanding of behavioural variations to the knowledge of specific pathological traits. As Pavone (2008, p. 11) observed, some aspects of genetic practices may:

9.1 Introduction

1. Encourage the research agenda to place greater emphasis on the genetic roots of common diseases at the expense of the studies on environmental and social factors.
2. Stimulate the redefinition of the traditional concepts of health, reproduction, and identity, with a greater emphasis on the genetic aspects of these concepts.
3. Endorse eugenics through selective reproduction and *therapeutic* abortion, especially through prenatal genetic diagnosis.
4. Support the switch of the medical focus from therapeutics to predictive medicine through genetic testing. Genetic diagnoses claim to be able to predict a disease long before the onset of symptoms.
5. Engender the formulation of new concepts of citizenship and political participation in which genetic risk and/or genetically "virtuous" behaviour become potentially discriminating factors.
6. Revolutionise preventive strategies: genetic diagnostics has the ability to establish particular risks for particular individuals. This could enable at-risk individuals to take preventive measures to avert or delay the onset of symptoms.
7. Promote the transformation of citizens into patients/consumers and increase the demand for medical information and medical care.

Furthermore, Phelan (2005) emphasised the dangers of geneticisation when he claimed that it could generate stigma. Genetics deals with the passing of traits from one generation to the next. Therefore, if genes are the basis of human identity and are strongly deterministic of behaviour, and if through genes it is possible to identify both desirable (healthy) and undesirable (pathological) traits, (Phelan argued that) further exploration and proliferation of access to genetic projects will exacerbate social stigmatisation. It will increase perceptions of differentness and perceived threats of pathological traits, which in turn should increase social distance and reproductive restrictiveness or selectiveness. Searching for ways in which these dangers can be reduced is a part of the sociological exploration of geneticisation.

9.1.4 Demedicalistion and Remedicalisation

One of the characters of medicalisation that Peter Conrad (2007, 2013) discussed is that it can be bi-directional—there can be remedicalisation as well as demedicalisation. As the progress of medicalisation continues, some issues may be demedicalised—no longer considered a medical problem, therefore requiring no medical intervention. Demedicalisation (an obverse of medicalisation) is a process of normalisation after a previous application of medical terms. Conrad (1992, 2007) claimed that demedicalisation refers to a problem that no longer retains its medical definition. Classical examples of demedicalisation include "gender dysphoria" or transexualism, masturbation, homosexualism, bisexualism, disability, and anorexia. Decades ago in western societies, homosexuality (same-sex relationships) and bisexuality (sexual feelings for both sexes) were considered social deviations and medical problems. Recently, they have been regarded as normal behaviours and there is a clamour for all societies to recognise homosexuality and bisexuality as normal sexual orientations. Many nations (including South Africa) now legalise homosexuality, while many nations in Africa still criminalise it. The rights of lesbian, gay, bisexual, transgender (LGBT), and intersex (having physical traits of both sexes) persons are also part of human rights recognised in many nations. Bisexuality and homosexuality are thus demedicalised and destigmatised. This is also applicable to masturbation, which was previously regarded as a medical problem. Moreover, services that are criminalised or prohibited in a medical setting are demedicalised (see Halfman 2012). If abortion is proscribed or outlawed in a state, it means that it is not in the domain of medical practice. This shows that the legal framework is a part of the driving force of medicalisation and demedicalisation.

Another dimension is remedicalisation. This indicates that an issue previously demedicalised can be remedicalised. The most common example of remedicalisation is male circumcision in western countries (sometimes referred to as the debate on the foreskin). Carpenter (2010) submitted that male circumcision became medicalised in the United States and Great Britain before World War II, but in the 1960s and 1970s it was demedicalised in Great Britain and the United States, respectively. Remedicalisation of the foreskin appears because of recent findings about its medical benefits, especially in HIV prevention. Studies have found that the removal of foreskin could reduce HIV transmission by 50–60% (see Auvert et al. 2005; Weiss et al. 2010; WHO/UNAIDS 2007). While male circumcision is generally high (especially among Muslim populations) in Africa, some African societies with a relatively low rate of circumcision are driving for remedicalisation in the context of HIV prevention.

Since medicalisation is a process involving people's constructions of reality, there is always room for a reconstruction either to demedicalise or remedecalise. Despite this two-way movement, medicalisation has significantly outpaced demedicalisation (Conrad 1992; Halfmann 2012). Demedicalisation and remedicalisation are usually achieved after some type of organised movement (of patients, women, gays and lesbians, people with disabilities, and proponents of alternative medicine) and research challenge medical definitions and control (Conrad 1992; Halfman 2012). Medicalisation depends on a cultural environment. For instance, among the Muslims and Jews, male circumcision is always a medical issue because it is religiously prescribed. Homosexuality and bisexuality also remain a prohibitive sexual pattern in many non-secular societies because heterosexual behaviours are culturally prescribed. As another example, while obesity has been medicalised in western societies, some communities in Africa are more sexually attracted to voluptuous women, or simply value the big-sized.

9.1.5 *Medical Enhancement*

The discourse of medical/human enhancement is one of the fundamental driving forces of medicalisation. It involves the application of medical intervention to a non-disease condition. Earlier presentations of enhancement were seen in fictitious films like *Cyborg* and *Terminator*. The reality now is that it is possible for humans to be wired or *cyberneticised* to improve capabilities and functions. Medical enhancement can be defined as any medical intervention directed to boost human capabilities beyond the species' typical level or statistically normal range of functioning (Daniel 2000). It is often difficult to arrive at a noncontroversial meaning of enhancement because it can be argued that eating a special kind of food or exercising might also be regarded as enhancement (Lin and Allhoff 2008). The case of food or physical exercise can be regarded as natural. The notion of medical intervention is included here to signify that it involves some human enhancement technologies and artificial measures. Therefore, enhancement implies nontherapeutic application of specific technologies (e.g., neuro-, cyber-, gene-, and nanotechnologies) to the human body to improve performance and function. Enhancement ranges from simple psychological and pharmacological interventions to the use of complex medical technology (e.g., genetic engineering).

Furthermore, Daniel (2000, p. 309) observed that while treatment includes services or interventions meant to prevent or cure (or otherwise ameliorate) conditions that are viewed as diseases or disabilities, enhancement involves interventions to improve conditions that are viewed as normal functions or features of members of the human species. The use of steroids to improve strength by a normal individual is an example of human enhancement. While Ritalin is used to treat attention-deficit/hyperactivity disorder (ADHD), in other words, to correct a deficiency, the use of Ritalin by students who do not have ADHD (to improve academic performance) amounts to human enhancement (Lin and Allhoff 2008, p. 253). Lin and Allhoff further observed that functional implants (computer chips and neural implants) in a healthy body constitute human enhancement as tools are supposed to be used externally by individuals, not implanted. Development of exoskeleton, anti-aging, life extension interventions, and cosmetic surgery (see Sect. 9.1.6.2) is associated with human enhancement. Ideas relating to eugenics and transhumanism (movement towards *homo-superior*) are also linked to human enhancement.

The implication is that human enhancement involves over-medicalisation, an application of medical technologies and possibilities beyond treatment and prevention of diseases or infirmities. If the trend continues, enhancement will lead to overdependence on medical technologies, even for basic human functions and other natural processes. There may be a continuous search and application of more *cosmetic* possibilities that would make many humans resemble artificial creations. Human dexterity and ingenuity may be meaningless in the face of enhancement. There have been a number of ethical concerns regarding safety, fairness, societal disruptions, and human dignity (Lin and Allhoff 2008). These ethical issues will be reserved for Chap. 10—the argument here is that enhancement is medicalising the human society.

9.1.6 Medicalisation: Beginning, During, and End of Life

The essence of this section is to provide examples of medicalisation at three stages of life. The three subsections will focus on medicalisation of pregnancy/childbirth, beauty, and death.

9.1.6.1 The Medicalisation of Pregnancy/Childbirth

Pregnancy and childbirth have been medicalised since at least the nineteenth century. The early classical works on the medicalisation of pregnancy/childbirth were advanced by Ann Oakley's *Becoming a Mother* (1979) and *The Captured Womb* (1984). While pregnancy and childbirth are supposed to be normal processes (or requiring little assistance), the whole process has now been medicalised, with every stage requiring medical intervention. Oakley (1979) observed that pregnancy is a state of health and not a disease. In most instances, the paternalistic approach is the norm with doctors making prescriptions and proscriptions. The medical profession often stresses the delicacy of pregnancy and childbirth, hence the expansion of professional obstetrics. The tendency nowadays is for doctors to attribute improved maternal outcomes to medical care without paying attention to overall socioeconomic development (Oakley 1979).

For instance, there are now a number of procedures due to medicalisation of child-wish including harvesting of gametes, induced ovulation and artificial insemination. A number of practices are also necessitated due to medicalisation of childbirth/pregnancy including, routine checks and measurements, disease screening (e.g., for HIV), caesarean section, vaginal examinations during pregnancy, shaving of the pubic hair during labour, prenatal genetic testing, selective reproduction, in vitro fertilisation, ultrasound monitoring of pregnancy and so on.

Furthermore, the colonisation of birth by medicine is a product of industrial societies as a result of heavy trust in technology, tests, and machines (Oakley 1979). The management of pregnancy and childbirth were formerly confined to the domestic sphere handled by fellow women until the growth of medicalisation. The process incorporates intervention in normal births such as routine intravenous infusions and electronic foetal monitoring (Johanson et al. 2002). While the obstetricians play an important role in complicated deliveries, Johanson et al. asserted that due to medicalisation, obstetrician involvement and medical interventions (including medically uninformed caesarean sections) have become routine in normal childbirth, without evidence of effectiveness. There is, therefore, the need to curtail the growing trends of medicalisation of pregnancy and childbirth.

9.1.6.2 The Medicalisation of Beauty: The Cosmetic/Aesthetic Revolution

There is an increasing medicalisation of beauty. Every part of the body (fingers, nails, hair, eyes, nose, legs, ears, neck, thighs, skin, mouth, chest, tummy, and particularly the private/sexual parts—the penis, vagina, and breasts) becomes medicalised in order to beautify or improve its image. A beautiful body is linked to its size, its structure, and its shape. The female body has been dominating in the contextualisation and conception of sexual bodies, beauty, and in the portrayal of human sexuality within the global world. The female body is, therefore, highly medicalised. There is a role of patriarchy. Cultural and global prescriptions and proscriptions are more common and stronger for women than men (Castro 2011). This signifies the patriarchal

9.1 Introduction

Table 9.2 Some common types of aesthetic/cosmetic surgery

Mammoplasty	Breast augmentation, reduction, or lift—for correcting the size, contour, and elevation of sagging breasts
Buttock augmentation	To augment the buttock—reshape, reduce the size, or make it firmer
Rhytidectomy	Face/neck lift—procedure to remove wrinkles and signs of aging from the face. It includes brow lift and chin augmentation
Rhinoplasty	Reshaping of the nose—to increase its projection, make it narrower, or reduce its size
Abdominoplasty/tummy tuck	Reshaping and firming of the abdomen
Liposuction/lipoplasty	Removal of fat deposits to reshape and redefine the contours of the body
Phalloplasty	Reconstruction of the penis, other procedure to make the penis longer/bigger/penile enlargement
Body modification	Surgical tattooing, piercing, implantation in parts of the body

basis of women's beauty which exacts more pressure on women to modify their physical look. The media also has a role in the medicalisation of beauty. The media representation of slimness as a sign of beauty generates the desire for the slim body figure and the freshness of the skin; women are expected to possess moderate hips, small or moderate breasts, decorate or paint (or tattoo) the body, make the breasts and the buttocks firm, maintain a flat tummy (stomach), have a soft/mellow voice, and have full lips and decorative nails. Achieving all these could involve medical intervention.

There is a revolutionary expansion of medicine to recreate the human body, a form of enhancement. Plastic or reconstructive surgery is meant to correct deformities; the focus here will be on aesthetic or cosmetic surgery, a kind of plastic surgery meant for beautification. The body can be medically manufactured or recreated; breasts could be firmed, reduced, or enlarged; the curves can be created or redressed; the tummy can be flattened; hips can be moderated and reshaped; face can be doctored (facelift); the nose can be reshaped, and so on. More individuals now opt for cosmetic procedures (see Table 9.2). While the table shows some surgical procedures, it should be noted that there are numerous non-surgical procedures with the use of injection and pills (e.g., cosmetic facial injection, lip and buttock enhancement, breast and penile enlargement pills, and laser hair removal). Unfortunately, not all procedures lead to a desired outcome.

A "beautiful body" is commoditised and thus becomes a new human desire. The global sexualisation of the body (defining parts of the body in their sexual essence) also promotes the medicalisation of beauty. Many individuals move from simple to advanced medical procedures to recreate their body parts. Africa is not left out, it accounted for 1.7 % of cosmetic surgeries performed in 2010 (ISAPS 2011). Since enhancement pills can be ordered without medical encounter, the use of non-surgical procedures remains largely undocumented. The rise of the medicalisation of beauty also holds enormous implications for human societies. Cosmetic enhancement can improve social relations and boost self-esteem. Many of the procedures can lead to adverse events. The use of unregulated pills and injections could amount to safety risks. More so, it can lead to unwarranted demand (bandwagon effects) of such procedures among healthy individuals. There is a growing obsession with medicalised beautification. For instance, in 2011 there were over nine million surgical and non-surgical cosmetic procedures in the United States and the trend has been growing over the years (ASAPS 2012).

9.1.6.3 The Medicalisation of Dying and Death

Dying and death have also been aggressively medicalised. There are varying related concepts such as natural, good, bad, assisted deaths, and, more importantly, clinical death. The modern image of death has spread with medical civilisation and has been a major force in cultural colonisation (Illich 1976), thereby shaping how individuals conceptualise death and respond to the process of dying. The image of death often signifies culturally conditioned anticipation of death at an uncertain date shaped by institutional structures, deep-seated myths, and the social character that predominates (Illich 1976). Among many cultures in Africa, death could be natural, accidental, or caused by evildoers (this relates to mystical beliefs), and it is often followed by some cultural rites. Through medicalisation, the physician now plays *significant* roles in the legitimation of death: predicting death or its risk, certification of death, and generally assisting and moderating the process of dying. Palliative care, including terminal sedation, is meant to assist the patient in the process of dying to make the process go more smoothly, dignified, and with less pain.

"Death by request" (i.e., euthanasia) is now a ranging phenomenon. Euthanasia (also called mercy killing) is a deliberate death but differs from suicide because it is part of medicalised practice and for medical reasons. It is the practice of ending the life of an individual who is suffering from a terminal illness or incurable disease/condition. It may be active (voluntary), such as by administration of a lethal drug, or passive, such as by withholding or withdrawing treatment or medical support (e.g., artificial ventilation, nutrition, respiration, and hydration) to hasten a terminally ill patient's death. Many countries, including the United States and United Kingdom, do not regard withholding withdrawal of treatment as euthanasia in cases of patients with poor prognosis. Active euthanasia could take the form of physician assisted suicide (PAS), when the physician delivers the means, and supports the patient to commit suicide. Another dimension of medically assisted death involves an advanced directive, especially a non-resuscitation directive. While non-resuscitation directives cannot be regarded as euthanasia, it is deliberate and the parties involved are aware of the fatal outcome. Like in the Netherlands and Belgium where euthanasia has been depenalised, there are a number of conditions to be fulfilled before it can be granted. In the Netherlands situation, it must be an informed decision of the patient, the action must be legitimised by two or more physicians and performed by a physician; the medical condition must be incurable or irreversible with suffering that cannot be alleviated and legal authorities must be informed (see Buiting et al. 2008).

Invariably, "good death" is gradually becoming a commodity, a new desire, which can be medically moderated. When the "death" at the societal level is easily recognised, it takes a lot of clinical effort and arguments to certify certain deaths or moderate the process of dying, such as for patients who are brain-dead or in a persistent vegetative state. There is also an intense debate about whether euthanasia (active or passive) is part of good or ethical medical practice. This is mainly because it seems to contradict the Hippocratic or ethical principle of non-maleficence and cultural/religious prescriptions in many countries.

From the foregoing, it is evident that everything is being pathologicalised. As Conrad (2013) observed, medicalisation is becoming global. While the process began in the western world, the trend is increasingly becoming evident in the developing world including Africa. Media hegemony from the western world is sending a lot of imitable medicalised signals to Africa. For instance, as previously mentioned, pharmaceutical products can be ordered online. In terms of geneticisation, a number of paternity disputes in Africa is being resolved through DNA testing. Many Africans are also opting for both surgical and nonsurgical procedures to augment various parts of their bodies. African is also witnessing, though slowly, a gradual demedicalisation of female cutting/circumcision. In short, globalisation of medicalisation is a new reality and thus a sociological analytical category, which requires further exploration especially in Africa where it is currently understudied.

9.2 Client-Practitioner Relations

Client-practitioner (also called doctor-patient) relations still remain a fundamental aspect of care. There are frequent encounters between the care seekers and caregivers in the process of health care, and the nature of such relations affect the outcome of care. The client-practitioner relationship refers to the ways in which health workers and lay people (also referred to as clients or patients) interact during a medical consultation (Gabe et al. 2004). Many factors such as the context of the consultation and communication styles influence the relationship. In the clinical realm, this relationship has been historically framed in terms of benevolent paternalism, until the 1960s which marked the rise of medical ethics and consumerism (Truog 2012). There has been a gradual shift from the domination of the doctors to the maximisation of inputs from the clients in medical care. The major thesis is that while the "physicians may be experts on the medical facts of a patient's condition, those facts are never sufficient to specify a course of treatment; clinical decisions must always include consideration of the values and preferences of the patient" (Truog 2012, p. 581).

A client is regarded as a situated being with experience, beliefs, values, and expectations. Such values and personal biography must be considered to ensure *appropriate* care. Man is thus not like a machine that the engineer can bolt and unbolt without any considerations. A client still retains his/her rights in the medical setting. Despite medical facts, a competent patient has the right to accept or reject medical interventions or participate in clinical trials. There is also the possibility of exploitation in medical encounters; this is why self-determination is crucial. Clients can make informed decisions on medical facts which need to be explained to them. Four models of client-practitioner relations have been discussed in the literature.

9.2.1 Models of Client-Practitioner Relations

Szasz and Hollender (1956) were the first to advance models of client-practitioner relationships based on activity-passivity (paternalistic model), mutual participation (shared model), and guidance-cooperation. Since then, client-practitioner relations have been a discourse not only in medical sociology but also in public health, bioethics, and other allied disciplines. It should be noted that while there are a number of practitioners involved in the care process, the focus here will be on the physician. It is important to study client-practitioner relations because it significantly affects the utilisation of health facilities, quality and outcomes of care, clients' satisfaction and because of ethical challenges that often arise in the course of such relationships. Client-practitioner relations is a domain of power relations, with the patients more vulnerable and at risk of medical malpractices from errors of commission or omission. Emanuel and Emanuel (1992) identified four models of client-practitioner relationships which will be discussed in subsequent subsections.

9.2.1.1 The Paternalistic Model

The paternalistic model stems from medical paternalism, a form of medical monopoly of decision and approach in the treatment of patients. This is the traditional approach in medical care before it underwent considerable transformation in the 1960s. The model places the patient in a passive and compliant role. This is why it is often referred to as the activity-passivity model. It is a feature of the sick role, where the patient's obligation is to seek competent help and cooperate with the physician (Parsons 1951). In the paternalistic approach, the treating physician weighs the benefits and risks of each option alone or in consultation with other physicians and makes a decision based on clinical judgment and experience (Charles et al. 1999). It is assumed that the client lacks the technical knowledge in medical care and should rely on the expertise of the physician who is positioned to serve the client's interest. This requires an absolute transfer of trust in service delivery.

This model is a typical notion of the *physician is always right*. He/she is a professional guided by professional principles. Therefore, the physician acts like a parent or guardian who directs and implements the best options available, regardless of the client's preferences. When assessing the values of the patients, the physician utilises universal and objective measures. In this case, the physician plays an authoritative role and could impose treatment if need be, so far as it promotes the well-being of the client. When there are tensions between autonomy and well-being or choice and health, the physician's choice will always take precedence (Emanuel and Emanuel 1992).

9.2 Client-Practitioner Relations

While there are ethical concerns regarding this model because it undermines the values, freedom, and autonomy of the clients, it could be appropriate in some instances. In the case of emergency or incompetent clients, the model is suitable in taking and implementing technical decisions based on available best practices regarding the medical condition. Apart from these extreme situations, paternalism has been heavily criticised. It may involve appropriation of power and arbitrary use of professional power by the physician.

9.2.1.2 The Informative Model

In the informative model, also called the informed decision-making model, the physician provides relevant factual information to the clients regarding his/her condition and therapeutic options. The information should be adequate to enable the client to select an appropriate course of therapy. The physician informs the patient of his or her disease state, the nature of possible diagnostic and therapeutic interventions, the nature and probability of risks, possible medical interventions, benefits and adverse events associated with the therapies, areas of medical expertise available or otherwise, and any uncertainties in knowledge (Emanuel and Emanuel 1992, p. 2221). The client then makes an informed decision thereby exercising control over medical care. The major duty of the physician is to cooperate with the clients by implementing his/her informed choices. In the informed model, the patient takes responsibility of therapeutic decision. It is assumed that with adequate information, the clients can make the best decision for themselves (Charles et al. 1999).

The values of the client determine the choice, but such values might be far from medical facts or best technical options. For instance, a client may turn down a blood transfusion because of religious values even when it is the most appropriate medical option. The informative model undermines the values of the physician. The physician assumes the role of a technical expert and provides truthful and comprehensive information. He/she has to respect the informed choices of the clients. One major grey area is that this model is only applicable to a competent client. Also about the nature of diseases, in many cases of acute or accident, there might not be an opportunity for explanations or interaction with clients. Most of those conditions require timely intervention (to save life).

In the era of consumerism accompanied by the advancement of informed consent (in bioethics), the model is the best for obtaining legal authority to proceed with medical intervention after documented informed consent. The informed consent transfers the legal obligation of care to the physician. In case of incompetent clients, the informed consent can be obtained from a legal guardian. Another major issue in the informative decision-making is time. A physician (especially a general practitioner) often has a limited amount of time with each patient. This might affect the amount of information offered and the opportunity for the client to adequately digest the information provided before making a decision. Limited time can be further constrained by limited knowledge. The physician can only offer therapy options known to him/her at a particular moment (Wirtz et al. 2006). The judgment of the client might also be affected by lay knowledge and beliefs.

9.2.1.3 The Interpretive Model

In this model, the physician makes the therapeutic decision or implements selected options, but in conformity with the values and aspirations of the clients. Emanuel and Emanuel (1992) observed that the physician provides the patient with adequate information on the nature of the condition and the risks and benefits of possible interventions. The client then relates his or her values in manners understandable to the physician who then interprets and provides medical interventions that best realise the specific values and aspirations of the client. In this model, the physician needs some form of cultural competence to be able to comprehend the patient as a situated sociocultural being in order to appreciate the inputs of the clients in the care process.

The corresponding model is the activity-guidance model in which the physician acts based on the guidance or information provided by the client. Before action is taken, the physician counsels the client. According to Charles (1999), the information that a patient might reveal to the physician includes aspects of health history, lifestyle, social context (e.g., work and family responsibilities and relationships), health and treatment-related beliefs and fears, and previous treatment (e.g., self-medication) used. This model is also appropriate for a competent client. It is open to misinterpretation because it could be difficult for the physician to have an emphatic experience with the patient—in terms of illness and sociocultural experiences. The first contact between the parties might be time consuming and produce some difficulties. Subsequently, through mutual understanding, decisions can be reached more easily.

9.2.1.4 The Deliberative Model

The deliberative model can also be referred to as shared, mutual participation or the negotiation model. "Deliberation" implies that the parties involved discuss various aspects relating to the medical condition and ensure mutual understanding of values and priorities which guide the course of action. In this case, the patients' values are open to development and revision through moral discussion, which might lead to mutual understanding (Emanuel and Emanuel 1992). Charles et al. (1997, p. 681) elaborated that the deliberative model involves: first, that at least two participants (physician and patient) be involved; second, that both parties share information; third, that both parties take steps to build a consensus about the preferred treatment; and fourth, that an agreement is reached on the treatment to be implemented.

Emanuel and Emanuel (1992) further observed that the physician acts as a friend or teacher. The fundamental role of the physician involves articulating and persuading the patient of the most admirable values as well as informing the client and implementing the client's selected intervention after mutual understanding. The stronghold of the model is the interactional nature which ensures that there is adequate involvement and input from the parties concerned. In many cases, the significant others might also have input in the decision-making process. This signifies the possibility of external influences which might add value to the decision reached.

This model is often favoured in medical encounters because of its two-way flow of information—both parties are active and share the responsibility for the action taken. The model is in variance with the informative or paternalistic models in which only one party takes responsibility of the decision.

In sum, it is important to note that in practice, there is no one clear-cut choice among the models as it is possible to combine elements from various models in one decision-making process. The important endpoint is often to reach a decision that will not compromise care or infringe on the rights of both the client and practitioner.

References

Abraham, J. (2007). Building on sociological understandings of the pharmaceutical industry or reinventing the wheel? Response to Busfield's "pills, power, people". *Sociology, 41*(4), 727–736.

Abraham, J. (2009). Partial progress: Governing the pharmaceutical industry and the NHS, 1948–2008. *Journal of Health, Politics, Law and Policy, 34*, 931–977.

Abraham, J. (2010). Pharmaceuticalization of society in context: Theoretical, empirical and health dimensions. *Sociology, 44*, 603–622.

ASAPS (The American Society for Aesthetic Plastic Surgery). (2012). Highlights of ASAPS statistics on cosmetic surgery. http://www.surgery.org/sites/default/files/2011-quickfacts.pdf. Accessed on 13 Sept 2012.

Auvert, B., Taljaard, D., Lagarde, E., Sobngwi-Tambekou, J., Sitta, R., & Puren, A. (2005). Randomised, controlled intervention trial of male circumcision for reduction of HIV infection risk: The ANRS 1265 trial. *PLoS Medicine, 2*, 11, e298.

Bell, S. E., & Figert, A. E. (2012). Medicalization and pharmaceuticalization at the intersections: Looking backward, sideways and forward. *Social Science & Medicine, 75*, 775–783.

Buiting, H. M., Gevers, J. K. M., Rietjens, J. A. C., Onwuteaka-Philipsen, B. D., van der Maas, P. J., van der Heide, A., & Delden, J. J. M. (2008). Dutch criteria of due care for physician-assisted dying in medical practice: A physician perspective. Journal of Medical Ethics, *34*, e12. doi:10.1136/jme.2008.024976.

Busfield, J. (2006). Pills, power, people: Sociological understandings of the pharmaceutical industry. *Sociology, 40*, 2297–2314.

Busfield, J. (2010). 'A pill for every ill': Explaining the expansion in medicine use. *Social Science & Medicine, 70*(6), 934–941.

Carpenter, L. M. (2010). On remedicalisation: Male circumcision in the United States and Great Britain. *Sociology of Health and Illness, 32*(4), 613–630.

Castro, A. L. (2011). Health and cosmetics: The medicalization of beauty. *RECIIS, 5*(4), 14–22.

Charles, C., Gafni, A., & Whelan, T. (1997). Shared decision-making in the medical encounter: What does it mean? (Or it takes at least two to tango). *Social Science & Medicine, 44*(5), 681–692.

Charles, C., Gafni, A., & Whelan, T. (1999). Decision-making in the physician-patient encounter: Revisiting the shared treatment decision-making model. *Social Science & Medicine, 49*, 651–661.

Conrad, P. (1992). Medicalization and social control. *Annual Review of Sociology, 18*, 209–232.

Conrad, P. (2005). The shifting engines of medicalization. *Journal of Health and Social Behavior, 46*, 3–14.

Conrad, P. (2007). The medicalization of society: On the transformation of human conditions into treatable disorders. Baltimore: Johns Hopkins University Press.

Conrad, P. (2013). Medicalization: Changing contours, characteristics, and contexts. In W. C. Cockerham (Ed.), Medical sociology on the move: New directions in theory (pp. 195–214). Dordrecht: Springer.

Daniels, N. (2000). Normal functioning and the treatment-enhancement distinction. *Cambridge Quarterly of Healthcare Ethics, 9*(3), 309–322.
Emanuel, E., & Emanuel, L. L. (1992). Four models of the physician-patient relationships. *JAMA, 267*(16), 2221–2226.
Filc, D. (2004). The medical text: Between biomedicine and hegemony. *Social Science & Medicine, 59*, 1275–1285.
Foucault, M. (2003). The birth of the clinic. London: Routledge.
Freese, J., & Shostak, S. (2009). Genetics and social enquiry. Annual Review *of* Sociology, *35*, 107–128.
Freidson, E. (1970). The profession of medicine: A study of the sociology of applied knowledge. New York: Doodd, Mead & Company.
Gabe, J., Bury, M., & Elston, M. A. (2004). *Key concepts in medical sociology*. London: Sage.
Gracia, J. R., Mackillop, J., Aller, E. L., Merriwether, A. M., Wilson, D. S., & Lum, J. K. (2010). Association between dopamine D4 receptor gene variation with both infidelity and sexual promiscuity. *PLOS ONE, 5*(11), e14162. doi:10.1371/journal.pone.0014162.
Halfmann, D. (2012). Recognizing medicalization and demedicalization: Discourses, practices, and identities. *Health, 16*(2), 186–207.
Hedgecoe, A. M. (2009). Geneticization: Debates and controversies. In *Encyclopaedia of Life Sciences (ELS)*. Chichester: John Wiley & Sons, Ltd. DOI: 10.1002/9780470015902.a0005849.pub2.
Illich, I. (1975). The medicalization of life. *Journal of Medical Ethics, 1*, 73–77.
Illich, I. (1976). *The limits of medicine: medical nemesis: The expropriation of health*. London: Marion Boyars.
ISAPS. (2011). International survey on aesthetic/cosmetic procedures performed in 2010. http://www.isaps.org/files/html-contents/ISAPS-Procedures-Study-Results-2011.pdf. Accessed 13 Sept 2012.
Johanson, R., Newburn, M., & Macfarlane, A. (2002). Has medicalisation of childbirth gone too far? British Medical Journal, *324*, 82–85.
Lin, P., & Allhoff, F. (2008). Untangling the debate the ethics of human enhancement. *Nanoethics, 2*, 251–264.
Lippman, A. (1991). Prenatal genetic testing and screening: Constructing needs and reinforcing inequities. *American Journal of Law and Medicine, 17*, 15–50.
Lippman, A. (1992). Led (astray) by genetic maps: The cartography of the human genome and healthcare. *Social Science & Medicine, 35*(12), 1469–1476.
Oakley, A. (1979). *Becoming a mother*. Oxford: Martin Robertson.
Oakley, A. (1984). *The captured womb: A history of the medical care of pregnant women*. Oxford: Blackwell.
Parsons, T. (1951). *The social system*. Glencoe: Free.
Pavone, V. (2008). *Genetic testing, geneticization and social change: Insights from genetic experts in Spain*. Paper presented in the Prime-Latin America Conference at Mexico City, September 24–26.
Phelan, J. C. (2005). Geneticization of deviant behaviour and consequences for stigma: The case of mental illness. *Journal of Health and Social Behavior, 46*(4), 307–322.
Szasz, T. (1970). *The manufacture of madness: A comparative study of the inquisition and the mental health movement*. New York: Harper & Row.
Szasz, T. S., & Hollender, M. H. (1956). A contribution to the philosophy of medicine: The basic models of the doctor–patient relationship. *Archives of Internal Medicine, 97*, 589–592.
Ten Have, H. A. M. J. (2012). Geneticisation: Concept. In *Encyclopaedia of Life Sciences (ELS)*. Chichester: John Wiley & Sons, Ltd. DOI: 10.1002/9780470015902.a0005896.pub2.
Truog, R. D. (2012). Patients and doctors—the evolution of a relationship. *The New England Journal of Medicine, 366*(7), 581–585.
Weiss, H. A., Dickson, K. E., Agot, K., & Hankins, C. A. (2010). Male circumcision for HIV prevention: Current research and programmatic issues. *AIDS, 24*(Suppl 4), S61–S69.

WHO/UNAIDS. (2007). *WHO and UNAIDS Announce Recommendations from Expert Consultation on Male Circumcision for HIV Prevention.* Geneva: UNAIDS.

Williams, S. J., Martin, P., & Gabe, J. (2011). The pharmaceuticalization of society? A framework for analysis. *Sociology of Health & Illness, 33,* 710–725.

Wirtz, V., Cribb, A., & Barber, N. (2006). Patient–doctor decision-making about treatment within the consultation–A critical analysis of models. *Social Science & Medicine, 62,* 116–124.

Zola, I. K. (1972). Medicine as an institution of social control. *Sociological Review, 20*(4), 484–504.

Chapter 10
Medical Pluralism: Traditional and Modern Health Care

10.1 Introduction

In all societies, there are alternative or complementary health care systems. However, in modern societies, biomedicine that claims to be evidence-based dominates the health systems. This is why other systems are often referred to as complementary or alternative medicine. The so-called complementary and alternative medicine (CAM) often predates modern medicine; it comprises ways or practices used in medical care before the introduction of modern medicine, but outlives modernisation. The term "medical pluralism" (in this context) is used to describe the coexistence of biomedicine and alternative medicine. Therefore, medical pluralism (MP) refers to "the coexistence in a society of differing medical traditions, grounded in different principles or based on different world-views" (Gabe et al. 2004, p. 183). In other words, MP can be defined as the adoption of more than one medical system or the use or integration of both conventional biomedicine and complementary and alternative medicine for health and illness.

Apart from modern medicine that is derived from scientific knowledge, there are other numerous medical traditions which are grouped as alternative and/or complementary medicine. This includes various forms of traditional medicine such as herbal medicine, acupuncture, chiropractic, and osteopathy. Alternative medicine refers to a medical tradition often devoid of systematic and scientifically verifiable evidence, which people sometimes use in the treatment and prevention of diseases. Alternative medicine is usually derived from historical and cultural traditions. On the other hand, complementary medicine is the phenomenon of the mix of modern and traditional medicines. In this case, traditional medicine is used alongside orthodox medicine. This is why complementary medicine is sometimes referred to as integrative medicine. The National Center for Complementary and Alternative Medicine (NCCAM 2012) defines CAM as a group of diverse medical and health care systems, practices, and products that are not generally considered part of conventional medicine. Conventional medicine (also herein called modern, western, orthodox, or allopathic medicine) is medicine as practiced by those who are formally trained in biomedical sciences. These people include the physicians, pharmacists, nurses, and other allied health professionals, such as physical therapists and psychologists.

Alternative medicine is usually derived from the cultural worldview of the people it serves. This is why there are countless types that are specific to particular ethnic and religious groups (e.g., Chinese, Korean, Yoruba, and Zulu traditional medicines). Cultural variation or multiplicity accounts for the variety of alternative medicines, which are mirrored in the country's pluralistic medical systems and beliefs surrounding the concepts of illness and health. The conception of health and illness often varies within the systems. Han (2002) observed that in pluralistic medical systems, there are divergent sickness labels and multiple interpretations of illness conditions. Pluralism also results from heterogeneous cultures with differential traditional care patterns.

Many people identify with alternative medicine because its existence provides options in health care. There is still a preference for alternative medicine among many individuals in both developing and developed countries. In most societies, there is competition between modern and alternative medicine in the care of the patients. Alternative medical practitioners often lay claim of expertise on various illness conditions. In most instances, they are closer to community members than the orthodox medical practitioners. And importantly, modern medicine has not been able to resolve all health problems, and alternative medicine often claims to fill the gap of medical possibilities. This is why they are still relevant.

Like other societies, African societies are not left out. Medical pluralism is a major feature of the health care system. Alternative medicine is osometimes called traditional medicine (TM). Here, some major issues in traditional and modern medicine will be discussed with African examples.

10.2 Traditional Medicine in Africa

There are as many traditional medicines (TM) as there are societies in Africa. Every ethno-religious group develops peculiar medical practices and beliefs based on historical and cultural development. TM is a comprehensive term used to refer to systems such as traditional Chinese medicine, Indian ayurveda, Arabic unani medicine, African medicine, and other forms of indigenous medicine (Alves and Rosa 2007). The WHO has come to recognise TM as a part of the care system in global health care. One of the first major WHO efforts in this direction was a meeting of African regional experts in Brazzaville in 1976 in which working definitions for TM and African traditional medicine were adopted. The meeting was followed by another one in Geneva in 1977 which aimed at fashioning strategies to promote traditional medicine. Since then, there have been several WHO reports on traditional medicine. Traditional medicine, also referred to as indigenous or folk medicine, is defined as "the sum total of the knowledge, skills, and practices based on the theories, beliefs, and experiences indigenous to different cultures, whether explicable or not, used in the maintenance of health as well as in the prevention, diagnosis, improvement or treatment of physical and mental illness" (WHO 2000, p. 1). Such knowledge and experience are passed from one generation to the next and could be preserved in writing or passed on orally.

Traditional medicine is considered an amalgamation of dynamic medical know-how and ancestral experience. Traditional African medicine is the sum total of all "practices, measures, ingredients and procedures of all kinds, whether material or not, which from time immemorial had enabled the African to guard against disease, to alleviate his [or her] sufferings and cure himself [or herself]" (WHO 1976, p. 3–4). The WHO African regional experts also define a traditional medical practitioner or traditional healer as a person "who is recognised by the community in which he/she lives as competent to provide health care by using vegetable, animal and mineral substances and certain other methods based on the social, cultural and religious backgrounds as well as the prevailing knowledge, attitudes and beliefs regarding physical, mental and social well-being and the causation of disease and disability in the community." From the foregoing definitions, some basic features of traditional medicine are evident.

1. **Traditional medicine uses physical materials in health care, which may include herbs and animal parts.** The major uniqueness here centres on the fact that such physical materials might not be refined. Herbal materials include crude plant material such as leaves, flowers, fruit, seeds, stems, wood, bark, roots, and other plant parts which may be fragmented or powdered, boiled, or consumed raw. Another category of physical materials include animal parts : a whole animal such as birds, reptiles, insects, and fish; and animal parts (e.g., leopard bones, antelope, buffalo or rhino horns, chameleon skin, deer antlers, testicles and penis of a dog, bear or snake bile) could be used to prepare concoctions and formulas to treat diseases. Alves and Rosa (2005) noted that animal byproducts (e.g., hooves, skins, bones, feathers, tusks) form important ingredients in the preparation of curative, protective, and preventive medicine. Other physical materials that could be used include sand, stone, water, and a number of derivatives from plants and animals.

2. **Traditional medicine has spiritual aspects**. This is a non-physical aspect of TM, which non-practitioners often regard as crude mystification. This is the realm of expression of magical powers and communication with the underworld. This is why lay people often refer to traditional medicinal practitioners as "witch doctors" with diabolic and terrestrial powers. The incantations, invocation of the gods, spiritual revitalisation, and supplications are the underlying foundation of the healing powers of traditional healers. Incantation or enchantment is a form of verbal invocation backed by spiritual powers, which can be used to create a spell or inject efficacy into a charm. Incantations can also be used for magical transformation of material and immaterial events with the use of metaphysical powers. In most African cultures, there is a metaphysical belief in the supernatural or ancestral beings who have links with worldly affairs. In most cases, the ancestors/spirits need to be worshipped, pleased, or atoned, sometimes with ceremonies or sacrifices.

3. **Traditional medicine is not scientific or amenable to science**. As previously mentioned, TM has both physical and spiritual aspects. Some of the physical aspects might be amenable to science because the plant and animal parts may

contain active ingredients that, according to biomedicine, could cure diseases. The spiritual aspect is less amenable to science. It sometimes consists of illogical actions and events, which account for the difficultly in establishing the link between the means and the ends. The "efficacious" power of incantations and prayers in healing cannot always be empirically explained. A series of incisions on the forehead to cure a headache, placing a sacrifice at the crossroads to cure infertility, or the offering of kolanuts to the gods for bountiful farm harvest are, in scientific explanations, mysteries, illogical and simply unscientific. The belief that disease or illness can be inflicted on a person by enemies, witches, ancestors, or gods (which is valid in traditional medicine) is also a mystery.

4. **Traditional medicinal methods are derived from the worldview of a society**. The worldview includes historical accounts and practices. Most of the ancestors and gods are believed to have existed at a point in time. The living can then relate with them to resolve the unknown, seek protection, or to gain (additional) powers. For instance, the Yoruba in southwestern Nigeria, as well as some peoples from Latin American countries and the Caribbean, believe in the existence of a god of thunder called *Sango*, who was once a king in the Oyo kingdom before his posthumous deification. He is seen as a source of thunder or lightning and could be invoked to resolve an unclear situation, punish evildoers, provide protection, or to make rain. Generally in Africa, the popularity of traditional healers is attributed to the fact that they take full account of the sociocultural background, historical events, beliefs of the people, and their implications for health and well-being. (Tella 1979).

5. **Traditional medicinal knowledge and practices are passed from one generation to the next**. Knowledge is passed on in writing or orally from father to son or practitioners to trainees. Healing knowledge is *jealously* guarded in certain families (Tella 1979). First, indigenous cultures are noted for their oral tradition and deep-rooted understanding of the sociocultural milieu. The practitioners are well versed in the names, eulogies, attributions, proscriptions, prescriptions, atonement patterns, and requirements of the ancestors and gods. For instance, in the Yoruba tradition, Esu is one of the gods with unique eulogies, atonement, and ritual requisites, which must be strictly followed to avert his wrath. These eulogies and patterns of atonement are embedded in oral traditions, which are learnt by heart and passed from one generation to the next.

6. **Traditional medicine is based on experience, not experiments**. Expertise in TM is derived from the accumulation of experiences in the cultural system of healing. This also involves the amassing of spiritual or metaphysical powers. Apart from having knowledge of herbs, the possession of metaphysical powers helps one relate to the ancestors and obtain (divine) prescriptions when necessary. The experience here signifies the extent of spirituality or metaphysical adventures. Traditional knowledge is derived from *cultural and metaphysical experiences* but not technical qualification. The experience is necessary because the gods usually reveal the cause(s) of illness to the practitioners through divine consultations (Taye 2009). There is no specific competency required, but recognition within the community.

10.2.1 Categories of Traditional Healers

There are a number of categories or specialties in traditional medicine. Often, the different specialties work together to ensure better health outcomes. Some of these specialties include herbalists, diviners, traditional birth attendants, traditional surgeons, traditional medicinal ingredient sellers, traditional bonesetters, traditional psychiatrists, and faith-based healers. The next few subsections will discuss these various specialties.

10.2.1.1 Herbalists

Herbalists are usually one of the most visible categories of the traditional healers. Herbalists mainly use herbs, that is, medicinal plants such as roots, stems, leaves, stem bark, flowers, fruits, seeds; whole or parts of animals such as snails, snakes, chameleons, tortoises, lizards, and so forth; inorganic residues such as alum, camphor, salt, and so on; and insects, such as bees and black ants (Adesina 2012). One or more combinations of these medicinal plants and animal parts are used to make preparations (e.g., medicine, concoction, ointment, and so on). Adesina (2012) further observed that such herbal preparations may be offered in various forms, including:

1. Powder, which could be swallowed or taken with pap (similar to drinkable maize pudding) or any drink. The powder could also be rubbed into incisions made on any part of the body with a sharp blade. There may be instructions on a specific number of incisions and a particular part of the body to be incised.
2. Preparation, soaked for some time in water or local gin, decanted as required before drinking; the materials could also be boiled in water, cooled, and strained. This form of preparation could also be used for bathing.
3. Preparation pounded with native soap and used for bathing; such "medicated soaps" are commonly used for skin diseases but could also be meant for ritual baths for protection or to ward off bad fate.
4. Pastes, pomades, or ointments in a medium of palm oil, shea butter, or olive oil. This could also be for daily use for protection against evildoers or to treat skin problems and other form of diseases.
5. Soup (usually called concoction) which is consumed by the patient. Such concoctions may be prepared with animal parts but may also include medicinal plants.

10.2.1.2 Diviners

This category of practitioners is perceived to have enormous metaphysical powers as they serve as a link between humans and the ancestors. They have inner sight to see the spirits and inner ears to communicate with them. As explained in Chap. 2, disease or illness in African cultures is often attributed to both mystical and supernatural causes. In such cases, there is need for special diagnosis and intervention. Diviners have the power to explain mystical and supernatural causes of illness. They explain the "unexplainable" problems or biomedically unexplained symptoms, and they also help by foretelling the future or human destiny with the help of the spirits and ancestors. The diviners mostly concentrate on diagnosing the unexplainable and other complex situations that cannot be treated with ordinary herbs. They need to reveal the hidden through mediumistic powers. They analyse the causes of specific events and interpret the messages of the ancestors.

Among the Yorubas, some diviners perform metaphysical consultation with a divination tray and chain. Through the mediumistic power, he/she hears revelations through the *orisa* (the gods) or spirits. The gods or witches would disclose what kind of atonement is required to cure inflictions. There are some diviners who are also versed in the use of herbs; they are called diviner-herbalists. Like the herbalists, such diviners know that traditional ingredients have certain recognisable effects on the human body when ingested, mixed, or applied in various ways (Hirst 2005). Diviners are essentially oracle or ritual specialists; they make use of enchantments and incantations and have the power of foresight or prophesy. For all cases of illness condition, diviners are usually the last resort.

Diviners do not only assist in health care, they are believed to be relevant in all aspects of social existence. They attend to various forms of problems affecting people, ranging from mate selection and marital relationships to occupational progress. They do all sorts of protective and preventive charms to void evil plots, avoid accidents or misfortunes and victimisation; they make all sorts of powerful charms for money rituals, traditional bulletproof charm, life prolongation, protection from evildoers, and punishment of social deviation (e.g., stealing, sexual assaults, and social injustice). Some of the diviners are also custodians of the deities in Africa. The diviners lead rituals and worship of the gods during which adherents or care seekers also pray and make requests from the gods.

10.2.1.3 Traditional Birth Attendants

Traditional birth attendants (TBAs) are also known as traditional, community, or lay midwives. A majority of TBAs are old mothers who have had multiple births and there are a number of men as well. They are primarily responsible for pregnancy-related issues including childbirth and child care. The WHO (1992) defines a TBA as a person who assists the mother at childbirth and initially acquires her/his skills by delivering babies by herself/himself and/or by working with other birth attendants. With the recognition of their roles in maternal health, some TBAs have undergone training through the modern health care sector to upgrade his/her skills by acquiring some basic best practices. Services could be delivered at the patient's home since the TBAs are well known in their communities and they are often called to assist women at the time of delivery.

In most societies in which resources are limited, more than half of pregnant women deliver at home without assistance from health care professionals (Wilson et al. 2011).

Over 80% of world maternal mortality occurs in developing countries. TBAs have been filling some of the gap in maternal care. Some of the TBAs also have knowledge of herbs. They attend to pregnant women in cases of pregnancy-related danger signs and take care of the newborn. Izugbara and Ukwayi (2003) observed that apart from delivery, TBAs also provide additional services such as abortion, child sex selection, family planning, and cures for infertility, STDs, serial miscarriage, and vaginal bleeding. Some of these maternal services are complicated at times, which is why it is essential that the TBAs are trained to use basic best practices in maternal care and know when to refer some maternal-related complications to the biomedical services.

Some women are attracted to traditional birth homes (TBHs) because their services are less expensive, provide required privacy regarding their conditions, and the women are confident in the "skills" of TBAs (Izugbara and Ukwayi 2003); however, many women still prefer home delivery, and the TBAs are the closest option for home delivery. While TBAs attend to over 50 million births annually, most of them do not possess the requisite standard skills to recognise, manage, and prevent pregnancy-related complications (WHO 1997). Due to the lack of prompt referrals of complicated cases to the modern facility, many TBAs contribute to delays subsisting maternal mortality in rural, poor, and illiterate communities (Umeora and Egwuatu 2010). If training is provided for the TBAs, they could serve as a major source of referrals in cases of complication during delivery. In many countries (including Ghana, DR Congo, and Zimbabwe), trained TBAs are gradually being incorporated into primary health care (PHC). This, however, is not universally accepted by the biomedical sector.

10.2.1.4 Traditional Surgeons

There are also traditional medicine practitioners who specialise in surgery. They have special skills in the use of local surgical knives and scissors. The most common duty of these local surgeons is traditional male circumcisions, usually performed in a non-clinical setting. In many African rural communities, male circumcision is a ceremonious ritual where males are initiated into manhood or another age-grade. The initiates gather after some traditional rites and the local surgeon starts the circumcision process. The local surgeon is also responsible for traditional tattooing and scarification or what is otherwise known as tribal marks (on the face or other parts of the body). A tattoo could be any form of inscription or drawing with the use of traditional knives. More so, Miles and Ololo (2003) and Wilcken et al. (2010) reported that itinerant traditional surgeons work throughout sub-Saharan Africa and perform many other procedures including tooth extraction, abortion, injections, incising and draining abscesses, uvulectomy, inguinal hernia surgery, non-invasive cataract luxation, and surgery on closed and open fractures.

Traditional surgeons have been heavily criticised. For instance, Miles and Ololo (2003) observed that cutting and injection equipment is not always cleaned properly and might be reused in rapid succession for many patients in a single clinic session. The re-use of unsterilised equipment could result in a number of health problems including tetanus, gangrene, contractures, abscesses, iatrogenic fistulae, and transmission of HIV, hepatitis, and other infectious diseases. Female and male circumcision is often performed for religious and cultural reasons. At times, traditional surgeons do not use recommended circumcision instruments (Peltzer et al. 2008). Despite movement to stop female circumcision (clitoridectomy), which has been equated to genital mutilation, many traditional surgeons continue to perform it. Traditional surgeons will continue to be an important source of circumcision for many males, especially in rural African communities (Wilcken et al. 2010). It will be beneficial to provide basic training in best practices for this category of care providers to avert complications that sometimes arise from their practices.

10.2.1.5 Traditional Medicinal Ingredient Dealers

A majority of the dealers of traditional medicinal ingredients are women who specialise in the buying and selling of plants, animals (or their parts) and insects, and minerals used in making herbal preparations and in ritual and sacrificial atonements. Usually, sections of major markets (or a number of stalls) are dedicated to the sale of medicinal ingredients. Like drugs are prescribed in modern medical practice, an herbalist may simply prescribe the ingredients to be used and how they will be used. The care seekers resort to the dealers to buy items required for the herbal preparation or concoction. Nowadays, some of the dealers, along with ingredients, sell basic herbal preparations and concoctions for immediate use. This accounts for the proliferation of herb sellers in African urban cities. They mainly sell herbs to cure common ailments, such as dysentery, malaria, and STDs; aphrodisiac herbs are also sold to treat sexual impotency or enhance sexual performance.

The dealers depend on the traditional hunters for the supply of animals, their parts, or byproducts for sale. It is common to find living and dead animals (e.g., birds, chameleons, snakes, snails, tortoises, monkeys, squirrels, antelopes, pangolins, etc.) and their body parts on display for sale. The poaching of animals for the medicinal trade is common in African countries. Endangered species are hunted because they are often required for medicinal purposes and yield more income for the poachers and medicinal dealers. An herbalist or diviner may require the tusk of an elephant, tongue of a lion, scales of a pangolin, skin/scales or tail of a python, kidney of a hippopotamus, the left eye of a leopard, and, at the extreme, the body parts of human beings for rituals. Ritualists, healers, diviners, and traditional medicinal users usually approach the traditional medicinal ingredient dealers to procure some of these items.

10.2.1.6 Traditional Bonesetters

Traditional bonesetters (TBSs) are specialised in bonesetting or traditional orthopaedic surgery, or the art of setting fractures and other orthopaedic injuries. Traditional bonesetters are those knowledgeable in the art and skill of setting broken bones in the traditional way, using their skill to see that bones unite and heal properly (Adesina 2012). In sub-Saharan Africa, community members still prefer native bonesetting to modern orthodox treatment (Dada et al. 2011; Udosen et al. 2006). For instance in Nigeria, more than 80 % of patients with fractures present first to traditional bonesetters (Dada et al. 2011). TBSs use traditional methods in bonesetting, which are not always consistent with the biomedical approach. They also use metaphysical powers to ensure fracture healing. Dada et al. noted that the origin of the practice is shrouded in mystery, but practitioners pass on the knowledge from one generation to another.

It is generally agreed that TBSs have made some contributions in the management of fractures, but their services are not devoid of some dangerous practices. They could serve as important referral links and could also benefit from basic training in modern orthopaedics to minimise harmful practices and consequently minimise complications and help refer complicated cases to the biomedical sector.

10.2.1.7 Traditional Psychiatrists

This is a specialty of traditional healers who care for those with various forms of mental disorders. A majority of the healers are diviner-herbalists, and they are able to use divination to understand the aetiology of the mental problem, especially in case of supernatural and mystical forces. They also administer herbs, concoctions, and other forms of preparations as therapy. Violent patients are treated with some level of violence, which ranges from flogging, chaining, and confinement to the administration of sedatives (Owumi 1996). The traditional psychiatrists often use different labels to describe what biomedical psychiatry categorises as psychotic disorders (Patel 2011). The traditional explanatory models conform to the traditional beliefs of the community. Most individuals in SSA still believe strongly in mystical causes of mental disorder, and traditional psychiatrists are considered better care providers in dealing with such mental illness. As there is still an unmet need for mental health services in most low- and middle-income countries, traditional psychiatry becomes the alternative therapy for patients and their families.

10.2.1.8 Faith-Based Healers

Faith-based healers (FBHs) are those who use religious principles in healing. Africa is a religious society. While traditional medicine is rooted in cultural beliefs, there was a gradual shift of religious beliefs with the advent of Christianity and Islam when many Africans converted to the modern religions. This subsection will briefly discuss faith-based healing as observable among Christians and Muslims. The healing practices are based on a spiritual connection with the Almighty God, who the adherents believe has solutions to all human problems. There is often general acclamation that *with God, all things are possible*. The same belief is applied in health care—that the all-powerful God can heal if one seeks for His intervention. Within religious circles, the FBHs emerged, using spiritual powers derived from a belief in God for health interventions. The spiritual healing focuses on the body, mind, and spirit. Ailment is most times viewed as a part of punishment for sinful endeavours.

Christian healers are prominent in health intervention. Modes of intervention differ from one denomination to another. The search for a spiritual intervention can be performed at the personal level or most times through consultation with religious leaders (e.g., pastors or bishops). Therapeutic intervention involves the casting of demonic powers that might be responsible for ailment, prayer sessions, spiritual bathing, sleeping in holy places, fasting, drinking of holy water, and applying of holy ointment. Alubo (1995, 2008) observed that spiritual healing takes place during open-air rallies and crusades, and such occasions are advertised in the mass media as opportunities for barren women to conceive, the bewitched to be freed, the demonised to be exorcised, and for others to be freed from other forms of affliction. The bedrock of religious intervention is the belief in the feasibility of miraculous healing with or without medical intervention. Thus some devoted Christians pray to God for healing in case of illness.

The Islamic healing process has its roots in the belief in Allah (God), who the adherents believe has power of healing without limitations. The Islamic healing practices can be categorised into three domains: Islamic religious text-based practices, Islamic worship practices, and folk healing practices (Alrawi et al. 2012). It was observed that each of the domains may further contain therapies such as spiritual healing, medicinal herbs, mind-body therapy, and dietary prescriptions. The Islamic healers (including imams and scholars) also draw from Prophetic prescriptions of use of natural medicinal products. Prayer sessions (or supplications) and Quranic recitation are held to secure the favour and mercy of Allah for salvation or delivery from all forms of affliction or ailments. Divine intervention in medical situations may be sought with or without the use of modern medicine.

10.2.2 *Determinants of Utilisation of Traditional Medicine*

The WHO has observed that in many Asian and African countries, a substantial majority of the population depends on traditional medicine for primary care. The traditional healers are available in large numbers, serving various communities, especially in resource-constrained societies where modern health care is limited. There is a growing demand for traditional or alternative medicine across African countries and even in western countries (Abdullahi 2011). Some of their medicines may be efficacious and, in fact, a few modern drugs are derivatives of the herbs used by the herbalists. It has been noted that over 100 countries now have some form of regulation for traditional medicine. With the resulting medical pluralism, people have a choice to make. With the heavy criticisms (see Sect. 10.2.3) of traditional medicine owing to some dangerous or unrefined practices, it is often assumed that people should rely more on the professionals with technical knowledge derived from evidence-based medicine.

10.2 Traditional Medicine in Africa

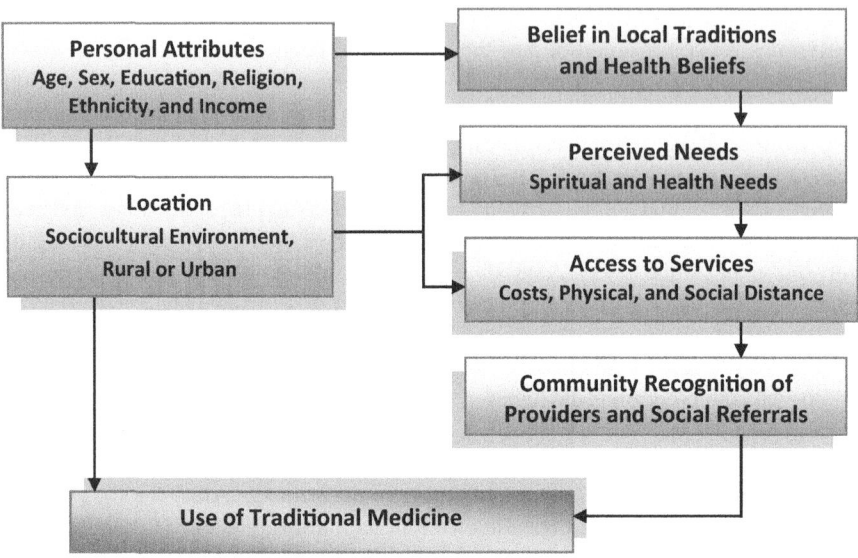

Fig. 10.1 Factors influencing use of traditional medicine

Figure 10.1 provides a basic framework, which shows factors influencing the use of traditional medicine.

Personal attributes often play a role in health care utilisation; the use of traditional medicine is not different. Factors such as age, education, and religion affect the utilisation of TM. The followers of traditional religion often rely on traditional medicine more than the followers of modern religions. While the use of TM cuts across all educational groups, its use is more prevalent among the less educated. Akighir (1982) observed that beliefs in mystical causes of psychiatric disorders were strong amongst uneducated people and those living in the more isolated rural areas. This may explain why people with less education use TM. More so, Sorsdahl et al. (2009) observed that the use of traditional healers was predicted by older age, race, unemployment, and a lower level of education. Figure 10.1 shows that personal attributes influence traditional health beliefs, which consequently determine perceived health needs.

Cultural beliefs also promote the use of traditional medicine. The belief in local traditions, especially the mystical and supernatural causes of illness, is strongly associated with the utilisation of TM. Such causes are believed to result in symptoms that cannot be explained by modern medicine; it is not uncommon for significant others to refer the ill to the traditional or spiritual healers. Cultural beliefs and subsequent use of traditional medicine are indications of cultural compatibility between parties. The traditional healers use incantations to seek the unknown from the gods while the faith-based healers use prayers and other spiritual means to resolve diabolic cases relating to illness. The cultural beliefs also dictate perceived needs both in terms of health and spiritual needs.

In most resource-constrained countries, there is limited access to modern health practitioners. Inadequate accessibility to modern medicines and drugs to treat and manage diseases in middle- and low-income countries, especially in Africa, contributes to the widespread use of TM, especially in poor households (Abdullahi 2011). Traditional healers usually reside in the community. The ratio of traditional healers to the population is far better than physicians to the population in many African countries (Abudullahi 2011). Moreover, traditional medicine is relatively less expensive to utilise. Apart from cultural preference, many poor households seek a more affordable and available health care option, which incidentally is TM. African countries continue to struggle to improve modern health services; unfortunately the high cost of allopathic medical health care and the expensive pharmaceutical products have become unavailable to a majority of people (Kofi-Tsekpo 2004), apart from a limited number of health care facilities. Figure 10.1 shows that access in terms of cost and physical and social distance also affects the utilisation of TM. Traditional healers reside in the community and might be aware of personal and historical antecedents of the community members. This explains (partly) why TM is patronised.

More importantly, the community recognition of traditional healers and social referral also promotes the use of TM. Once an individual is recognised in the community as competent to provide some service, referrals and acceptance are likely to increase. The practice of TM is based on the indigenous knowledge (Weisheit 2003) and, thus, traditional healers are an integral part of the local culture and are appreciated as key and sustainable sources of care. As such, they will continue to be relevant in health care; this is why the WHO acknowledges traditional medicine as a part of primary health care (PHC), to increase access to care and preserve knowledge and resources. The major issue is to provide basic training to the traditional practitioners to ensure a number of best practices. While this has been the argument over the years, there have been a number of shortcomings militating against the successful integration of traditional medicine into the mainstream of conventional medicine.

10.2.3 Shortcomings of Traditional Medicine

There have been a number of criticisms against traditional medicine. These criticisms are usually made in comparison to modern medicine. The criticisms also limit the full incorporation of TM into the modern medical system in many countries. When TM is integrated, its practitioners usually provide primary care, often under the supervisory role of conventional medical practitioners. The major criticisms are as follows:

1. **Traditional medicine is not entirely amenable to science.** As mentioned earlier, TM has both physical and spiritual parts. While the physical aspect may be made compatible with scientific practices, the spiritual part may not. The prayers, incantations, and supernatural and mystical beliefs are not within the realm of science. This implies that TM cannot be entirely evidence-based. It is difficult to (objectively) test the efficacy or demonstrable effects of incantations or prayers and make it a valid bio- or sociomedical prescription.

2. **Within traditional medical practice, there is no regulation of entry and exit.** While conventional medicine is based on technical qualification, TM is not. Knowledge is usually passed from one generation to another; a substantial part of the knowledge is orally preserved. There is an abundance of fake healers or those who lay questionable claims of therapeutic powers whose activities are difficult to curtail. Some of them lay claims that cannot be verified.
3. **A majority of the traditional medical practitioners still use traditional procedures and equipment.** Most of the herbal products are consumed raw, and most times there is a problem of measurement. The same herb that is meant for drinking could also be for bathing. Endangered animal parts may be required and hunted.
4. **From a biomedical point of view, traditional medical practice is devoid of procedural and objective diagnosis.** The dominant practice is devoid of a medical model of disease that is based on the establishment of pathogens responsible for a disease condition. A traditional healer may only need to consult with the deities to diagnose what could be wrong with an individual. Only those in the same spiritual world (with a similar power) can replicate the procedure.
5. **There is no standardisation of practice.** The deities differ from community to community. The mode of diagnosis or therapy might not be similar. Procedures vary from one healer to another. Ten healers may mean ten deities and ten different procedures. This has made it problematic to accommodate a number of variations of traditional techniques in a unified, conventional medical practice.
6. **The physical environment might be poor, equipment not sterilised, and personal hygiene might not be guaranteed.** In TM, most activities are carried out in a non-clinical or poor medical setting, which could also be detrimental to the well-being of their clients.
7. **While ethical issues cut across all medical practices, those in TM are cruder and highly unwholesome.** For instance, traditional healers sometimes engage in medicine murder, or the killing of human beings in order to use their body parts to prepare medicine (see Ashforth 1998; Bhootra and Weiss 2006; Salisbury and Roberts 2012; Vincent 2008). Basically, professional ethics are not a priority in TM compared to conventional practice.
8. **There is a need for more research on the safety of use of some herbal therapies in terms of both short- and long-term events.** This is because there are no standardised procedures for efficacy or toxicity tests of most traditional medicine products.

10.3 Modern Health Care in Africa

The remaining part of this chapter will focus on modern health care in Africa. It provides a brief historical account of modern medicine in Africa, a discussion of the components of modern health care systems, categories of modern health professionals, political organisation of health systems (utilitarian, capitalist, socialised and socialist, and two-tier heath care systems), levels of health care delivery (primary, secondary, and tertiary), and challenges of health care delivery in Africa.

10.3.1 A Brief Historical Note

The origin of modern medicine can be traced to the Scientific Revolution in western societies, which touched all aspects of life and triggered industrial development and, consequently, advancement in medicine, its organisation, and medical technology. Before modernisation, western countries also had mystical explanations of illness and death. Before the so-called modernisation, Egypt had one of most advanced medical systems based on advanced medical practices, technological progress, and public health (Thoral 2012). Generally, the 19th century marked the rise of modern medicine; there was scientific breakthrough in chemistry, physics, microbiology, pharmacology, medical technology, and equipment, followed by new evidence-based ideas of epidemiology, bacteriology, and virology. One of the remarkable social advancements was the dissipation of metaphysical and theological explanations of diseases and illnesses with scientific explanation. The birth of the germ theory or medical model of disease became prominent. The principle of antisepsis, development in surgery and nursing practice, and many more were products of modernisation. More importantly, the emergence of the enlightenment era, which promoted rationalism and empiricism, encouraged groundbreaking research and discoveries in medicine. Hence the medical transformations still continue.

The history of modern medicine in Africa is linked to colonialism. One major event is the scramble for Africa during the 1884–1885 Berlin conference in which African territories were partitioned among the imperial powers (including Britain, France, Portugal, Germany, Belgium, Spain, and Italy). While these nations exacted political control on African nations, they also brought with them a number of development activities, partly through the works of the missionaries. One of these activities was the introduction of modern medical practice. The inception of western medicine in Africa was in the service of the colonial agents and to facilitate the colonial interests; care for the colonial agents who were meant to open up Africa for trade and exploitation of resources (Burke-Gaffney 1968; Ityavyar 1987).

The physicians were part of the colonial team and offered medical treatment primarily to European explorers, missionaries, and colonial administrators and their families. In Nigeria, like in many other colonised African nations, the first generation of health facilities by the colonial state were located in cities and towns near the Atlantic Coast and were only for Europeans, and later for Africans employed by them (Ityavyar 1987). In the then-colonial state, social amenities were also accessible close to regions where the exploitation of resources was concentrated. The transportation system and educational development reflected the colonial priorities shaped by exploitative interests. Before the extension of the coverage of modern health care, other members of the population relied on traditional medicine for health care (Burke-Gaffney 1968).

Ityavyar (1987) observed that some provision of medical services was achieved because of pressures coming from the nationalist movements after the First World War for the colonialists to provide more amenities for local communities. The physicians also participated in the wars of colonisation and religion through medical evangelism. A great deal of the early provision of medical facilities for Africans was owed to the missionary enterprise. Selected medical students were trained for missionary work in Africa and missionaries were taught elements of medical practice (Burke-Gaffney 1968). The spread of modern health care began by locating a hospital along with a church and a school with every colonial post. A majority of the primary health posts established by the missionaries were concentrated near the populations who were the targets of evangelism (Ademiluyi and Aluko-Arowolo 2009).

Western medicine was not formally introduced into Nigeria until the 1860s, when the Sacred Heart Hospital was established by Roman Catholic missionaries in Abeokuta (now the capital of Ogun State in southwestern Nigeria) (Library of Congress 1991). The 1860s also marked the beginning of colonisation of Nigeria (specifically, Lagos). The missionaries played a central role not only in terms of the provision of health facilities but also manpower development. Missionaries opened teacher training colleges, nursing and midwifery schools, and training schools for other paramedicals, which were most needed for Nigeria's incipient health care system (Ityavyar 1987, p. 491). The first crops of indigenous medical officials were products of missionary scholarship. The religious missions were a major supplier of modern health care facilities in Nigeria, as missions accounted for about 40 % of hospital beds after independence from British colonialism in 1960 (Library of Congress 1991). It was further reported that by that time, the number of mission hospitals exceeded government hospitals in number: 118 mission hospitals compared with 101 government hospitals. Later, there was the colonial health development plan that led to the establishment of the University College of Ibadan in 1948 (now the University of Ibadan) with University College Hospital (UCH) in 1952. The objective of UCH was to facilitate manpower development in health care.

The experiences in Ghana (then the Gold Coast), Uganda, Tanganyika and Zanbibar (both now Tanzania), Kenya, and Sudan are similar to that of Nigeria. Modern health care was introduced to make Ghana hospitable to colonialism (Twumasi 1981). Health problems such as malaria and yellow fever constituted a great challenge for the Europeans. As described in 1821 when the British displaced the Dutch to take over the Gold Coast, the place was not very hospitable because of prevalent diseases. The 19th century marked the beginning of urban-centred health facilities and services in Ghana. The British Colonial Administration built hospitals in commercial and administrative centres, the few postal agencies were given anti-malarial drugs to distribute to government clerical officers, and clinics were located in cities and principal towns where colonists engaged in commercial and mining activities (Twumasi 1981). The missionaries and colonists also started providing basic medical training to the local population as some of them were employed to assist in nursing as well as in dispensaries and laboratories. It was observed that colonialism or the colonial exploitation of resources would have been impossible without the introduction of modern health services to protect the colonialists and local allies. In Uganda, the colonialists founded a hospital in 1897, and in Kenya, the colonial medical department was first organised in 1905 (Burke-Gaffney 1968).

The beginning of modern health services in North Africa (especially Morocco, Tunisia, and Algeria) is a bit different from what happened in SSA. The French colonialists classified North Africa as part of the tropics. Modern health care services were meant to support the colonial army responsible for the conquest of the colonial territories and maintenance of colonial order (Thoral 2012). The then-Arabic traditional medicine had some notable physicians (e.g., Avicenna in the 11th century and Averroes in the 12th century), who influenced the development of western medicine (Thoral 2012). It was further observed that in the early days of French colonialism in North Africa before scientific revolution in western medicine, the French assimilated some traditional Arabic medicine and exploited some medicinal ingredients for use in France. The process of medical encounters between French and non-European medical systems passed through a number of overlapping steps (Thoral 2012). The first was exploration and appropriation, which signified interest and direct borrowing from traditional non-European medicine. The second was exploitation of medical natural resources to improve health conditions in Europe. The last was subordination and imposition of modern health services, which happened in the later years of colonialism (late 19th and 20th centuries).

The settler colony of South Africa (SA) was more hospitable than the west coast. The political resistance and colonial policy of discrimination in SA led to social demarcation between the colonialists/white settlers, Africans, and other groups. The social polarisation also reflected in the provision and utilisation of modern health services (see Rensburg and Ngwena 2005). There have been white settlers (who battled with local indigenes of rights to their possessions) since 1652, before formal colonial rule from 1806 (Coovadia et al. 2009). In the early days of European encounters, the traditional healers served the African communities and the imported labourers while the European trained medical practitioners provided health services to the Europeans. An era of subjugation of the traditional healers started in the early 19th century and was followed by a period of marginalisation and indignation of traditional medicine in the late 19th century when orthodox medical practice became professionalised (Coovadia et al. 2009). Throughout the colonial and apartheid years, non-European communities were poorly served with modern medical services (see Rensburg and Ngwena 2005). The resulting health inequality was obvious and impaired the livelihood of the non-European people. The government of SA is still battling to resolve the historical health inequalities between the minority whites and the non-white majority.

The development of modern medicine through research and training has been progressive from the colonial to the postcolonial era. This is apart from medical reforms and concerted efforts to improve population health. More importantly, colonial evidence-based medicine or medical research also began during the same period. One subject of such significant research focused on the most deadly disease of the tropics—malaria. Ronald Ross, after establishing the vector agent of malaria, mosquitoes, through his research in India (from 1882–1899), made a research tour of Africa (especially West Africa) (Burke-Gaffney 1968). The interest in medical research led to the establishment of the Liverpool and London Schools of Tropical Medicine in 1898 and 1899, respectively, and the Wellcome Tropical Research Laboratories in Khartoum (Sudan) (through the generous donation of Henry S. Wellcome) in 1902, devoted to specialised training and research in tropical diseases (Abdel-Hameed 1997; Burke-Gaffney 1968).

Colonial contact marked the beginning of the coexistence of modern and traditional medicine, especially from the 19th century when full control of the colonies, the development of modern medicine, and subsequent subjugation of TM began. As there was inequality in the ability to access modern health services, the local population continued to rely heavily on traditional practitioners. The denigration of traditional medicine was a major feature of the colonial era. The missionaries also added their voice to "downgrade" the practice of traditional medicine. The new converts of the new religion were discouraged from utilising traditional medicine as the healers were known as "fetish healers," "magical men," and "witch doctors" (Twumasi 1981). There was obvious conflict of superiority between the two systems: the modern medical system often claimed to be systematic and evidence-based in diagnosis and treatment, thereby criticising TM as a primitive practice full of mysteries and witchcraft. With gradual cultural change and new religion, the local population began to accept the limited health services provided by the colonial government. Unfortunately, the pattern of health inequality created in terms of rural and urban centres, still persist.

The period after colonialism was fraught with a lot of health reforms based on further development of modern medical practices. Some of the reforms also affected traditional medicine as a number of countries were battling to incorporate TM (or complementary medicine) with modern medical practice. In the postcolonial era, modern medicine has been the mainstay in heath care in Africa. All the countries invest efforts to improve the provision of modern medical care.

10.3.2 The Components of the Modern Health Care System

A health care system consists of all organisations, people, and actions with the primary intent to promote, restore, or maintain health (WHO 2007, p. 2). It involves all levels of care (see Sect. 10.3.4) and efforts that could promote health whether educational, preventive, or control activities. Primary care at the home level is also considered to be a significant part of the health system. This implies that health care systems go beyond bureaucratic or formal structures. WHO (2007, p. 3) has identified six major components (see Fig. 10.2) of the health care system including:

1. **Service delivery**: the culture of service is the bedrock of a health care system. Health care is important to human functioning. Therefore, every society deserves good health services, which are effective, safe, and of a good quality, "when and where needed, with minimum waste of resource."
2. **Health workforce**: the driving force of the system involves trained or competent, committed, and efficient individuals who are motivated to deliver good health services "to achieve the best health outcomes possible, given available resources and circumstances." There is a need for a fair distribution of a sufficient workforce with an appropriate mix of professionals.

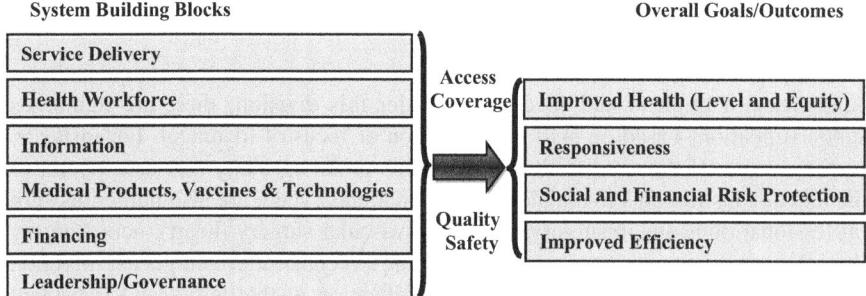

Fig. 10.2 WHO health system framework. (Source: WHO 2007, p. 3)

3. **Health information**: another vital component is a health information system that is functional and well-defined, to ensure "the production, analysis, dissemination and use of reliable and timely information on health determinants, health systems performance and health status." There should be appropriate feedback mechanisms, and actions should be based on available information or evidence.
4. **Medical products, vaccines, and technologies:** equitable distribution of essential medicinal products, vaccines, and technologies is also a vital component of a health system. The four major assurances in the use of products should include quality, safety, efficacy, and cost-effectiveness.
5. **Health financing** : this involves ways of raising adequate funds in manners that will remove financial barriers to accessing care. A good health financing system should guarantee affordability and attract adequate financing through budgeting and risk-pooling systems (e.g., insurance and welfarism).
6. **Leadership and governance:** this implies an effective and efficient course of action in order to harness available resources and provide strategic frameworks, regulations, and policies. Governance involves decision-making and priority setting on which other components of the system are built.

The modern health care system is bureaucratised as a system of coordinated units linked together by the goal of care and service. Each of the coordinated units engages in specialised functions that contribute to care and support the patients or service users. Other issues that will be discussed here include categories of the health workforce, the political organisation of health care, level of care, and challenges facing modern health services in Africa.

10.3.3 Categories of the Health Workforce

There are numerous professionals in the modern health care system. The general classification of health care professionals is often based on skills and skill specialisation. Such classification is not necessarily hierarchical, although sometimes it is. Modern health care practitioners can be grouped into the following five broad categories.

10.3.3.1 Medical

The physician (medical doctor) is grouped here. The medical division includes generalist practitioners and specialists. Under this division, there are numerous subclassifications based on skill specialisation or focus of treatment. For instance, surgery is one of the subdivisions here, which is the specialty that uses operative manual and instruments to diagnose or treat patients. There are also numerous sub-professional divisions in surgery, like cardiovascular surgery (heart), neurosurgery (brain), and orthopaedic surgery (bone fracture), reconstructive surgery (correction of deformities), cosmetic surgery (for beautification of the body), and transplant surgery (replacement of organs). Apart from the surgeons, there are other physicians classified based on the organ of specialty, nature of activities, disease, or age of patients. The specialty professionals include (among others) paediatricians (children), geriatricians (the elderly), cardiologists (heart), oncologists (cancer), gynaecologists and obstetricians (female reproductive system: pregnancy and childbirth), pulmonologists (respiratory tract), dermatologists (skin), psychiatrists (mental health), and radiologists (uses imaging to diagnose and treat disease visualised within the human body). Within each of these specialties, there are other subspecialties. Normally, the first contact in the modern health system is the general practitioners or primary care physicians who may then refer the care seeker to the appropriate specialty if specialised care is required.

10.3.3.2 Dentistry

This specialty of medicine is often classified separately from other medical divisions. It is a specialised division which focuses on oral health; it involves the study, diagnosis, prevention, and treatment of diseases and conditions of the oral cavity, including associated biological structures. The WHO regards oral health as a state of being free from mouth and facial pain, oral and throat cancer, oral infection and sores, periodontal (gum) disease, tooth decay, tooth loss, and other diseases and disorders that limit an individual's capacity in biting, chewing, smiling, speaking, and psychosocial well-being. The general practitioners of dentistry are called dentists. The specialty also has a number of subspecialties, which include dental public health (promotion of dental health through community efforts), endodontics (focuses on dental pulp and periradicular conditions), dental surgery (engages in surgical intervention in oral health), oral radiology (use of imaging in oral health), and periodontics or periodontology (focuses on tissues or structures of the teeth). Dental cavities or tooth decay and later loss of teeth affect almost all adults worldwide. There is a high level of unmet needs for dentistry.

10.3.3.3 Pharmaceutical

This division consists of professionals (usually called pharmacists) who are in charge of effective use of medication or medicament. The division manages medicament prescriptions, safety, and disbursement of medications. Major health facilities often have pharmacies where drugs can be obtained; pharmacies or drug stores are also located across cities. Pharmacists are vital members of the health care system. There are also growing specialties in pharmacy which include hematology/oncology, infectious diseases, ambulatory care, nutrition support, drug information, critical care, paediatrics, and many others. The major categories of pharmacists include community pharmacists, those who operate drug stores or pharmacies in the community and dispense based on prescription or prevailing legal regulations; and hospital or clinical pharmacists, who practice in the hospital setting and contribute in the management of medical cases. Clinical pharmacists often work together with physicians. Their roles may include the development of a therapy plan (drug choice, dose, route [intravenous, oral, or rectal], frequency, and duration of therapy), as well as monitoring of drug adherence and adverse events.

10.3.3.4 Nursing

The International Council of Nurses (2010) defined nursing as encompassing autonomous and collaborative care of individuals of all ages, families, groups, and communities, sick or well, and in all settings. This includes promotion of health, prevention of illness, and the care of ill, disabled, and dying people. Nursing is a major feature of modern health care systems. The nurse, with a definite scope of care activities, often works in close collaboration with the physician. Midwifery also forms a part of this category. The International Confederation of Midwives (2011) defines a midwife as a responsible and accountable professional who works in partnership with women to give the necessary support, care, and advice during pregnancy, labour, and the postpartum period, to conduct births under the midwife's own responsibility, and to provide care for the newborn and the infant. It is further stressed that the roles of a midwife also include preventive measures, the promotion of normal birth, the detection of complications in mother and child, accessing medical care or other appropriate assistance, and carrying out emergency measures. Nurse and midwife are not synonymous; one can be a nurse but not a midwife and vice versa. It is possible to be a nurse-midwife (i.e., to have both qualifications). There are also many specialties in nursing categorised based on disease and age of patients, and so forth. The specialties include (among others) psychiatric, geriatric, neonatal, oncological, surgical, paediatric, cardiac, critical care, and surgical and forensic nursing.

10.3.3.5 Allied Health Professionals

Allied health professionals (AHPs) can also be referred to as health associate professionals (HAPs). They normally include other categories of health workers apart from those previously discussed. The central roles of the AHPs include delivery of health or related services pertaining to the identification, evaluation, and prevention of diseases and disorders; dietary and nutrition services; and rehabilitation and health systems management, among others (ASAHP 2012). They also contribute to the care of patients; some of them (e.g., paramedics) provide primary care and help in the rehabilitation of patients. Physical therapists may provide rehabilitative training for patients in need. Some of them are administrative workers who help in the management or administration of a health care system. There is usually a large number of AHPs (maybe up to 60 % of the workforce) in a typical health organisation. A large body of them are part of the various categories of assistants (nursing, laboratory, and pharmaceutical assistants); others include technicians, dental hygienists, diagnostic medical sonographers, dietitians, radiographers, respiratory therapists, and some health social scientists (including health or clinical psychologists, marriage or family therapists, hospital social workers, occupational therapists, environmental health officers, and speech therapists, among others).

The five aforementioned categories represent those who have direct input in the management of care seekers. The other-ranks also play supportive roles to ensure adequate running of the health care system. This category of workers includes security personnel, cleaners, and (ambulance) drivers. Also part of this category are volunteers who often serve as links between the hospital and the community. Some of these volunteers are also trained in basic care, especially in the case of an emergency. Community health workers (CHWs) are also part of this category; they are often trained to grant primary care within the community or play supportive roles in the hospital.

The success of care delivery lies in the teamwork of these categories of workers. The medical category often provides the lead role in the management of the care seekers. The physician, however, heavily depends on the input from other categories of professionals (e.g., input from a pharmacist for an appropriate therapy plan, radiologist or radiographer for a certain diagnosis, laboratory assistants for test results, physical therapists for follow-up management of fractures, and, more importantly, on the care provided by the nurses for effective treatment of patients). This collaboration among the various categories is absolutely necessary. Due to interdependence, and in some cases intermingling roles, conflict can arise. The patterns of interprofessional cooperation and conflict among health workers have been part of the research focus of medical sociology. It is important to study such teamwork and conflict and their impact on job satisfaction and health care delivery (see Gjerberg and Kjølsrød 2001; Hendel et al. 2007; Krogstad et al. 2004; Lichtenstein et al. 2004). Apart from the composition of professionals who are the driving force of health care delivery, political principles also affect the organisation of delivery systems.

10.3.4 Political Organisation of Health Care Systems

In Chap. 1, health politics and policy was briefly discussed as part of the topical description of medical sociology. The organisation of health care in relation to access to care is determined by national objectives that might differ between countries. As a consequence, health care is organised in various ways in different countries of the world. In essence, the political and economic systems provide a basis on which health care is also organised. One of the central political goals is to maintain justice (in terms of fairness, equity, desert, and merits) in the allocation of resources including health care resources. As observed by Povar et al. (2004) and Breyer (2009), there are a number of pressing issues that affect access to health care and thus there is need for political efforts to ensure justice in health care. First, health care resources are finite; their allocation requires hard choices. Second, powerful economic and sociopolitical forces simultaneously shape the rationing of health care. Third, the question of justice, limits, rationing, need, medical necessity, and quality are still unresolved in the distribution of health care resources.

Whether health is seen as human right or a social, natural, or common good, the theories on justice in health care such as the libertarian (capitalism/free-market health care), the utilitarian, the egalitarian (socialist and socialised system), and the two-tier system or mixed economy provide the basis for organising access to health care in terms of the political frameworks that inform the system. The realm of politics provides the arena for evolving a principle of distributive justice which can also be applied to ensure equal opportunity in health care (Daniels 2000, 2001). The most critical principle is justice, which Rawls (1971) expanded as fairness. Nations or governments try to work out the best possible strategies to ensure fairness in health care distribution. Economic and sociopolitical forces in each nation determine how health care is organised, accessed, and rationalised. The essence of this section is to briefly explain some of these political principles.

10.3.4.1 Utilitarianism

The utilitarian stance advocates that in case of scarce health resources or an imbalance between demand and medical care, the greatest good for the greatest number must be the principle. Health care must be served in a way that a substantial majority must benefit from health resources. The utilitarian stance focuses on the maximisation of beneficiaries and benefits. Publicly funded health care is directed towards the coverage of common diseases that affect the majority, with the less common ailments being cared for with other available means. Many insurance policies are geared towards the common medical predicaments, so that the majority will benefit with common disease burden alleviated. Certain criteria (e.g., age, medical history, nature of disease) may be set to accommodate the majority of community members in accessing specific care. For instance, "age" may be a criterion in decisions on the limitation of treatment; minors, youth, and adults may be the primary focus of the health care systems where they constitute the majority in the society, while the aged may have limited access to health care. Utilitarianism often presents a technical means of maximising profits because primarily treating the common ailments usually requires less financial burden.

10.3.4.2 Libertarian (Capitalist/Free-Market) Health Care

Libertarian (capitalist/free-market) health care is one of the common principles in health care organisation. The fundamental creeds of free-market health care are efficiency, equity, and freedom of choice. The libertarian health care system is the type that is free of government (imposed) regulations and where services and costs are determined by supply and demand. More importantly, every individual has freedom to choose from numerous available options and payment plans. This type of system is organised and managed by private individuals with the mission to provide appropriate services to their clients. Since most companies are motivated by profit, it is assumed that they would provide the best services to attract patronage in order to maximise profits. In essence, the health sector is deregulated to allow for private players, and offers unlimited services and choices for members of the society (see Herzlinger 2004a).

Deregulation of the health sector might also involve the elimination of government restrictions on the production and sale of pharmaceutical products. The government should minimise oversight and licensing functions to create more entries of experts and production of health goods in order to increase supply (Herzlinger 2004a, b). Sustained and increased supply should create competition which will eventually reduce market prices of health care. Government-sponsored health insurance schemes do not have a place in a libertarian system; rather the insurance world accommodates an influx of providers that are equipped with the best practices for efficient delivery of services in order to attract as many customers as possible. The consumers also reserve the right to switch from one provider to the other and determine the kind of desirable coverage. In practice, the government may provide a limited intervention to support the needy in accessing health care. For instance, in the United States, managed care was instituted to provide basic support such as Medicare for the aged and people living with disabilities, and Medicaid to support poor households.

One of the core tenets of free-market health care is self-determination or self-responsibility. The individual is responsible for selecting health care services and health insurance based on their own or informed risk assessment (see Herzlinger 2004a, b). Individuals may decide to access cosmetic surgery and any other "luxury" care if there are felt needs and resources to do so. In a regulated care system, certain luxury or expensive care might be limited. Due to the personal cost of health care, individuals are likely to minimise health costs by reducing risk behaviours. Government subsidy may lead to poor management of risks and unnecessary use of health services. More so, in a free-market system, the individuals also select providers that best serve their interests and needs.

The libertarian system has been heavily criticised. One major feature of a capitalist society is social stratification/inequality. This signifies that there are social differences which translate to differential capacities and capabilities in the society. For instance, there are poor people, people living with disabilities, the unemployed, the aged, youth and children, and undocumented migrants; these groups are vulnerable and may lack adequate capacity to access appropriate health care. In the developing world, where the poor constitute the majority, a free-market system partly accounts for limited access to care. As it is, health is *objectified*, *commoditised*, and sold to those who can afford it. Health insurance companies may provide selected services and coverage in order to maximise profits. Such kind of discrimination in coverage is evident in most capitalist health systems.

10.3.4.3 Egalitarian, Socialist, or Socialised Health Care

Another system is egalitarian (socialist and socialised) health care which is based on the need principle. While the goals of both socialised and socialist health care are the same, there is a conceptual difference between the two systems. The socialist system is an overall socioeconomic and political system that involves government regulation of all spheres of life. Such socioeconomic principles also reflect in health care. Socialised health care signifies that the state does not practice socialism but engages some of the principles of socialism in health care in order to provide equal access to all regardless of socioeconomic status. Here, egalitarian, socialist, or socialised health care will be used interchangeably. In such systems, there is a collective, social obligation to provide equal access to health care for all. It is also a form of a system that provides universal access to care (universal health care) which is based on humanitarian solidarity.

Humanitarian solidarity is a form of social relation which implies close links in the society. Humanitarian solidarity also implies a high level of "material" solidarity in terms of the distribution of resources—a situation in which the needs of the less privileged in the society are met. Since there is a polarisation of the society into upper, middle, and lower classes with different capacities, abilities, and vulnerabilities, combining resources will enable the less privileged to be served according to their needs. The government provides an avenue for the collection of taxes and redistribution by providing health care for all. When humanitarian solidarity is related to a health care system, it connotes a situation where everyone contributes according to their ability to the *pool* (of resources) in order to ensure equitable provision and distribution of the health services to all without discrimination on the basis of any social factors such as income, gender, age, education, geographical location, residential status, and so on. It is an advanced form of *risk-sharing* at the societal level. A progressive taxation system is implemented in many western countries to ensure adequate resources for the provision of social amenities including health services. Health care is considered a common good rather than a for-profit market good.

A socialised health care system is the basis for universal health care in the United Kingdom, Cuba, France, and Canada. Everybody contributes to health funds according to their ability and the services are shared according to need. This is fundamental *risk- and burden-sharing* at the societal level. Health care needs should be met equitably and efficiently, and require a commitment to social solidarity as a fundamental value. It has been argued that health care services should only reflect differences in health care needs and not individual or group differences (see Daniels 2001). In other words, there should be equal benefits to all. Once health care reflects group difference, this implies discrimination which is not ethical. This will ensure that those in the lower and upper classes both have considerable equitable access to health care services as a basic human necessity.

In a socialised health care system, *fair burden* is a fundamental principle. Individuals should not bear undue brunt; therefore, the costs and burden of meeting health care needs is spread across individuals in the society by a progressive tax system. With this, the poorest in the society will bear fair burden according to their capacity. Moreover, a socialised health care system provides *universal coverage*. The major barriers to accessing health care such as inadequate financial capacity, unemployment, old age, and so forth will thus be eventually overcome. Another issue that is related to universal access is *comprehensive benefits*, a situation in which a health care system is strengthened to cover almost all services that might be required by the citizens. A health system may be regarded as just when health services cover the full range of health care needs. There should be preventive, diagnostic, therapeutic, chronic, and long-term care, as well as acute, home, and hospital care and treatment for mental and physical illness.

An early attempt at a socialist medical system in Africa was in Tanzania from 1961 to the early 1980s, during the political leadership of Julius Nyerere (see Bjerk 2010; Weaver and Kronemer 1981). Tanzania made some progress in health care provision (see Acharya 1981), but in general African socialism was a failed endeavour and was later abandoned (in the early 1980s) to give way to private enterprise. Socialised health care may fail because it limits freedom of choice. There is often strict legislation which outlaws private players. The unidirectional method of seeking care puts more pressure on the health system. Many patients end up on a waiting list to access medical care. There are often limited choices or sometimes no choices at all. Socialised medicine often promotes inefficiency. There is often bureaucracy since everybody has to turn to a government-run system. In a system where there is no (healthy) competition, innovation in care is deterred. One major setback is the close link of care with government expenditure. The link implies that a cut in public spending means a drastic overall fall in the quality of care. In the era of economic recession which necessitates reduction in government spending, there is a common fate of reduced quantity and quality in government-administered social amenities including health care. In socialised medicine, fair burden does not mean or translate to fair treatment. Patients' satisfaction with services may be undermined at the expense of free access to care.

10.3.4.4 Two-Tier or Pluralistic System of Health Care

A two-tier (or pluralistic) system of health care is a kind of hybrid system of health care. In a mixed economic system, there is the possibility to combine both socialist and free-market principles in the provision of health care. In this case, the system allows for both publicly and privately administered health care to run concurrently, giving the members of the public a choice. This is the most prevalent system of health care in Africa. The private system may offer more advanced and expensive general and specialised services while the government provides basic services or primary health care. In some instances, the government may provide some free services, such as maternal and child health care or free HIV treatment. In most African countries, an insurance system is not available or is limited. Like in Nigeria, less than 10 % of the population is covered by insurance. The majority still relies on out-of-pocket payment to access health care.

Bloom and Standing (2008) observed that economic crises tend to lead to state and institutional failures in access, delivery, and regulation of health care provisions in developing countries. Many individuals resort to self-treatment or medically unregulated traditional medicine for care. In a pluralistic system, there seems to be a wide door for all kinds of health care. One of the key observations by Bloom et al. (2011) is that the majority obtain health care from the informal sector with the attendant problem of efficacy and safety. Bloom and Standing (2001, 2008) identified two other dangers in the pluralistic system. First, there could be rampant *marketisation* of health goods and services at all levels accompanied by *deprofessionalisation* and provider pluralism. Second, there is a blurring of the boundaries between what is public and what is private and a multiplicity of actors and institutions, formal and informal, involved in health care production. A public practitioner can at the same time provide private services. In the public health sector, care seekers may still have to pay for some services. More so, a pluralistic system as practiced in Africa creates room for the influx of unregulated practitioners. Despite this combination of (political) principles in health care, access to health care in Africa is still a major challenge. Before discussing some specific challenges, it is important to examine how health care is organised in terms of levels of care.

10.3.5 Levels of Health Care Delivery

The health care delivery system is organised in levels but linked with a coordinated referral system. There are three dominant levels of care, primary, secondary, and tertiary. Figure 10.3 shows a pyramid illustrating the levels of care in a bottom-up referral sequence of care. The primary care level is responsible for a substantial majority of health cases through basic care, including education and preventive activities. Cases that require further care may be referred to the secondary health facilities where specialised care is offered. The last level of referral is the tertiary level in which more advanced care is available. While the sequential flow is an ideal situation, studies have indicated that many patients frequently bypass primary health care facilities in favour of higher-level hospitals to get better care despite spending a substantial amount of additional time and money (Audo et al. 2005; Kruk et al. 2009; Kahabuka et al. 2011), mainly because of a perceived low quality of care at the lower health care units.

10.3.5.1 Primary Health Care

The proper institutionalisation of primary health care (PHC) in most countries started after the International Conference on Primary Health Care in Alma-Ata, held in the then USSR in 1978, with a major goal of ensuring "health for all" by 2000.

10.3 Modern Health Care in Africa

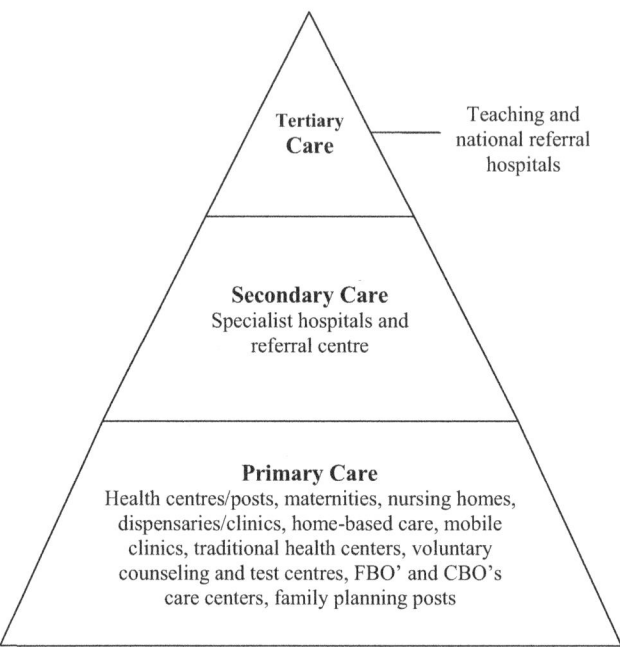

Fig. 10.3 Pyramid showing the levels of care

Unfortunately, the period has passed without achieving the goal. It is also becoming obvious that the health-related Millennium Development Goals (MGDs) might not be met by 2015, especially in many developing countries (Amzat 2009). In any case, the primary concern here is to briefly discuss PHC as a level of care. The WHO (1978, p. 3–4) simply conceived PHC as essential health care that is developed based on community peculiarities, relies on sustainable and appropriate health technology, promotes community engagement and participation in decisions about health services provided at affordable costs, encourages self-care and empowerment of community members, and serves as the first level of contact with the health care system which brings health care as close as possible to where people live, work, and play. It is thus a community-centred approach in health care provisioning.

The major issues around PHC extend beyond the provision of a physical structure (often called a primary health care centre) to the philosophy underlining the PHC system. In most developing countries, PHC has been erroneously reduced to the provision of a physical structure called a PHC facility. Provision of primary care is not the only philosophy of the PHC system. The framework of PHC incorporates public health practices. It includes health education, adequate nutrition, maternal and child health care, basic sanitation and safe water, basic vaccination against lethal disease, family planning services, prevention and control of locally endemic diseases, treatment of common diseases and injuries, and the provision of essential drugs (WHO 1978, 2008). PHC also includes appropriate human resources such as physicians, nurses, midwives, auxiliaries, and community workers, where applicable, as well as traditional practitioners suitably trained as participants in the health team to respond to the expressed health needs of the community (WHO 1978).

Practically, primary care (as a level of care) is provided at health posts, village health centers, primary health care centers, clinics, dispensaries, and health offices located within the community. It is also provided by primary care physicians, general practitioners, family physicians, or a non-physician primary care provider such as a medical assistant, nurse, midwife, community health worker, village health worker, rural medical aid, trained birth attendant, or traditional healer, depending on the location or country. A majority of the providers have wide knowledge of various health conditions and are meant to serve as sources of referrals to another level of care when further care is required. In most African countries, the PHC centres/posts are managed by local or district authorities or, in short, the closest level of government to the people. For instance, in Nigeria, PHC is the responsibility of the local government authority, which is the third tier of the federating units. Like in many countries, they are supported by voluntary agencies such as non-governmental organisations (NGOs), both local and international, and faith- and community-based organisations.

10.3.5.2 Secondary Health Care

The secondary health care (SHC) centres offer more advanced and specialised care compared with the PHC. In ideal cases, SHC accepts referrals from primary care providers. Some SHC centres are specialised in certain fields of care like children specialist hospitals or eye hospitals while others have various departments that offer various specialised care. The allied health professionals are commonly found from the secondary level of care and above. Invariably, the SHC facilities normally offer more clinical care of a higher quality by more skilled and competent staff than those found in most PHC facilities. It is possible that certain procedures such as specialised surgical interventions may not be available; these often require referral to the tertiary health care centers. The SHC facilities are usually equipped with laboratory and other diagnostic techniques suitable for medical, inpatient, and outpatient activities. They often manage patients until the patient can return home or to the PHC providers for further primary care.

10.3.5.3 Tertiary Health Care

Tertiary Health Care, or THC, is the apex of the health care system with the provision of sophisticated diagnostic, therapeutic, and rehabilitative services. THC is provided by teaching hospitals, which also provide advanced medical training. The tertiary care or teaching hospital, in most cases, is attached to a university with a large amount of manpower. THC is also provided by national referral hospitals, which apart from serving the national population can also accept international referrals. The national referral hospitals also provide what is sometimes called quaternary care (this may be a fourth level of care) by providing uncommon diagnostic and surgical interventions. The teaching and referral hospitals provide leadership in medical research, clinical standards, and treatment protocols. In most African states, the teaching and national hospitals are administered by the national government. In many of these countries, there are also a number of accredited private hospitals which also offer tertiary care.

10.3.6 Challenges of Health Care Delivery in Africa

Africa is confronted with a heavy burden of disease and the modern health care system has been the mainstay in the management of health conditions. Before highlighting some specific challenges, it is important to refer to King (1966) who described medical care in developing countries. King (1966) averred that social determinants (especially poverty-related issues; see Chap. 4) had a huge adverse influence on population health in developing countries (especially Africa). After several decades, King's propositions that poverty-related issues, limited access to health care, and shortage of health care manpower were highly prevalent still deserve urgent attention. Here, the focus is on the challenges facing the delivery of modern health care. Across Africa, the problems are quite similar. Some major challenges of health care delivery are discussed here.

1. **High level of poverty:** this is a significant factor affecting health care delivery systems. First, poverty is a major social determinant of health or a fundamental cause of illness (see Sects. 3.6.2 and 4.3). Poverty has multiple adverse influences on health. It is responsible for a high prevalence of disease because it accounts for poor nutrition, social maginalisation, poor living conditions, and (more importantly) low access to health care. Poverty limits the financial capability of individuals to access appropriate health care. It also stymies the effectiveness of basic health care (especially preventive services). The malnourished or those who lack basic hygiene or who reside in unhygienic environments are constantly exposed to health hazards. In addition, poor people have an increased risk of non-communicable diseases due to an unhealthy lifestyle (e.g., poor nutrition and smoking). This has been a major challenge to health care delivery in Africa.
2. **Low level of education:** education and health literacy are important in health care delivery (see Sects. 3.6.4 and 4.4). Many people lack basic knowledge of preventive health care or find it difficult to comprehend health information. Low literacy also leads to health misconceptions and health beliefs which restrain access to health care. Many people still decline to have their newborn vaccinated because of a low level of understanding and literacy.
3. **Inadequate access to health care:** access to health care is limited in Africa both in terms of affordability and, more importantly, availability (see Sect. 4.9). There is a limited supply of health services and provision of facilities. Rural areas are usually underserved. There might be no health facility or the distance might be too far. In places with underdeveloped transportation networks, community

members have to rely on any available alternative care service, usually from traditional practitioners or untrained "health workers."

4. **Insufficient political prioritisation of health:** Some African governments only pay lip-service to health care prioritisation. The health budget is often very low when compared to health needs. A substantial amount of funds available are through foreign aid. For instance, artemisinin-based combination therapy for treatment of malaria and antiretroviral therapy are prioritised by international donor agencies, but African governments often make very little contribution.

5. **Inadequate human resource for health:** there is a constant shortage of health professionals of various categories in Africa (see WHO 2006). First, there are limited training facilities for certain medical specialties. Some Africans trained abroad may have limited facilities to work within Africa. Even where there are adequate capacities, a majority are brain-drained to the western countries for "greener pastures," thereby perpetuating the shortage of manpower in Africa. Another dimension of the shortage of manpower reflects in the rural-urban dichotomy with the rural areas bearing a greater shortage. Many health facilities in African rural areas are not manned by qualified personnel. This explains the low quality of care in rural areas.

6. **Poor motivation of health workers:** this could be part of the reason for the outward migration of health workers and other professionals from Africa. The work environment is often poor coupled with low remuneration and poor work infrastructures. Strike action by health professionals to demand improved work conditions is a yearly occurrence in many African countries. These strikes are often accompanied with adverse consequences, especially for the service-users. Poor motivation leads to limited input which leads to general poor service outcomes.

7. **Inadequate health insurance scheme:** the essence of health insurance is to provide a platform for risk-pooling mechanisms to redistribute the financial burden of catastrophic health expenditures. Health insurance should reduce the high level of out-of-the-pocket payments for health care, improve access to health care, and protect against financial risk of ill-health. Health insurance has been described as a major strategy of ensuring universal access to health care (WHO 2010). Unfortunately, many countries in Africa do not have an effective insurance scheme in place; where available, the coverage is very limited with many individuals in the informal sector or the rural population left out. Only about one-tenth of people in sub-Saharan Africa have access to formal social protection, including health or accident insurance (WHO 2010, p. x). Due to the lack of an insurance scheme, individuals with serious illnesses may have to pay exorbitant fees for health care, which most times may not be affordable and could push people to financial catastrophe.

8. **Poor governance or corruption:** apart from a low level of political will, the inappropriate use of resources is another major challenge. Corruption is common and high in many African countries. The small amount of available resources are not judiciously utilised with substantial funds and materials subverted by health officials and political administrators (see UNDP 2011). The WHO (2007)

noted that there is rampant corruption in medical products and technology procurement systems, unreliable supply systems, unaffordable prices, and irrational use of resources. UNDP (2011, p. 6) corroborated that common corrupt practices in the health sector include absenteeism, theft of medical supplies, informal payments, fraud, weak regulatory procedures, improperly designed procurement procedures, diversion of supplies in the distribution system for private gains, and embezzlement of health care funds. The general poor political governance also reflects in weak governance of health development across Africa (see Kirigia and Kirigia 2011).

References

Abdel-Hameed, A. A. (1997). The Wellcome Tropical Research Laboratories in Khartoum (1903–1934): An experiment in development. *Medical History, 41*(1), 30–58.

Abdullahi, A. A. (2011). Trends and challenges of traditional medicine in Africa. *Afr J Tradit Complement Altern Med, 8*(S), 115–123.

Acharya, S. N. (1981). Perspectives and problems of development in Sub-Saharan Africa. *World Development, 9*(2), 109–147.

Ademiluyi, I. A., & Aluko-Arowolo, S. (2009). Infrastructural distribution of healthcare services in Nigeria: An overview. *Journal of Geography and Regional Planning, 2*(5), 104–110.

Adesina, S. K. (2012). Traditional medical care in Nigeria. http://www.onlinenigeria.com/health/?blurb=574. Accessed 30 July 2012

Akighir, A. (1982). Traditional and modern psychiatry: A survey of opinions and beliefs amongst people in Plateau State, Nigeria. *International Journal of Social Psychiatry, 28,* 203–209.

Alrawi, S., Fetters, M. D., Killawi, A., Hammad, A., & Padela, A. (2012). Traditional healing practices among American Muslims: Perceptions of community leaders in southeast Michigan. *J Immigrant Minority Health, 14,* 489–496.

Alubo, S. O., (1995). *Medical professionalism and state Power in Nigeria.* Jos: Centre for Development Studies, University of Jos

Alubo, O. (2008). Ontological response to illness. *Jos Journal of Social Issues, 6,* 1–16.

Alves, R. R. N., & Rosa, I. L. (2005). Why study the use of animal products in traditional medicines? *Journal of Ethnobiology and Ethnomedicine, 1,* 5. doi:10.1186/1746-4269-1-5.

Alves, R. R. N., & Rosa, I. L. (2007). Biodiversity, traditional medicine and public health: Where do they meet? *Journal of Ethnobiology and Ethnomedicine, 3,* 14. doi:10.1186/1746-4269-3-14.

Amzat, J. (2009). Assessing the progress towards Millennium Development Goals in Nigeria. In A. O. Olutayo, I. S. Ogundiya, & J. Amzat (Eds.), *State and civil society relations in Nigeria* (pp. 290–309). Ibadan: Hope Publications.

Association of Schools of Allied Health Professionals (ASAHP). (2012). The definition of Allied health professionals. http://www.asahp.org/definition.htm Accessed 20 Aug 2011.

Ashforth, A. (1998). Reflections on spiritual insecurity in a modern African city (Soweto). *African Studies Review, 41*(3), 36–67.

Audo, M. O., Ferguson, A., & Njoroge, P. K. (2005). Quality of health care and its effects in the utilisation of maternal and child health services in Kenya. *East African Medical Journal, 82,* 547–553.

Bhootra, B. L., & Weiss, E. (2006). Muti killing: A case report. *Medicine, Science, and the Law, 46*(3), 255–259.

Bjerk, P. K. (2010). Sovereignty and socialism in Tanzania: The historiography of an African State. *History in Africa, 37,* 275–319.

Bloom, G., & Standing, H. (2001). Pluralism and marketisation in the health sector: Meeting health needs in contexts of social change in low and middle-income countries, IDS Working Paper No. 136, http://www.ntd.co.uk/idsbookshop/details.asp?id=614. Accessed 21 Aug 2012.

Bloom, G., & Standing, H. (2008). Introduction: Future health systems: Why future? Why now? *Social Science & Medicine, 66*, 2067–2075.

Bloom, G., Standing, H., Lucas, H., Bhuiya, A., Oladepo, O., & Peters, D. H. (2011). Making health markets work better for poor people: The case of informal providers. *Health Policy and Planning, 26*, i45–i52

Breyer, F. (2009). Health care rationing and distributive justice. In M. Baurmann & B. Lahno (Eds.), *Perspectives in moral science* (pp. 395–410). Frankfurt: Nomos Verlag.

Burke-Gaffney, H. J. O'D (1968). The history of medicine in the African countries. *History of Medicine, 12*(1), 31–41. doi:10.1017/S0025727300012746.

Coovadia, H., Jewkes, R., Barron, P., Sanders, D., & McIntyre, D. (2009). The health and health system of South Africa: Historical roots of current public health challenges. *Lancet, 374*, 817–834.

Dada, A. A., Yinusa, W., & Giwa, S. O. (2011). Review of the practice of traditional bone setting in Nigeria. *African Health Sciences, 11*(2), 262–265.

Daniels, N. (2000). Accountability for reasonableness. *BMJ, 321* (7272), 1300–1301.

Daniels, N. (2001). Justice, health and health care. *American Journal of Bioethics, 1*(2), 3–15.

Gabe, J., Bury, M., & Elston, M. A. (2004). *Key concepts in medical sociology*. London: Sage Publications.

Gjerberg, E., & Kjølsrød, L. (2001). The doctor-nurse relationship: How easy is it to be a female doctor co-operating with a female nurse? *Social Science & Medicine, 52*, 189–202.

Han, G. (2002). The myth of medical pluralism: A critical realist perspective. *Sociological Research Online, 6*, 4. http://www.socresonline.org.uk/6/4/han.html. Accessed 12 Nov 2012.

Hendel, T., Fish, M., & Berger, O. (2007). Nurse/physician conflict management mode choices: Implications for improved collaborative practice. *Nursing Administration Quarterly, 31*(3), 244–253.

Herzlinger, R. E. (2004). Consumer-driven health insurance: What works. In R. E. Herzlinger (Ed.), *Consumer-driven health care* (pp. 74–101). San Francisco: Wiley.

Herzlinger, R. E. (2004b) Health care productivity. In R. E. Herzlinger (Ed.), *Consumer-driven health care* (pp. 102–126). San Francisco: Wiley.

Hirst, M. (2005). Dreams and medicines: The perspective of Xhosa diviners and novices in the Eastern Cape, South Africa. *Indo-Pacific Journal of Phenomenology, 5*(2), 1–22.

International Confederation of Midwives (ICM). (2011). ICM international definition of the midwife. http://www.internationalmidwives.org/Portals/5/2011/Definition%20of%20the%20Midwife%20-%202011.pdf. Accessed 20 Aug 2011.

International Council of Nurses. (2010). Definition of nursing. http://www.icn.ch/about-icn/icn-definition-of-nursing/. Accessed 20 Aug 2012

Ityavyar, D. A. (1987). Background to the development of health services in Nigeria. *Social Science & Medicine, 24*(6), 487–499.

Izugbara, C. O., & Ukwayi, J. K. (2003). The clientele of traditional birth homes in southeastern Nigeria. *Healthcare for Women International, 24*(3), 177–192.

Kahabuka, C., Kvåle, G., Moland, K. M., & Hinderaker, S. G. (2011). Why caretakers bypass Primary Health Care facilities for childcare—a case from rural Tanzania. *BMC Health Services Research, 11*, 315. doi:10.1186/1472-6963-11-315.

King, M. (1966). Introduction. In M. King (Ed.), *Medical care in developing countries: A primer on the medicine of poverty and a symposium from Makerere*. Nairobi: Oxford University Press.

Kirigia, J. M., & Kirigia, D. G. (2011). The essence of governance in health development. *International Archives of Medicine, 4*, 11. doi:10.1186/1755-7682-4-11.

Kofi-Tsekpo, M. (2004). Institutionalization of African traditional medicine in health care systems in Africa. *African Journal of Health Sciences, 11*(1–2), i–ii.

Krogstad, U., Hofoss, D., & Hjortdahl, P. (2004). Doctor and nurse perception of inter-professional co-operation in hospitals. *International Journal for Quality in Health Care, 16*(6), 491–497.

Kruk, M. E., Mbaruku, G., McCord, C. W., Moran, M., Rockers, P. C., & Galea, S. (2009). Bypassing PHC facilities for childbirth: A population-based study in rural Tanzania. *Health Policy Plan, 24*(4), 279–288.

Library of Congress. (1991). Nigeria: History of modern medical services. http://lcweb2.loc.gov/cgi-bin/query/r?frd/cstdy:@field(DOCID+ng0074). Accessed 7 Aug 2012

Lichtenstein, R., Alexander, J. A., Mccarthy, J. F., & Wells, R. (2004). Status differences in cross-functional teams: Effects on individual member participation, job satisfaction, and intent to quit. *Journal of Health and Social Behavior, 45*, 322–335.

Miles, S. H., & Ololo, H. (2003). Traditional surgeons in sub-Saharan Africa: Images from south Sudan. *International Journal of STD & AIDS, 14*, 505–508.

NCCAM. (2012). What is complementary and alternative medicine? http://nccam.nih.gov/health/whatiscam. Accessed 30 July, 2012

Owumi, B. E. (1996). Traditional practitioners: Healers and healing practices. In E. A. Oke & B. E. Owumi (Eds.), *Readings in medical sociology* (pp. 223–233). Ibadan: RDMS.

Patel, V. (2011). Traditional healers for mental health care in Africa. *Global Health Action, 4*, 7956. doi:10.3402/gha.v4i0.7956.

Peltzer, K., Nqeketo, A., Petros, G., & Kanta, X. (2008). Traditional circumcision during manhood initiation rituals in the Eastern Cape, South Africa: A pre-post intervention evaluation. *BMC Public Health, 8*, 64. doi:10.1186/1471-2458-8-64.

Povar, G. J., Blumen, H., Daniel, J., Daub, S., Evans, L., Holm, R. P., Levkovich, N., McCarter, A. O., Sabin, J., Snyder, L., Sulmasy, D., Vaughan, P., Wellikson, L. D., & Campbell, A. (2004). Ethics in Practice: Managed care and the changing health care environment: Medicine as a profession managed care ethics working group statement. *Annals of Internal Medicine, 141*(2), 131–136.

Rawls, J. (1971). *The theory of justice*. Cambridge: Harvard University Press

Rensburg, H. C. J., & Ngwena, C. (2005). Health and health care in South Africa against an African background. In W. C. Cockerham (Ed.), *The blackwell companion to medical sociology* (pp. 365–391). Massachusetts: Blackwell Publishers Ltd.

Salisbury, S., & Roberts, L. (2012). The practice of ritual killings and human sacrifice in Africa. *The Human Rights Brief*. http://hrbrief.org/2012/09/the-practice-of-ritual-killings-and-human-sacrifice-in-africa/. Accessed 15 Oct 2012

Sorsdahl, K., Stein, D. J., Grimsrud, A., Seedat, S., Flisher, A. J., Williams, D. R., & Myer, L. (2009). Traditional healers in the treatment of common mental disorders in South Africa. *Journal of Nervous and Mental Disease, 197*(6), 434–441. doi:10.1097/NMD.0b013e3181a61dbc..

Taye, O. R. (2009). Yoruba traditional medicine and the challenge of integration. *The Journal of Pan African Studies, 3*(3), 73–90.

Tella, A. (1979). The practice of traditional medicine in Africa. *Nigerian Medical Journal, 9*(5–6), 607–612

Thoral, M. (2012). Colonial medical encounters in the Nineteenth Century: The French campaigns in Egypt, Saint Domingue and Algeria. *Social History of Medicine, 25*(3), 608–624.

Twumasi, P. A. (1981). Colonialism and international health: A study in social change in Ghana. *Social Science & Medicine, 15B*, 147–151.

Udosen, A. M., Otei, O. O., & Onuba, O. (2006). Role of traditional bonesetters in Africa: Experience in Calabar, Nigeria. *Annals of African Medicine, 5*(4), 170–173.

Umeora, O. U. J., & Egwuatu, V. E. (2010). The role of unorthodox and traditional birth care in maternal mortality. *Tropical Doctor, 40*(1), 13–17.

United Nations Development Programme. (2011). *Fighting corruption in the health sector: Methods, tools and good practices*. New York: UNDP

Vincent, L. (2008). New magic for new times: Muti murder in democratic South Africa. *Tribes and Tribals. Special, 2*, 43–53.

Weaver, J. H., & Kronemer, A. (1981). Tanzania and African socialism. *World Development, 9*(9/10), 839–849.

Weisheit, A. (2003). Traditional medicine practice in contemporary Uganda. *Indigenous Knowledge (IK) Notes, 54,* 1–4.

WHO. (1976). *African traditional medicine: Report of the regional expert committee*. AFRO Technical Report Series, No. 1. Brazzaville

WHO. (1978). *The Alma Ata conference on primary health care*. Geneva: WHO.

WHO. (1992). *Traditional birth attendants: A Joint WHO/UNFPA/UNICEF Statement*. Geneva: WHO.

WHO. (1997). *Coverage of maternity care: A listing of the available information* (4th ed). Geneva: WHO.

WHO. (2000). *General guidelines for methodologies on research and evaluation of traditional medicine. WHO/EDM/TRM/2000.1*. Geneva: WHO.

WHO. (2006). *The World Health Report 2006– working together for health*. Geneva: WHO.

WHO. (2007). *EverybodyÊ¼s business: Strengthening health systems to improve health outcomes: WHO's framework for action*. Geneva: WHO

WHO. (2008). *The world health report 2008: Primary health care now more than ever*. Geneva: WHO.

WHO. (2010). *The World Health Report 2011– The world health report: Health systems financing: The path to universal coverage*. Geneva: WHO.

Wilcken, A., Keil, T., & Dick, B. (2010). Traditional male circumcision in eastern and southern Africa: A systematic review of prevalence and complications. *Bulletin of the World Health Organization, 88,* 907–914. doi:10.2471/BLT.09.072975.

Wilson, A., Gallos, I. D., Plana, N., Lissauer, D., Khan, K. S., Zamora, J., MacArthur, C., & Coomarasamy, A. (2011). Effectiveness of strategies incorporating training and support of traditional birth attendants on perinatal and maternal mortality: Meta-analysis. *BMJ, 343,* d7102

Chapter 11
Towards a Sociology of Bioethics

11.1 Introduction

Bioethics is a distinctive field of study and practice, although in practice it involves transdisciplinary approach. It has links with law, public policy, historical studies, the popular media; the disciplines of philosophy, religion, literature, medicine, biology, ecology; and population studies and social sciences (Callahan 2004, p. 279). Health social sciences (in particular) are relevant in the consideration of the bioethical agenda. The essence of this chapter is to promote the understanding of bioethics and stress the relevance of sociology to the bioethical agenda. The idea is not to provide a comprehensive examination of bioethics as a field or an in-depth analysis of topics in bioethics but to explore some of the critical areas of bioethics in order to provide (sociological) understanding of the core issues (as background for students) in the field. This should also expose how sociology could contribute to the social dimensions of the bioethical agenda.

Bioethics has been defined in various ways. One definition is that it is a multidisciplinary endeavour focusing on the study and regulation of the moral, legal, social, and philosophical perplexities in health care and the development and application of science and technology in human life. The critical focus of bioethics is "conflict of interest" that often arises from biomedical sciences in relation to human life or survival. In other words, "bioethics is a field that ranges from the anguished private and individual dilemmas faced by physicians or other healthcare workers at the bedside of a patient, to the terrible public and societal choices faced by citizens and legislators as they try to devise equitable health or environmental policies" (Callahan 2004, p. 280). Moral questions often come with the application and development of sciences. Such dilemmas could be the question of what is right or appropriate in the context of care, allocation of resources, formulation of policies, research development, and application of technologies. Bioethics often starts with a critical assessment of the prevailing circumstances and consideration of the limits of scientific practices in relation to human values.

Providing a more encompassing definition, Reich (1995) defined bioethics as the systematic study of the moral dimensions—including moral vision, decisions, conducts, and policies—of the life sciences and health care, employing a variety of ethical methodologies in an interdisciplinary setting. One major addition to Reich's definition is the issue of *vision*. Bioethics does not only relate to the rightness or appropriateness of the present moral conduct but also with the historical and future evolutionary and sociocultural implications. Invariably, the implications of biomedical conduct for the future generations are part of the essential focus of bioethics.

It is important to note that bioethical practice is usually prescriptive through assertion of values and moral judgments (Turner 2009). In order to make moral judgments, bioethicists need to understand the ethical issues emanating from a particular moral dilemma. In addition, bioethicists require some understanding of the institutional structures, social arrangements, and normative patterns in the social worlds within which ethical issues emerge (Turner 2009). These sociocultural, normative, and institutional issues are mostly within the confines of sociological studies. As noted earlier (see Sect. 1.1), sociology deals with understanding social relations and institutions, stressing on the social norms, order, and facts. The social facts or realities, norms, and culture constitute the basis of human morality. Therefore, sociological insight and input are crucial in bioethics if the ethical conundrums presented by science (in general) and medicine (in particular) are to be successfully resolved in practice.

Sociology of bioethics deals with the application of sociological insights, perspectives, and methods to the understanding of the moral dimensions of the life sciences and health care. Sociologists can provide input in ethical deliberations because of their in-depth understanding of the patterns of social relations and cultural beliefs. The only caution is that while sociology (like other social sciences) often tends to provide universal ideas, the views of moral relativism and particularism are central, especially in clinical bioethics. In bioethical practice, what is universally appropriate may defy an individual's choice, which must be respected. Despite the universal contents, in practical terms morality varies from one individual to another. The use of moral relativism is applicable in the cultural context *and* at the individual level in bioethical practice. For instance, while cosmetic surgery may be good for person A, it might not be for both person B and the community as a whole because of the differential preference and costs involved. It explains the difficulty in arriving at a collective sentiment regarding access to a particular form of care.

In addition, medical sociology holds a lot of crosscutting interests with bioethics. The issues regarding organisation of health care (see Sect. 10.3.4); social determinants of health (see Chap. 4); allocation of health resources, health policies, and politics; cultural context of scientific conducts; and health practices among others are approached by the fields from different perspectives. The major difference lies in the prescriptiveness of bioethics by focusing on how to ensure justice among various groups and thereby making some form of ethical recommendations. In relation to ethical discourse, medical sociology focuses more on the sociocultural context responsible for (re)production of population health and social implications of policies and related issues. Having made some clarifications about bioethics and the sociology of bioethics, it is important to examine the history and changing notions of bioethics.

11.2 On the History and Notions of Bioethics

Moral predicaments are as old as human history and are a part of human existence. At every point in time, there are regulations governing human interactions and hard choices have to be made. Bioethics as a discipline was recognised at a period when there were increasing ethical issues due to emerging scientific possibilities (which raise some apprehensions). Specifically, Callahan (2004) observed that the 1960s particularly marked the era of extraordinary technological progress in biomedicine. The 1960s saw the advent of kidney dialysis, organ transplantation, medically safe abortions, the contraceptive pill, prenatal diagnosis, the widespread use of intensive-care units and artificial respirators, a dramatic shift from death at home to death in hospitals or other institutions, and the first glimmerings of genetic engineering (Callahan 2004, p. 280).

This surge in new medical possibilities and applications generated moral contestations, which led to new voices and movement regarding the *limits of science*. There is no debate that not all scientific engagements are humane and should be applied without limits. Within the application of innovation, how can the rights of the citizen be protected, and how to ensure safety and avert societal disruptions? As a human endeavour, moral ethics (applied in social relations, politics, or economics) have been a part of the concerns of the fathers of philosophy (e.g., Aristotle, Socrates, Plato, Kant, Epicurus, and Aquinas). The Hippocratic Oath is all about medical ethics, regulating the conducts of medical professionals to conform to the value of care. Despite this historical antecedence, the development of bioethics as a discipline is a recent development.

Bioethics flourished from the 1970s, especially with the works of Van Rensselaer Potter (1911–2001), which were landmarks in the development of the discipline. But before Potter, recent developments revealed that Fritz Jahr (1895–1953), a German teacher and theologian, is credited as the first to use the term "bioethics" in his paper "Bio-ethics: A Panorama of Ethical Relations of Man Toward the Animal and the Plant" in 1927. It was further observed that during some 20 years of his publishing activity (1927–1947), Jahr authored 18 papers in which ethical discourse was frequently featured (Muzur and Rinčić 2011). Jahr's initial conception of bioethics was based on the acceptance of moral obligations to all living beings (including plants and lower animals, especially in relations to humans). Jahr (1927) submitted that every living being should be respected as such and cannot be destroyed arbitrarily and worthlessly, as they all (plants and animals as well as people) have rights. This was a pioneer promotion of the right to life of animals and plants in relation to humans, particularly with the advocacy of animal rights. In his 1927 paper, Jahr made a striking remark that has formed a fundamental thrust in bioethics in the 21st century: that every living being should be respected essentially as an end-in-itself and should be treated as such (the influence of Kantianism is evident in the statement). As it will later be observed, *respect* for persons and non-tolerance of the instrumental use of persons are now core ideas in bioethics (see Sect. 11.4.2).

The most widely read history of bioethics, however, began in the 1970s with the works of Potter, who is also credited to have (re)-coined the term "bioethics" in 1970. This development presents a bi-location of the origin of the concept of bioethics. Perhaps because his papers were published in English, they were more widely read than Jahr's. Potter re-coined *bioethics* to describe the need to bridge science and human values by combining the science of biology (*bio*) and the study of human value systems (*ethics*) (Potter 1970, 1971, p. vii), and he stressed that he was proposing a new discipline. In 1971 Potter published the first major book in the new discipline—*Bioethics: Bridge to the Future.* The conception of bioethics by Potter (1971) provided elaborate notions of bioethics as a bridge between present and future, science and values, nature and nurture/culture, and man and nature. By relating bioethics to a bridge between the present and the future, Potter implies that there is need to regulate the emergence of any scientific knowledge that is potentially detrimental to the future survival of mankind (Ten Have 2012). This will require development of utopia frameworks—what "ought to be or ideal patterns" which will enable bioethics to provide directions towards the attainment of future goals of mankind. Potter averred that science should proceed with wisdom combined with the values of humility and respect (Potter 1971). The wisdom is required to guide scientific practice towards the survival of mankind. A combination of biological and cultural adaptability is inevitable for human survival; bioethics should also provide the wisdom to always link the two. That is why Potter submitted that scientific knowledge of nature will only be useful if it relates to long-range goals of the society (Ten Have 2012).

In the beginning, Potter was more interested in ecological ethics, which was why he viewed bioethics as a bridge to the future—a practice that would moderate sustainability in scientific practice, that is, without compromising the future. Potter expressed concerns about the dehumanisation of science and the need for a new discipline that would help re-establish ecological balance and protect ecological resources (Muzur and Rinčić 2011). Ecological bioethics clearly has a long-term goal that is concerned with the need to preserve the ecosystem in a form that is compatible with the continued existence or survival of the human species (Potter 1988, p. 74; Potter and Potter 1995). It is important to note that within the interest of human survival, Potter also aligned the new discipline to issues of poverty, security, pollution, politics, and human development (Ten Have 2012, p. 64).

Potter (1988) proposed a fusion of medical and ecological bioethics when he observed that the term "bioethics" has been mostly used to focus on individuals and medical issues; he proposed "global bioethics" to signify the encompassing term. He observed that global bioethics is thus "biology combined with diverse humanistic knowledge forging a science that sets a system of medical and environmental priorities for acceptable survival" (Potter 1988). Potter's definition of global bioethics then provides room for broad issues relating to value systems or morality as it affects human survival. Ten Have (2012) noted that Potter's definition is reflected in the *Universal Declaration on Bioethics and Human Rights*, concerned with health care, the biosphere, and future generations, as well as social justice.

Fig. 11.1 Varieties of bioethics

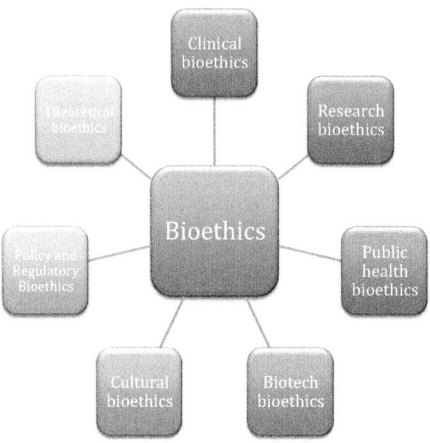

11.3 Varieties of Bioethics

The concise description of bioethics will involve a brief elaboration of its major aspects. This will give a general overview of the core areas that have developed over the years. Callahan (2004) described four major aspects, while three other aspects (public health, research and biotech bioethics) that are not well captured in Callahan's description are added. Figure 11.1 shows the various aspects of bioethics. The next seven subsections will describe these aspects.

11.3.1 Theoretical Bioethics

There is a need for a systematised knowledge of morality in a way that will guide not only empirical investigation but also practical evaluation and application of moral values in bioethics. Hence there are series of invocation of moral theories in bioethics. Many bioethicists specialise in theoretical analysis and application of theories to ethical discourse. This aspect is one of the core areas that has developed with close links to philosophy. The discussion of moral ethics requires adequate philosophising to create a systemised body of theoretical or epistemological stance upon which subsequent specialists can rely. Therefore, there are a number of theoretical underpinnings in bioethics. It is important to note that modern bioethics was born in the West and the earlier prominent theoretical perspective reflects the traditions of Western moral philosophy, political, and social theories (Chattopadhyay and De Vries 2008).

The development of ethical theories is thus necessitated to provide a systematised philosophical basis of medical science, ethics of health care, and research involving human subjects. The objective of an ethical theory is to provide an adequate normative framework for processing and resolving moral problems (Beauchamp 2003) not only in Western societies but at the global level. Some of those ethical theories include

Kantianism (deontological-based theories), utilitarian/consequentialism, Marxism, libertarianism (right-based theories), virtue ethics (character-based theories), ethics of care, feminism, personalism (person-centred theories), and communitarianism (community-based theories). Apart from the numerous middle-range theories, there is also a growing application of religious doctrines in ethical deliberations. This is why theologians and philosophers are among the core specialists in theoretical bioethics. The theories often provide various arguments that are sometimes vague in guiding moral judgments in practical incidents. However, the three major derivatives from some of the theories are "rights, duties and norms." The rights of an individual in any situation, the professional duties of the scientists, and the normative regulations are the core guiding priorities of most of the theoretical underpinnings. African philosophy also provides streams of moralities that conform to the norms and values of the African people. This helps to provide a relative basis in the consideration of ethics in the African context.

11.3.2 Clinical/Health Care Bioethics

This area usually concentrates on moral perplexities arising from client-practitioner relations and practices. The Hippocratic Oath is the origin of the guiding professional ethics in medical practice. There have been some modifications to the Oath following attendant contentions regarding its modern applicability. While the Oath provides historical ethical guidelines, the emerging trends induce moral problems that are often complex and require deliberation within health care settings. Unlike theoretical bioethics that provides general explanations, clinical bioethics focuses on the individual case to determine an appropriate clinical/care decision. There is often tension between the professional construction of facts and that of the patients, as well as the desires of the parties. Such cases might require hard decisions (e.g., withdrawal of treatment and abortion) that must be guided by professional ethics, normative values, and personal choices of the patients. The normative framework also includes the legal codes, which mediate medical practice. The interplay of these guiding principles serves to build a method of resolving ethical apprehensions in clinical cases.

The questions of health care ethics do not only stop at the level of the hospital but also within the norms of society. For instance, a request for an abortion must be considered within the legal rules of the society—whether the law prescribes or proscribes it, whether professional ethics prescribe abortion as care or harm to the embryo, whether the patient understands the implications of the procedure or has a *tenable* reason for requesting abortion. In this case, there are many issues that interplay to arrive at an ethical decision. The same applies to the request for euthanasia by a patient (see Sect. 9.1.6.3). Aside medical requests, clinical ethics also include the consideration of values in client-practitioner relations. The handling of information, truth telling, confidentiality, and patterns of interaction and control of medical malpractice are the core of clinical ethics. The exchange of information in a medical setting could involve sensitive disclosures. For instance, how will the physician disclose to a patient with a terminal disease that death is imminent and medicine is helpless, and that the condition is irreversible? Does the physician have a right to inform a partner of a person living with HIV of the risk of HIV without the permission of the patient? Sometimes, respecting patient's choices could be problematic because of overindulgence or uneasy requests. In other words, are there limits to a patient's involvement in care? How can the physician handle incompetent patients (with a mental problem or in a vegetative state) without compromising their own moral values? Can the values of parents be applied to their underage children, especially when those values are against biomedical norms? Is it ethical to withhold or withdraw treatment from a newborn with spina bifida or because of perceived non-clinical benefits or established poor prognosis? The vital issue involves how to handle a particular patient without compromising personal, social, legal, and medical rules/norms.

Furthermore, there are countless moral perplexities that are generated in the day-to-day medical practice. This is why many medical institutions are setting up health care ethics committees and institutional review boards (IRBs) to deliberate on appropriate ethical decisions that should guide medical practice and research (see Sects. 11.6.1 and 11.6.2). This aspect of bioethics gains prominence because of some extreme cases that often find their way into the media spotlight, thereby generating global discussions. The cases of Piergiorgio Welby (an Italian poet with muscular dystrophy in 2006) and Tony Nicklinson (with locked-in syndrome in 2012) whose requests for euthanasia led to legal battles and media magnification of ethical discourse.

11.3.3 Research Bioethics

Research bioethics is also a prominent aspect which involves the regulation of moral uneasiness in scientific research in a way that will not compromise both the goals of science and human values. While many ethical issues could be generated in all research endeavours, particular interest here is on those involving human subjects. The fundamental crux is how to ensure moral science as being against "jungle" science where all practices prevail irrespective of their implications. Sometimes scientists want to generate empirical facts and solutions without considering the limits, long-term implications, and the rights of the (human) participants. For instance, stem cell research (SCR) has generated some ethical concerns despite its promises to revolutionise medical practice, especially in transplantation medicine. Some SCR involves the use of human embryos, but many bioethicists consider the embryos as potential humans and argue that they should not be used as research materials. Some discuss whether it is right to create embryos or use leftover embryos from in vitro fertilisation (IVF) for research (see Devolder 2005). Embryos can be created to benefit patients with certain illnesses and injuries. There have been some clamours to explore other sources of cells (e.g., those from adult and xenogeneic cells, and therapeutic cloning) with less serious ethical concerns.

This aspect of bioethics also focuses on clinical trials by analysing ethical concerns at all the phases of clinical trials. Some of the areas of ethical concern include, among others: recruitment and protection of participants (including vulnerable subjects), methodological/scientific requirements, informed consent, risks and benefits, control of adverse events, handling of samples, community protection, obtaining of ethical clearance, and commercialisation of research results. The involvement of human subjects in social science empirical activities signifies the need to consider ethical issues. It also requires obtaining informed consent, minimisation of harm to the study population, maintenance of confidentiality about the research participants, protection of privacy, and other rights of the research participants. The question of human dignity cuts across all forms of research. The bottom line is that all empirical activities must be within ethical constraints. The interest and dignity of those involved must be upheld and research must not "impress" the donors, enhance promotions (in academics), or advance human knowledge while unethical practices pervade and cause harm (physical, psychological, or social) to the human subjects.

Another fundamental issue is whether there should be a limit in scientific research or whether scientists should be allowed to proceed with any possible enquiry without minding the social and medical implications. The research about human cloning poses fundamental ethical concerns. Human genome/genetic research is also raising a number of concerns yet to be fully resolved. Generally, it is advocated that human subjects should be regarded as moral agents and subjects in any research with fundamental rights, which must be protected beyond any scientific interests. The concern about research malpractice (see historical cases such as Nazi human experimentation and the Tuskegee Syphilis Study [1932–1972]) that resulted in many deaths and injuries formed a part of the basis for the development of ethical guidelines such as the Nuremberg Code in 1948, the Helsinki Declaration in 1964, the Belmont report in 1974, and CIOMS (Council for International Organizations of Medical Sciences) Guidelines in 1993. This also accounts for the development of institutional review boards (IRBs) to regulate the conduct of scientific research within the limits of ethics (see Sect. 11.6.2). Like other continents, Africa has been a site for a number of unethical experimentations and clinical trials (e.g., Depo-Provera trial, Zimbabwe; sterilisation experimentation, Namibia; Trovan trial, Nigeria; and a number of HIV/AIDS-related trials in Southern Africa) (see Kaler 1998; Lurie and Wolfe 1997; Washington 2006).

11.3.4 Biotech Bioethics

The development of technology is one of the driving forces of new possibilities in life sciences and medicine. The use of technology here refers to advanced technologies such as neuro-, cyber-, gene-, and nanotechnologies that make human enhancement, reproductive technologies (IVF, sex selection, and prenatal genetic testing), tissues engineering, and other hi-tech practices in life sciences possible. The reference includes therapeutic and nontherapeutic applications of such technologies. Bioethicists are interested in these areas because the application of these technologies has the potential for serious implications in human societies and for individuals. The pace of discovery in biotechnology is very rapid with considerable possibilities to alleviate human suffering but is not devoid of medical and social risks.

While the initial considerations are usually the potential benefits of biotechnologies, it incites caution and fear that humanity is gaining too much power and too little choice over human evolution and destiny (McLean 2012). This could result in societal disruption or normlessness. The possible worst-case scenarios could be terrifying in relation to human survival in the long run. The controversies about the development and use of genetically modified (GM) food, the possibilities of life extension, and transhumanism (belief that human nature is improvable with the use of applied sciences) are proliferating. The questions of safety, equity, respect for nature, societal disruption, and human dignity in the application of advanced technologies are yet to be fully resolved (Gordijn 2005; Lin and Allhoff 2008). The ELSI (ethical, legal, and social implications) approach in technology assessment is the major methodology used in this aspect of bioethics.

Furthermore, transgenic biotechnology, the practice of transferring genetic materials from one species to another, presents a number of possibilities in medical practice. In transferring genetic traits, it is possible to have various combinations such as plant-animal-human, animal-animal, and animal-human (Robert and Baylis 2003). The use of xenogeneic (animal) cells in SCR is a typical illustration. Additionally, scientists can produce animals carrying human organs, which can be used in transplantation to humans (referred to as xenotransplantation) (see NCB 1996). The critical ethical issues are apparent: whether it is morally and biological safe to create and use transgenic animals as sources of live organs and tissue for transplantation into human beings, and to use such xenotransplants in human beings. While there are promises through transgenic biotech in prevention and treatment of diseases and disabilities, some dangers are also imminent, including effects on human behaviour (could be more animalistic), disruption of human genetic makeup, reduced susceptibility (which could lead to more animal diseases among humans), and other latent/unintended sociocultural impacts. While Robert and Baylis (2003) alluded to the notion of moral confusion regarding social and ethical obligations to novel interspecies beings, Glenn (2003) submitted that there is a need to harness the potential benefits in transgenic biotechnology to alleviate human suffering. In general, the repercussion of the growing utilisation of biotechnology forms a central concern of this aspect of bioethics.

11.3.5 Public Health Bioethics

The primary goal of public health is to improve population health. Public health concentrates on organised efforts/interventions to address community health needs (Kass 2001). The focus is on the community rather than the individual. The starting point is the assumption that every individual has a right to health care and the resources necessary for health. This is why addressing the fundamental causes/social determinants of illness is an elemental aspect of public health. It is understandable that the community barriers to accessing care have to be addressed in order to improve population health. Another central aspect of public health practice is the assessment of health services in line with the objectives of health systems. The foregoing shows that public health is a community-based (not hospital-based) approach to improving human health. Public health raises a number of moral problems, hence it requires an ethical framework. Therefore, the essence of public health bioethics is "to provide practical guidance for public health professionals and to highlight the defining values of public health, values that differ in morally relevant ways from values that define clinical practice and research" (Kass 2001, p. 1176).

Public health professionals conduct research within the community to examine factors promoting health or otherwise with the aim of controlling both positive and negative factors. One way of improving community health is through the dissemination of health information, which will enable individuals to make informed choices regarding their health. More so, public health professionals sometimes create or enforce health-related regulations and legislation including mandating screening, treatment, immunisations, and environmental sanitation (Kass 2001). The two major strategies involve changing people's behaviour (to stimulate positive behaviour and create demand for required health services) and changing their communities (by managing community factors and creating supply of health services). Activities of the professionals also need to be guided in a way that will ensure moral conduct without transgressing the boundaries of the entrenched acceptable values of the communities.

With particular reference to Kass (2001) and Callahan and Jennings (2002), some of the critical areas of ethical concerns include:

1. How to assess the limits of the goal of public health within the limits of community interests/values;
2. How to ensure equitable distribution of community benefits from public health programs within the community and across communities;
3. Ensuring that scientific principles guide the development and implementation of health intervention which should be based on available evidence;
4. Assessing the effectiveness of public health programs. Monitoring and evaluating health programs are necessary components of a good public health program;
5. Assessing the potential burden of health interventions and how to minimise such burden;
6. Despite the goal of health risk reduction, it is important to control invasive practices within the community;
7. How to limit the effects of structural and economic inequalities on health by addressing socioeconomic indicators in order to prevent adverse health outcomes;
8. How to guide health advocacy and moderate information dissemination. Information empowers the people with required knowledge and assists in making informed decisions;

9. Empower vulnerable groups/communities to attain conditions necessary for health. A target segment is the risk group or vulnerable population in order to maximise the benefits of health programs;
10. And uphold the rights of individuals in the community and for the community as a sociopolitical entity, especially through social legitimation of activities and conformity to the principle of non-maleficence.

11.3.6 Policy and Regulatory Bioethics

This aspect of bioethics deals with the enactment of rules (including legal framework) guiding the general practice of medicine and biosciences. Callahan (2004) submitted that regulatory bioethics ordinarily seeks laws, rules, policies, and regulations that will guide general practices, and its aim is practical rather than theoretical, with a focus on the general population rather than the individual. For instance, it involves the development of legal and medical definitions of clinical conditions such as clinical death (Callahan 2004). The development of a code of ethics and practices, for instance in the use of human biomedical research, and hospital rules for do-not-resuscitate (DNR) or advance directives regarding withholding and withdrawal of treatment are also a part of the preoccupation of the regulatory bioethics.

Callahan further noted that this aspect encompasses the development of policies designed to allocate scarce health care resources or to protect the environment. For instance, it requires structured guidelines and procedures for allocating organs for transplantations. This is important in maintaining justice in the allocation of scarce resources within the hospital or at the national level. Another important example in this area is triage, or the selection of patients for treatment based on the severity of their condition, in the hospital. The hospital needs to set general rules to guide the health workers on prioritisation of cases so that patients who deserve emergency attention are considered before others.

Generally, the domain of rules in health care administration also falls within this aspect. At a general level, health care policies and reforms are critically evaluated to assess moral concerns regarding access and related issues that will affect population health. The aim is often to generate a policy discourse, influence policies, or advance policies that will promote population health. Regulatory bioethics also extend to the debate regarding various aspects of health systems—whether socialised, capitalist, or a two-tiered system—and how to protect the public from insurance regulation of services.

11.3.7 Cultural Bioethics

The socio-spatial environment often affects the construction of morality. This is why morality is relative and dynamic. Cultural relativity necessitates the consideration of personal values and priorities in ethical decisions and deliberations. The cultural context of practice is important in offering appropriate care and respecting the beliefs of the individual. This aspect of bioethics considers the ethical issues in relation to the cultural milieu. The attempt is to situate ethics within cultures in a way that will not compromise care and scientific sensibilities. This is why ethical decisions are not fixed and universal. The cultural context regulating the provision of abortion services in Tunisia is different from that of Kenya or Zimbabwe. For instance, the influence of religion is vital in ethical decision-making in North Africa because the region consists of predominantly Muslims who operate within the limits of Islamic laws. Additionally, the Catholic church has played important roles in ethical decisions, both theoretical and practical.

Therefore, apart from specific cultural norms, "religion" is important in bioethics, hence the development of theological bioethics. It is not uncommon for non-secular critique to regard cloning as "playing God" or embryonic research as "playing with human lives," since embryos are regarded as humans. There are cultural differences in the explanation and attitude towards issues such as disclosures of terminal diagnosis, reproductive technology, child adoption, SCR, therapeutic cloning, organ transplantations, and euthanasia (Rehmann-Sutter et al. 2006). The preoccupation of this aspect is the examination of cultural context in the production of morality, especially in terms of what is permitted, prescribed, and proscribed, and the (cultural) rationalisation behind the morality. Another important point in the foregoing is that cultural context also generates what is considered to be an ethical problem. While abortion, homosexuality, and artificial insemination by donor have been normalised in many western cultures, they are still seen as moral problems in many African cultures. This is why Rehmann-Sutter et al. (2006) further noted that biomedical developments carry with them social and cultural meanings that must be taken into account in order to understand and resolve bioethical dilemmas. Apart from making relevant contributions in other aspects of bioethics, social science especially, sociology and anthropology are particularly relevant in this aspect.

11.4 Bioethical Agenda: Some Areas of Moral Perplexities in Health Care

It has been repeatedly mentioned that the core thrust of bioethics is the understanding of moral conundrums in biosciences. The discourse centers on whether some practices are moral or hold adverse ethical, legal, and social implications (both short- and long-term). The concern is also about social/societal disruption, a breakdown of social life or order. The essence of this section is to present more core areas of ethical discourse at three stages relating to human life: before birth, during life, and at the end of life. The aim is also to provide more illustrations that will generate further understanding. While the illustrations complement previous ones, they are not exhaustive. This presents some starting points for building a proper engagement in the bioethical discourse.

11.4.1 Moral Conundrums in the Process of Childbirth

The focus of this section is on some moral anxieties which are evident before birth or in the process of conception. There are countless medical possibilities that generate ethical discourse across cultures including use of assisted reproductive technology, prenatal genetic testing, abortion, sex selection, surrogate motherhood, sperm or gamete donation, and selective reproduction (including eugenic practices), among others. Medicalisation of pregnancy/childbirth, which also generates some concern, has been previously discussed (see Sect. 9.1.6.1).

The application of reproductive technology presents a number of moral issues. There have been some arguments over the overmedicalisation of the female body due to limitless interventions on the female body or feminisation of infertility. Some feminists argue that reproductive function or biological reproduction is one of the major sources of oppression against women. In developing countries, parents without children have low social status, and women, in particular, are viewed as "culprits." There are growing reproductive possibilities to assist those who have a child-wish. Surrogate motherhood and sperm or gamete donations are among the options sometimes applied through in vitro fertilisation (IVF). Surrogate motherhood or mothering by proxy is the practice that requires a woman to carry a pregnancy and delivers the child for another couple or persons (see Purdy 2006). The surrogate mother (some of them prefer to be called gestational carriers) may provide the egg that will be fertilised or a fertilised egg may be placed in her womb to carry the pregnancy to term and consequently deliver the baby on behalf of a couple or another person. As Purdy observed, surrogate motherhood separates sex and reproduction, marriage and reproduction, and motherhood and childhood. Since a monetary reward is usually provided for the "service," mothering (in this case) is a transaction bound by legal contracts and obligations. The practice could help to alleviate infertility. It helps some women avoid the risk of pregnancy, eliminate work disruption due to pregnancy, prevent some genetic diseases, and help same-sex couples and unmarried individuals to fulfill their wish for a child (Purdy 2006).

There have been a number of moral concerns regarding mothering by proxy, which include the notions of transactional motherhood or contractual pregnancy, baby-selling, exploitation, disruption of family patterns, and arbitrary separation of mother-to-child bond. The process could also involve artificial insemination, or sperm or gamete donation. At times, these biological resources are provided for monetary gain. The question is whether is it is morally right or wrong to sell sperms or gamete and whether a (free) donation is ethical since it obscures the biological affinity of the offspring (as the true biological father or mother may not be known to the child). The question is also whether it really matters to accept and promote social parenthood instead of biological parenthood. Some concerns are also raised regarding sex selection and selective reproduction. In cases of gender inequality, some individuals prefer a certain sex of a child to the other. Many couples desire to determine the sex of a child for social reasons (because of the value of a male or female child in the community) or to select due to specific genetic or biological reasons. The practice of eugenics also involves ethical conundrums because of selections based on some physiological or genetic characteristics. Some ethicists term the deliberate selection of traits as a manifestation of discrimination and moral perversion of reproduction as a gift of nature. Many experts accept prenatal genetic testing to detect future health risks of a foetus and view medically indicated abortion as a preventive option. On the other hand, many others reject such genetic screening with a claim that it amounts to genetic reductionism and could accrue medical risks to the foetus and lead to abortion (termed as a termination of life).

11.4.2 Ethics During Life: Respect for Persons

How to ensure respect for persons or personhood is perhaps the most significant ethical concern throughout a lifetime and in all medical interventions. The illustration here will present an ethical discourse during lifetime in relation to personhood. The human agents deserve and expect respect in all medical interventions. There are three major aspects of respect in medical encounters, which include the person, body, and values. While it can be argued that the body and values are integral parts of the person, they are mentioned separately to signify that they represent distinct issues. The most fundamental issue is that a human person should not be used as a means to an end. The human person has the highest intrinsic value in the application of technologies and medical care (Amzat and Grandi 2011). This is why there are debates on the consideration of the human person in bioethics. The central thesis is that the "human person is a subject, not an object as are the things of the world." Janssens further elaborated that the human person should have opportunities for self-determination as a moral agent, deciding on all his or her doings in conscience and consequently in a responsible way. More so, "the human person is a subject in corporeality. Our body forms part of the totality that we are: what concerns our human body affects our person" (Janssens 1990, p. 94, 1999).

Medical encounters and health care (in general) present with a variety of issues that emphasise the notions of the human person. For instance, in medical encounters, it is important to note some of the core value expectations of the patients/clients; the wishes and values of human persons should be considered or prioritised during medical encounters. The human person should not be reduced to a medical condition or discriminated due to a medical condition. It also involves whether the application of biotechnology and medical practices are good for the human person and considers the implications for human safety and survival. In the use of body products such as blood in the biobank or medical information, there must be confidentiality and conscientious use in a way that will protect personal/human values. The exchange of information between the physician and the client should involve truth telling, appropriate disclosures, and trust. The use of informed consent in research and medical interventions has become a legal and ethical requirement. Informed consent ensures that the client understands his/her medical condition and entrusts the physician with his or her body to proceed with medical intervention.

Apart from information issues, any intervention involving the body should be devoid of medical malpractice, including all forms of harassment and exploitation. An example is the process of procurement of an organ in transplantation medicine. There have been serious concerns regarding several "market" where vulnerable people sell their organs. The question is whether organ sale transgresses the respect for bodily integrity both for the seller and the buyer. More so, the idea of personalist consideration also seeks to promote fairness and equality in the allocation of medical resources.

Furthermore, in terms of personhood, the Kantian tradition proposes that rationality confers personhood to humans. In this case, those with mental incapability may be regarded as non-persons. The term "person" is often considered from a moral point of view. The moral status of the person is a discourse with divergent arguments. The typical scenario is whether unconscious individuals should be given a full moral status like other conscious persons.

11.4.3 Ethics in End-of-Life Care

Towards the end of life, a number of ethical concerns could be generated in care. One of the major issues could be a request for death, which has been previously examined (see Sect. 9.1.6.3). The issue of euthanasia dwells on the sanctity and preservation of life in the face of medical challenges. Apart from euthanasia, caring for terminally ill patients presents a number of moral challenges. Palliative/terminal sedation, advance directives, organ harvesting, obtaining consent from incompetent patients, terminating life-sustaining treatment/devices, and limits of intensive care are among issues with reoccurring ethical challenges. More importantly, in treating dying patients, who are often frail and vulnerable, physicians must meet a high standard of professional and ethical conduct, which includes respecting the autonomy and wishes of the patients, considerate truth-telling, setting of treatment goals, providing for symptom control, continuing attentive care, and accompaniment throughout the course of the illness (Latimer 1998, p. 1741). Unfortunately, the basis for and course of action are sometimes contentious.

One important measure in end-of-life care is palliative/terminal sedation, which is meant to lower the consciousness of the patient as a relief from pain. This is done in the case of irreversible decay of bodily and mental capacities, refractory symptoms, suffering, and pain. Such sedation is often granted upon request by the patient but when the patient has no capacity to decide, it becomes problematic to act. Can the family members decide on such vital care on behalf of the patient? For some patients that are "competent," it is also possible that the experience of pain might positively influence the decision. While it has been argued that palliative sedation is a medical intervention that should be considered as part of a continuum of palliative care, some argue that it could shorten the life of the patient (Maltoni et al. 2012). Although the goal of palliative sedation is never to end life, it is sometimes referred to as "slow death," thereby negating the principle of non-maleficence. Some related

Fig. 11.2 Four principles of bioethics

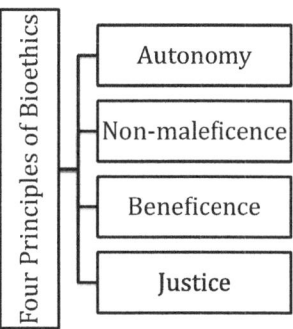

instances also include ethical considerations of aggressive treatment and the use of life-supporting interventions despite poor prognosis during end-of-life care (see Baumann et al. 2011).

The discourse of "good death" is common to both bioethics and the sociology of dying and death. The quest for good death is a value among many individuals. Good death often reflects a peaceful death devoid of suffering and pain and, at times, death at home in the hands of the family network. There is contention on whether the prolongation of life in the face of refractory symptoms with artificial measures (e.g., artificial ventilation) is within the appropriate values of the patient. Additionally, while organ retrieval (from non-heart-beating patients) could save other people's lives, it is still contentious whether it reflects the value of good death for the patients from whom organs are harvested. More importantly, there is no uniformity of actual time after the heart stops beating to retrieve organs. Some ethicists observe that there could be a subjective judgment by the physician to "impulsively" retrieve organs from a patient who could be resuscitated. More pressing is that there is no uniform definition of death, especially in cases involving brain death. It is possible to maintain or restart the functioning of the heart and lungs after the brain has stopped functioning with the use of medical technologies. The concept of social death is also relevant here (see Sect. 1.5.10). The quest for uniform criteria is necessary to declare death for ethical, medical, legal, and social purposes.

11.5 Understanding Principlism in Bioethics

In the course of the development of bioethics, especially in the late 1970s, four fundamental principles of ethical guidelines emerged to guide medical practice. The four principles (shown in Fig. 11.2) include respect for autonomy, non-maleficence, beneficence, and justice. The historical origin of the principles can be traced to the Hippocratic Oath. While there has been some criticisms of these principles, especially in terms of adequacy and sufficiency in guiding moral judgments, they still stand in providing general guidelines (Beauchamp 2001). Many bioethicists often recommend that the four principles should be considered to be universal, and

11.5 Understanding Principlism in Bioethics

in their *prima facie* nature (see Dawson and Garrard 2006; Gillon 1994). The debate is whether the principles are sufficient to guide moral norms in clinical ethics or should be ordered (as shown in Fig. 11.2) and generalised. Nevertheless, the essence of the principles is to provide a framework to direct moral decision-making in health care. The overall goal is to ensure respect for human persons, promote freedom and choices, and prevent medical malpractice. The principles will be briefly examined in the next four subsections.

11.5.1 Autonomy

"Autonomy" is the first of the principles, derived from the Greek *autos* (self) and *nomos* (rule or governance), literally meaning self-rule (Beauchamp and Childress 2001, p. 57). This principle negates the notion of medical paternalism (see Sect. 9.2.1.1) but promotes self-determination and responsibility in the course of treatment. This indicates respect for privacy, individual choices, freedom of will, and self-actualisation without coercion or undue interference from external forces/agents. The only basis of interference on the part of the physician is to provide adequate technical information that would aid personal choices. The concept presumes that the patients have freedom of reason and choice and should be independent by acting in judicious manners that conform to their lived experiences.

As ethics is projected as aiming for a good life with and for others in a just society (Ricoeur 1999), it should be subjectively constructed and interpreted by individuals based on personal criteria. As mentioned previously, persons are not like things of this world but are blessed with the rationality to act in accordance with personal preferences, which invariably form the prerequisite for the actualisation of a good life. The concept of autonomy confers a sense of responsibility to the patients. The concept also provides the basis for informed consent, which should be sought from the patient before commencement of treatment or participation in research. In general, the assumption that the patient has the capacity for rational choices might be incorrect in some situations. This notion could hinder the progression of best choices as perceived by medical professionals.

11.5.2 Non-maleficence

The second principle is non-maleficence, which implies that there should not be any infliction of harm on the patient. "Do not do harm" is a fundamental responsibility of the physician. Beauchamp and Childress (2001, p. 117) explained that the basic moral attributes include: do not kill or incapacitate and do not cause pain, suffering, or offence. The essence of care is to promote positive experiences and activities that will alleviate pain or suffering. The infliction of harm could be a result of errors of omission (breach of duty) or errors of commission (activities that are substandard).

There is a general rule that negative actions that expose the patients to suffering or risk of death constitute harm. The meaning of "harm" is still not definite. There are issues that generate a debate regarding the principle of non-maleficence. Such issues include abortion, euthanasia, withholding, and withdrawal of treatment. The question is whether these issues could be regarded as medical care or rationalised/legitimised harm in a medical setting. Apart from physical harm, there could also be other dimensions including emotional and psychological harm, which are not easy to measure objectively.

11.5.3 Beneficence

"Doing good" is also a major principle in bioethics. This involves the implementation of actions that will enhance or promote the health of patients. Medical action must be beneficial to the patient. Beauchamp and Childress (2001) observed that there is no clear difference between beneficence and non-maleficence. While the physician is required to avoid inflicting harm on patients, he/she is also required to ensure actions take place that will lead to recovery. This is a duty-based approach in care. Some of the moral rules include: protection of rights, prevention of harm, alleviating conditions that could cause harm, and providing assistance to high-risk persons or those with disabilities.

It is often problematic to decide on the criteria that will be used in promoting the well-being of the patient since health is not only about medical well-being but also includes social and psychological well-being (see Veatch 2012). For example, if amputation is medically beneficial, what about the quality of life in terms of personal and social well-being? A medical decision to amputate might also affect aesthetic and economic well-being. Therefore, there is a need to balance the benefits and harm in all ramifications, even while the physician pursues the best medical measures that could produce the best outcome (Veatch 2012).

11.5.4 Justice

The notion of justice is often applied to an individual relative to others in the society or examined to access the general conditions of health services. It implies that fairness and equality must be prioritised in the allocation of finite resources. In terms of justice, issues such as access to health care and health insurance are paramount. Generally, there are three aspects of justice: fair distribution of scarce resources (distributive justice), respect for people's rights (rights based justice), and respect for morally acceptable laws (legal justice) (Gillon 1994, p. 185). Distributive justice refers to "fair, equitable, and appropriate distribution determined by justified norms that structure the terms of social cooperation" (Beauchamp and Childress 2001, p. 226). In this sense, "justice" goes beyond equal treatment and focuses on equal prioritisation of needs as there are many different health care needs in a society. Justice also involves situations in which the rights of individuals are respected and protected within the social and legal context.

There are often conflicts of interest in the prioritisation of health care needs due to limited funds for health care. The conflicts centre on how to distribute health care facilities, limit some services in favour of the others, and control social determinants of health and enact public policies in health care. For instance, providing incentives to the vulnerable populations (especially the poor) will promote access to health care and thereby reduce the mortality rate of the country. There should be a responsive minimisation and mitigation of the effects of personal attributes (e.g., class and gender) in access to health care. The doctrine of justice plays a pivotal role, especially within relational context. There are numerous criteria for justly allocating health care resources that can be morally justified but not all can be fully met simultaneously (Gillon 1994). Responsive commitment (by the stakeholders) to the needs of the population and morally acceptable tenets are the hallmarks of ensuring a just health care system.

The four principles have been widely defended as moral guidelines, especially as a North American ideology of bioethics. While the four principles have been popularised, it is also important to note that there are a number of criticisms with respect to ordering the principles and their perceived absoluteness in ethical considerations. More importantly, the European tradition promotes different bioethical principles which include autonomy, dignity, integrity, and vulnerability (see Rendtorff 2002). The European principles were generated after a multidisciplinary research study involving many EU countries which led to the Barcelona Declaration of 1998 of the four European principles of bioethics. Briefly, *autonomy* is described as having a capacity for moral insight, self-rule, and self-responsibility free from coercion; *dignity* is the capacity of being human with infinite value, thus deserving honour and respect; *integrity* simplifies the coherence and wholeness of life which should be free from harm; and *vulnerability* means the protection of those whose autonomy, dignity, and integrity are capable of being threatened, especially because of their peculiar circumstances. The declaration was that autonomy, dignity, integrity, and vulnerability constitute vital values in European culture and therefore should serve as reflective guidelines in bioethics (Rendtorff 2002).

11.6 Structures in Bioethical Deliberations

While there are moral codes, it is often pertinent to institute structures that will apply the codes and inform moral decisions. This is why health care/clinical ethics committees and review boards are instituted. These are regulatory agencies with the specialised function of evaluating biomedical circumstances and moral implications with the purpose of resolving cases and playing advisory roles. In cases where there are no ethics institutions, the physician still holds paternalistic power to make appropriate moral implications based on prevailing sociomedical and legal contexts. The development of ethics committees is recent in Africa and many medical institutions still lack such a committee. On the other hand, institutional review boards (IRB) are still at the early stage of recognition. The following two subsections will briefly examine casuistry as a responsibility of clinical ethics committees and the roles of IRBs in the management of research protocol.

11.6.1 *Casuistry: Health Care Ethical Case Deliberation*

Following the rising incidence of moral uneasiness in medicine, there is a need to draw specific practical strategies of resolving issues to produce ethical decisions. This gives rise to the development of health care ethics committees to deliberate and make prescriptive recommendations on the appropriate course of action for the treating physician. The method used by the health care ethics committee is called casuistry. Casuistry, "a term derived from the Latin word meaning *event or occurrence* and in later Latin, *case*," is now applied in bioethics (especially health care/clinical ethics) as the "method of analysing and resolving instances of moral perplexity by interpreting general moral rules in light of particular circumstances" (Jonsen 2004, p. 374). The committee usually consists of a number of experts including (but not limited to) medical, legal, cultural, and theological experts who examine a particular case with the goal of making recommendations. In a previous elaborate definition, Jonsen and Toulmin (1988, p. 257) defined *casuistry* as a method of case deliberation "using procedures of reasoning based on paradigms and analogies, leading to the formulation of expert opinion about the existence and stringency of particular moral obligations, framed in terms of rules and maxims that are general but not universal or invariable, since they hold good with certainty only in the typical conditions of the agent and circumstances of the case."

Case deliberation is important because there are no universal procedures or regulations applicable to all cases. The primary features of any case deliberations are relativism, particularism, and specificity. While these features are sacrosanct, the committee might be guided by a general procedure. For instance, the Nijmegen Method of ethical case deliberation is one of the most elaborate methods which takes into consideration most of the issues that might enhance appropriate action prescriptions. The issues identified in the Nijmegen Method includes: the moral problem in the case, the available facts on the case (including medical, nursing, patient's views, social, and organisational dimensions), values (including well-being and autonomy of the patient and responsibility of health care professionals), and decision-making (recapitulation of the moral problem, unknown details, arguments, decision, and evaluation) (Steinkamp and Gordijn 2003, p. 240). Due to the aforementioned features, there is a reasonable methodological plurality across health care organisations or countries and thus also on the values and factors leading to the formulation of ethical decision. Health care ethics committees focus on moral issues during the course of care while IRBs or research ethics committees focus on ethical guidelines in scientific investigations.

11.6.2 Institutional Review Boards

An institutional review board (IRB), also called an ethical review board, is usually instituted to examine, approve, monitor, and review biomedical and behavioural research involving humans with the aim of ensuring appropriate practices and scientific standards. For instance, some clinical trials could have risks for the participants (including permanent injuries and fatal consequences) (see Geissler and Molyneux 2011; Jegede 2009; Washington 2006). In evaluating any research protocol, an IRB considers the following issues:

1. The procedure and methodology are scientifically appropriate. This is to ensure that the basic phases of research are followed and the design takes research limitations into consideration.
2. The fundamental rights of the human subjects are adequately protected. Most of these rights are those reflected in the declaration of human rights. That is, humans are not used like "things" in the course of the research.
3. The risk-benefit analysis is examined to ensure that risk is drastically minimised, and there could be accrued benefits (not necessarily to the participants) but to the society either in the short- or long run.
4. The informed consent and confidentiality protocols are applied appropriately. While this could reflect as part of human rights, the emphasis is worthwhile in bioethics. The use of inducement and coercion are appropriately minimised.
5. The selection of participants is just and equitable and there is no discrimination on the basis of participation or non-participation. Importantly, vulnerable groups are protected. The right to withdraw at any stage of the research should be guaranteed.
6. There are appropriate mechanisms or structures to control both predictable and unpredictable events in the course of the study. This usually involves the management of adverse events in the course of the research.
7. The use of data and research outcomes conform to set standards in line with the set research goals and the interest of the participants, the organisations (involved), and the society at large.

The aforementioned issues (usually considered) are not exhaustive and may vary from one research protocol to another. It is now becoming mandatory for all research (especially those studies involving human subjects) to obtain an ethical approval from the IRB before proceeding with the implementation of the research.

Conclusively, it is evident that there is need to consider humans as situated or social agents in the course of moral understanding and ethical decision-making. In this area, sociology holds promise to synergise efforts and moderate course of action with sociological insights (from empirical, theoretical, and practical knowledge). This role might be defining for bioethics as humans are largely social beings.

References

Amzat, J., & Grandi, G. (2011). Gender context of personalism in bioethics. *Developing World Bioethics, 11*(3), 136–145.

Baumann, A., Claudot, F., Audibert, G., Mertes, P., & Puybasset, L. (2011).The ethical and legal aspects of palliative sedation in severely brain-injured patients: A French perspective. *Philosophy, Ethics, and Humanities in Medicine, 6*, 4. http://www.peh-med.com/content/6/1/4.

Beauchamp, T. M. (2001). Principlism and its alleged competitors. In J. Harris (Ed.), *Oxford reading in philosophy: Bioethics* (pp. 479–493). Oxford: Oxford University Press.

Beauchamp, T. M. (2003). Ethical theories and bioethics. In T. M. Beauchamp & L. Walters (Eds.), *Contemporary issues in bioethics* (6th ed.). New York: Wadsworth.

Beauchamp, T. M., & Childress, J. F. (2001). *Principles of biomedical ethics* (5th ed.) Oxford: Oxford University Press.

Callahan, D. (2004). Bioethics. In S. G. Post (Ed.), *Encyclopedia of bioethics* (278–287) 3rd ed. New York: Macmillan Reference USA.

Callahan, D., & Jennings, B. (2002). Ethics and public health: Forging a strong relationship. *American Journal of Public Health, 92*, 169–176.

Chattopadhyay, S., & De Vries, R. (2008). Bioethical concerns are global, bioethics is Western. *Eubios Journal of Asian and International Bioethics, 18*(4), 106–109.

Dawson, A., & Garrard, E. (2006). In defence of moral imperialism: Four equal and universal prima facie principles. *Journal of Medical Ethics, 32*(4), 200–204.

Devolder, K. (2005). Creating and sacrificing embryos for stem cells. *Journal of Medical Ethics, 31*, 366–370. doi:10.1136/jme.2004.008599.

Geissler, P. W., & Molyneux, C. (Eds.). (2011). *Evidence, ethos and experiment: The anthropology and history of medical research in Africa*. New York: Berghahn Books.

Gillon, R. (1994). Medical ethics: Four principles plus attention to scope. *British Medical Journal, 309*, 184–188.

Glenn, L. M. (2003). Biotechnology at the margins of personhood: An evolving legal paradigm. *Journal of Evolution and Technology, 13*, 35–37.

Gordijn, B. (2005). Nanoethics: From utopian dreams and apocalyptic nightmares towards a more balanced view. *Science and Engineering Ethics, 11*(4), 521–533.

Jahr, F. (1927). Bioethics: A panorama of the human being's ethical relations with animals and plants. *Kosmos* Nr. 24 Translated by José Roberto Goldim/2005.

Janssens, L. (1990). Personalism in moral theology. In C. E. Curran (Ed.), *Moral theology: challenges for the future* (pp. 94–107). New York: Paulist.

Janssens, L. (1999). Particular goods and personalist morals. *Ethical Perspectives, 6*(1), 55–59.

Jegede, A. S. (2009). Understanding informed consent for participation in international health research. *Developing World Bioethics, 9*(2), 81–87.

Jonsen, A. R. (2004). Casuistry. In S. G. Post (Ed.), *Encyclopedia of bioethics* (374–380) 3rd ed. New York: Macmillan Reference USA.

Jonsen, A. R., & Toulmin, S. E. (1988). *The abuse of casuistry: A history of moral reasoning*. Berkeley and Los Angeles: University of California Press.

Kaler, A. (1998). A threat to the nation and a threat to the men: The banning of Depo-Provera in Zimbabwe, 1981. *Journal of Southern African Studies, 24*(2), 347–376.

Kass, N. E. (2001). An ethics framework for public health. *Am J Public Health, 91*(11), 1776–1782.

Latimer, E. J. (1998). Ethical care at the end of life. *Canadian Medical Association Journal, 158*(13), 1741–1747.

Lin, P., & Allhoff, F. (2008). Untangling the debate the ethics of human enhancement. *Nanoethics, 2*, 251–264.

Lurie, P., & Wolfe, S. M. (1997). Unethical trials of interventions to reduce perinatal transmission of the human immunodeficiency virus in developing countries. *New England Journal of Medicine, 337*, 883–885.

References

Maltoni, M., Scarpi, E., Rosati, M., Derni, S., Fabbri, L., Martini, F., Amadori, D., & Nanni, O. (2012). Palliative sedation in end-of-life care and survival: A systematic review. *Journal of Clinical Oncology, 30*(12), 1378–1383.

McLean, M. R. (2012). A framework for thinking ethically about human biotechnology. http://www.scu.edu/ethics/publications/submitted/mclean/biotechframework.html. Accessed 16 Nov 2012.

Muzur, A., & Rinčić, I. (2011). Fritz Jahr (1895–1953)—the man who invented bioethics. *Synthesis Philos, 51*(1), 133–139.

NCB (Nuffield Council on Bioethics). (1996). *Animal-to-human transplants: The ethics of xenotransplantation*. London: Nuffield Council on Bioethics.

Potter, V. R., & Potter, L. (1995) Global bioethics: Converting sustainable development to global survival. *Medicine & Global Survival, 2*(3), 185–191.

Potter, V. R. (1970). Bioethics: The science of survival. *Perspectives in Biology and Medicine, 14*, 127–153

Potter, V. R. (1971). *Bioethics: Bridge to the future*. Englewood Cliffs: Prentice-Hall.

Potter, V. R. (1988). *Global bioethics: Building on the Leopold Legacy*. East Lansing: MSU Press

Purdy, L. M. (2006). Surrogate mothering: Exploitation or empowerment? In H. Kushe & P. Singer (Eds.), *Bioethics: An anthology* (pp. 90–99, 2nd ed.). Oxford: Blackwell Publishing.

Rehmann-Sutter, C., Düwell, M., & Mieth, D. (2006). Introduction. In C. Rehmann-Sutter, M. Düwell, & D. Mieth (Eds.), *Bioethics in cultural contexts: reflections on methods and finitude* (pp. 1–10). The Netherlands: Springer.

Reich, W. T. (1995). Introduction. In W. T. Reich (Ed.), *Encyclopedia of bioethics* (p. 3: 2nd ed.). New York: Macmillan Reference.

Rendtorff, J. D. (2002). Basic ethical principles in European bioethics and biolaw: Autonomy, dignity, integrity and vulnerability– towards a foundation of bioethics and biolaw. *Med Health Care Philos, 5*(3), 235–244.

Ricoeur, P. (1999). Approaching the human person. *Ethical Perspectives, 1*, 45–54.

Robert, J. S., & Baylis, F. (2003). Crossing species boundaries. *American Journal of Bioethics, 3*(3), 1–13.

Steinkamp, N., & Gordijn, B. (2003). Ethical case deliberation on the ward: Comparison of four methods. *Medicine, Health Care and Philosophy, 6*, 235–246.

Ten Have H. A. (2012). Potter's notion of bioethics. *Kennedy Institute of Ethics Journal, 22*(1), 59–82.

Turner, L. (2009). Bioethics and social studies of medicine: Overlapping concerns. *Cambridge Quarterly of Healthcare Ethics, 18*, 36–42.

Veatch, R. M. (2012). *The basics of bioethics* (3rd ed.). Boston: Pearson.

Washington, H. A. (2006). *Medical apartheid: The dark history of medical experimentation on Black Americans from colonial times to the present*. New York: Doubleday.

Chapter 12
A Sociological Study of Health Problems in Africa

12.1 Introduction

Africa bears the major brunt of major fatal diseases. As it has been previously acknowledged, while discussing health problems in Africa one must consider the political economy of health, social construction of illness, determinants of health, health beliefs, access to care, medical pluralism, and other related issues, which have been adequately examined in the previous chapters. This chapter presents some selected major health problems in Africa—the malaria problem in Africa, the sociocultural context of HIV/AIDS, and the state of maternal and child health (MCH). This chapter will provide some pragmatic discussions that will further help to situate some of the conceptual and theoretical issues explained in the previous chapters. In doing so, the chapter will make reference to the five regions in Africa—North, West, Central/Middle, East, and Southern Africa. Figure 12.1 shows the regions and countries in Africa. SSA includes all the regions except North Africa (Saharan Africa).

12.2 The Malaria Problem in Africa

Malaria is a major population health challenge in Africa. Like other diseases, there are a number of social correlates of malaria. Malaria is a life-threatening parasitic disease. Malaria, or "ague" as it is otherwise known, has a very long history. The word "malaria" comes from an Italian phrase "mal aria," and it literally means "bad air" (MacArthur 1952). The earliest description of malaria as a human disease is found in a document prepared by the Emperor Huang around 2,700 BC (Wellcome 2002). However, Hippocrates (460–370 BC) is acclaimed as the first malariologist because he classified the fever now known to be malaria. After the recognition of the malaria parasite by Charles Louis Alphonse Laveran (1845–1922) in 1800, some scientists including Patrick Manson (1844–1922), a Scottish medical doctor and Ronald Ross (1857–1932) suspected mosquitoes as the malaria vector (Wellcome 2002). Later, Ronald Ross (1857–1932) worked on the lifecycle of malaria and submitted that an infected mosquito could transmit it (Wellcome 2002).

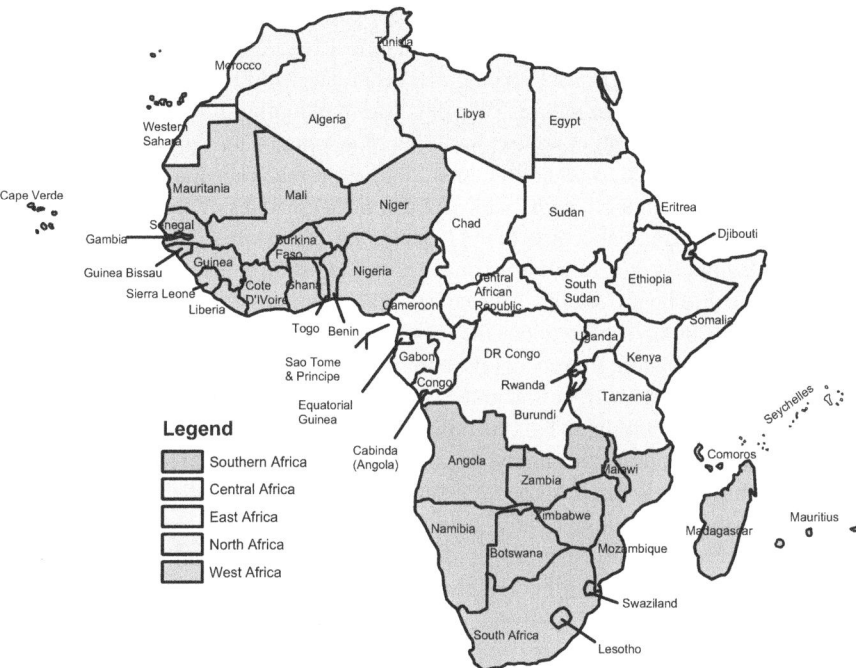

Fig. 12.1 Map of Africa showing regions and countries

The vector of malaria is the female anopheles mosquito, which sucks human blood to facilitate its egg production. Therefore, the mode of transmission is through the bite of an anopheles mosquito. Malaria takes the lives of up to 700,000 people per year, 90 % of whom live in sub-Saharan Africa (SSA), and causes about 300 million people to fall ill (WHO 2012a). It is important to note, however, that the under-five children are the most vulnerable malaria risk group. Generally, everyone (children and adults) living in malaria-endemic areas are at risk of malaria. However, 85 % of malaria-related deaths occur among under-five children, who have not yet acquired the semi-immunity which adults residing in endemic areas may have developed.

The human malaria infection is caused by four different species of protozoan parasites of the genus Plasmodium: *Plasmodium Falciparum*, *Plasmodium vivax*, *Plasmodium ovale*, and *Plasmodium malariae* (Wellcome 2002). *Falciparum* is the most dangerous and toxic of the family. It is further observed that *P. Falciparum* migrated with Africans to other parts of the world (Wellcome 2002). It was further reported that until the 19th century, malaria was not found in Northern Europe, North America, and Russia, but transmission in Southern Europe was intense, while Africa, especially SSA, excluding South Africa, is malaria-endemic.

Since malaria is usually perceived and defined through its symptoms and signs, it therefore becomes highly pertinent to discuss the manifestation of this deadly disease. Malaria is classified into two major clinical types. The first classification of malaria is referred to as simple, uncomplicated, moderate, or non-severe type, otherwise known as mild malaria. Symptoms of mild malaria include fever, nausea, vomiting, diarrhea, headache, cough, chills, muscle pains, and lassitude. Mild malaria might develop into complicated or severe malaria, which is life-threatening. It is important to note that malaria has symptom complex, implying that some of its signs and symptoms could also be attributed to other ailments. Since mild malaria usually presents with fever, in malaria-endemic countries like Africa, most episodes of fever are treated as malaria cases, especially because of inadequate diagnostic kits. Therefore, diagnosis is often presumptive in nature, based on the signs and symptoms perceived. In some cases, there could be misdiagnosis because of the symptom complexity of malaria.

The WHO (2008a) reported that *Plasmodium falciparum* malaria is usually very severe and is responsible for most of the cases of malaria-related death. The inability of most people to take swift action in the case of a severe malaria attack could mean a fatal consequence within 48 h of the onset of illness. This is why procrastination of treatment is dangerous. Accordingly, one of the Roll Back Malaria (RBM) objectives at the community level is to improve prompt recognition of malaria by caregivers and to assist them in taking effective action within 24 h of the onset of illness.

Malaria is often described as a disease of poverty or underdevelopment. Mosquitoes usually breed in poorly planned neighborhoods. Because of the poor housing facilities, there might be poor sanitation systems resulting in water logging, which serves as a breeding site for mosquitoes. Most windows and doors might not be screened to prevent mosquitoes from entering the homes. The poor usually have little or no access to information and education about public health. They might not have basic knowledge of insecticide-treated bed nets (ITNs) or available drugs. Most of the available treatment and preventive measures may also not be affordable to them.

12.2.1 Community Understanding of Malaria

In Africa, there are various cultural explanations of malaria which are divergent from the biomedical explanations. Such explanations involve cultural constructions informed by the prevailing beliefs and knowledge about malaria. Heggenhougen et al. (2003) observed that the perception of malaria may vary by culture, shaped by such factors as educational level, social status, religious beliefs, and location (urban or rural). Understanding these local notions of malaria is crucial in malaria control. This is why Heggenhougen et al. (2003) further noted that malaria control efforts should consider multidimensional human contexts that create and support varying notions of malaria because of their profound consequence for prevention, treatment, and control. The notion is often understood by examining the perceived causes, modes of transmission, symptoms, vulnerability, and other related beliefs about malaria. Many local communities still hold a number of misconceptions which are detrimental to control efforts (Amzat 2011). There is attribution of malaria to incorrect etiologic agents such as dust, heat, palm oil, stress, evil spirits, and other mystical factors. This causal attribution is not peculiar to malaria; it forms a part of the general disease explanation in many African communities (see Sect. 2.7).

Adera (2003), in a study conducted in Ethiopia, reported misconceptions of the mode of malaria transmission as respondents mentioned dirt, nature, mud, and water. Similarly, Comoro et al. (2003) reported that in some parts of Tanzania, the common perceived cause of *degedege* (local concept for malaria) among the under-five children was an evil spirit. Hence urinating on the child who suffers from *degedege* and fuming him/her with elephant dung are the usual traditional remedies. If the mode of transmission of malaria is well understood at the community level, it will help to promote the use of appropriate preventive measures. Unfortunately, some mothers of under-fives and pregnant women (who are the most vulnerable) do not understand the mode of transmission of malaria (Amzat and Omololu 2009). Due to wrong causal perceptions, the perceived mode of transmission is still misconceived, thereby attributing it to cuddling and other forms of physical contact (Jegede et al. 2005). Understanding the human context and general cultural milieu in relation to malaria would direct intervention at the community level.

12.2.2 Malaria Prevention and Treatment

The control of mosquito breeding sites is still poor in many African communities. For instance, Opiyo et al. (2007), in a study in Kenya, found that despite knowledge that the removal of water containing borrow pits controls mosquitoes breeding, most community members do not translate such knowledge into action. One major step in malaria control is environmental sanitation to curtail the breeding of mosquitoes. Moreover, the use of ITNs is a major preventive measure; it helps to avoid contacts with mosquitoes. The consistently high prevalence of malaria in SSA signifies that there is still low usage of preventive measures. An increase in the use of preventive measures would reduce morbidity and mortality due to malaria. In 2000 the ITN was launched in Abuja, Nigeria (the goals set often referred to as the Abuja target). It was projected that there would be considerable ITN coverage (of 60 % in 2005) of pregnant women and under-five children. The use of ITNs is still generally low as no nation in SSA met the Abuja target. Opiyo et al. (2007) observed that most people have adequate theoretical knowledge of how to prevent malaria but with a gap between theoretical knowledge and practical household malaria prevention.

A considerable percentage of households in SSA do not own ITNs despite harbouring pregnant women and under-five children who are most vulnerable to malaria. In Nigeria, more than 80 % of respondents had never purchased any form of ITN (Onwujekwe et al. 2005), while a report submitted that less than 20 % of households own ITNs (Amzat 2011; WHO 2011). Even where there is a high level of knowledge regarding the benefits of ITNs (in Ghana), it does not translate to a high level of usage (De La Cruz 2006;). However, there has been progress in some countries. In Malawi, ITN coverage of under-five children was 8 % in 2000, increased to 38 % in 2004, and up to 60 % in 2010 (AU 2006; WHO 2011). Also in Togo, almost 50 % of children sleep under an ITN (AU 2006), while in Mali, the percentage of households owning at least one ITN is up to 80 % (WHO 2011).

In general, the percentage of households owning at least one ITN in SSA is estimated to have risen from 3 % in 2000 to 53 % in 2012 (WHO 2012a). It is further reported that the use of intermittent preventive treatment during pregnancy (IPTp) ranged from 4 % in Namibia to 68 % in Zambia. This shows that while there has been progress in many countries which led to a decline in the estimated malaria cases and deaths, many countries are still far behind in control efforts. Additionally, in general the rates of decline are still low compared with the set targets (both Abuja and MDG targets).

There have been community action plans in many SSA countries (e.g., Senegal, Mali, Kenya, and Tanzania) which have helped in reducing the burden of malaria (WHO 2002). It is important to note that home management of malaria (HMM) has been the cornerstone of malaria management at the community level. The idea of scaling up HMM signifies an expansion of a preexisting community idea but with the supportive resources (e.g., diagnostic tools and new drugs) needed for proper malaria management. Such expansion and improvement have been demonstrated in Burkina-Faso, Nigeria, Ghana, and Uganda and have been found to be an effective strategy in malaria control (Gyapong and Garshong 2007). However, self-treatment and presumptive treatment, which do not follow established guidelines at the community level, have been implicated in the development and spread of drug resistance. The development of drug resistance led to the demise of Chloroquine but unfortunately resistance has also been established for ACT. Even at the health facility, the percentage of cases confirmed with diagnostic tools is less than 20 % (WHO 2011).

From the foregoing discussions, there are still a number of community factors that need to be addressed in order to ensure effective malaria control. There is a need to improve local understanding of malaria, especially by addressing some misconceptions. Creating more access to effective preventive and treatment measures is also vital. It is still imperative to promote knowledge of the ITN and demonstrate its effectiveness in malaria control in many local communities. Ensuring appropriate case management both at home and at the facility level is essential in reversing the trends of drug resistance. If the aforementioned measure is coupled with political will, increased funding, and proper management of available resources, there could be further considerable decline in the burden of malaria.

12.3 Sociocultural Factors in the Spread of HIV/AIDS

HIV/AIDS has existed long before the first diagnosis in the United States in 1981 (Sharp and Hahn 2011), and it is now a major health problem in all countries of the world. The major mode of transmission remains sexual intercourse, which is also a major risk factor for many other diseases (see Sect. 3.3.1.4). Other modes of transmission include all practices that involve the exchange of body fluids. Globally, 34 million people were living with HIV at the end of 2011 (UNAID 2012a). Meanwhile, SSA is the hardest hit by AIDS, with nearly 1 in every 20 adults (4.9 %) living with

HIV and accounting for 69 % of the people living with HIV worldwide. UNAIDS (2012b) estimated that there are 23.5 million people living with HIV/AIDS in Africa, with a particularly high prevalence in Southern Africa. In 2011 HIV/AIDS accounted for about 1.7 million deaths worldwide—70 % occurred in SSA. While the number of deaths is still huge, it represents almost a 24 % decline compared with that of 2005 (UNAIDS 2012b). Despite the progress made, new infections continue to occur, but at a declining rate; there was more than a 50 % reduction among adults (15–49 years) in many countries between 2001 and 2011 (UNAIDS 2012b). One major factor in the decline includes the increasing treatment coverage of those living with HIV.

The prevalence rate among the youth is still a major source of concern. Population Reports (PR) (2001) observed that more than half of all new infections occur among young people. The physical, psychological, and social attributes of the youth make them particularly vulnerable to HIV/AIDS (PR 2001). This is because the youth constitutes persons who are preparing to start sexual relations or have just started it, are inexperienced, and thus are highly vulnerable to high-risk sexual behaviour. Generally, there is a high prevalence of non-consensual sex among youth (Finger 2004). It is in this vein that Jackson (2002) observed that young people are the most critical age group to reach for HIV/AIDS prevention.

Since the 1980s, HIV/AIDS has wreaked tremendous havoc on the socioeconomic development in Africa as well as other continents. The average life expectancy has drastically declined to about 47—without AIDS it would be around 60 + years (Mukherjee et al. 2003). The pandemic has consumed a large part of funds that would have been used in development projects. The AIDS epidemic exacts enormous negative effects on most salient economic indicators—family income, food production, security, education, and health care (Amzat 2010). AIDS accounts for increasing pauperisation as more people living with the virus die, leaving economic vacuums, especially in agriculture which is a dominant occupation in Africa. AIDS is thus a developmental tragedy of our time (Amzat 2010).

As noted earlier, the pattern of sexual relationships in the community is a major factor influencing the level of prevalence of HIV/AIDS. Sexual behaviour has a sociocultural context, as well as other structural factors influencing HIV vulnerabilities. This section will examine some sociocultural factors influencing the prevalence of HIV in Africa. This section therefore involves an examination of some sociocultural correlates which interplay in Africa to account for the epidemiologically high burden of HIV/AIDS.

12.3.1 Gender Inequality

In previous sections (see Sects. 3.6.3 and 4.2), gender has been discussed as a factor in health and illness behaviours and a social determinant of health. Also relevant is the theoretical discussion of feminism (see Sect. 6.5). This section will further extend these arguments, especially in relation to gender inequality context as an adverse factor in HIV transmission in Africa. The central argument is that women bear the brunt of gender inequality which increases their level of vulnerability to HIV infection. In SSA, six out of ten people living with HIV/AIDS are women. Young women are partly at higher risk of sexual violence because of their economic dependence on men (Amzat 2010:4). Poverty affects more women than men because women are often denied adequate access to education and paid employment. Due to low economic security and poverty in particular, a number of them enter into sex work, or frequently engage in sex in exchange for material favours from male partners.

In African contexts, gender norms that are related to femininity can prevent young women from accessing HIV information and services (WHO 2009). In most cultures in Africa, young girls are supposed to maintain modesty and are not generally permitted to discuss sexualities in the open. The cultures of shyness and silence are socially prescribed and enforced. Norms of femininity prescribes submissiveness to the male partner. Hence it is often considered a cultural and moral aberration for a wife to discuss sexuality or negotiate sexual issues with her partner. In general, women have limited decision-making power in all household matters. This social passiveness within the household is responsible for women's low status in the community. Women's social relevance is marked by domestic and reproductive roles. Gender norms related to masculinity can encourage men to have more sexual partners and older men to have sexual relations with much younger women (WHO 2009). The "sugar daddy syndrome" is a typical illustration whereby older rich men have sexual relations with young ladies mostly in exchange for material benefits. While such a syndrome exposes men to HIV, it puts young girls at even more risk. The syndrome creates a sexual network of many individuals who are unknown to each other. The spiral could expand to the point in which an individual in the network gets infected and spells a common destiny of HIV to all members of the network, unless preventive measures are effectively utilised.

The low status of women also promotes gender-based violence including rape. Forced sex can contribute to HIV transmission due to resultant tears and lacerations (WHO 2009). More so, physical, psychological, and economic domination are symbols of oppression, powerlessness, and submissiveness, which subsequently reduce the ability to negotiate sexual rights. Despite the contextual predisposition of women to HIV, those women living with the virus tend to suffer more from stigmatisation, discrimination, and social rejection. They are viewed as sexually promiscuous and are blamed for their condition. Even when both partners are HIV-positive, there is tendency to blame the female as the vector of HIV transmission (Mbonu et al. 2009).

12.3.2 Polygyny

Polygyny is a marriage pattern in which a man marries more than one wife; a practice has been implicated in the prevalence of HIV. A polygynous union may involve a sexual network of three individuals to as many as possible (it could be up to five, ten, or more). This necessitates sexual fidelity or safe sex among a number of people to avert vulnerability to STDs including HIV. The negative scenario is that if one of them should contract HIV, others are automatically at risk of HIV. In most cases, additional wives are married without exact knowledge of their sexual history. As more wives (with unknown sexual histories/HIV status) join the marital network, the higher the vulnerability to HIV infection. Polygyny is widely practiced in Africa, especially in rural areas and different religious groups.

Beyond the hypothetical negative scenarios, research has found that polygyny is associated with high transmission of STIs (including HIV) mainly because it involves a multiplication of sexual partners or a concurrent sexual partnership (Bove and Valeggia 2009). Polygynous union may be characterised by marital instability due to divorce and remarriage, and some women may have extramarital affairs because of inadequate satisfaction with their sexual life (Hattori and Dodoo 2007). Another study indicated that junior wives in polygynous unions are more likely to be HIV-positive than spouses of monogamous men (Reniers and Tfaily 2012).

12.3.3 Harmful Cultural Practices

A number of African societies still engage in some harmful cultural practices which also influence the prevalence of HIV. Some forms of widowhood rites have been implicated in the spread of HIV. For instance, widow inheritance is a widespread cultural practice in SSA that has been postulated as contributing to the risk of HIV transmission (Agot et al. 2010; Mabumba et al. 2007). Widowhood inheritance, also called levirate marriage, involves the marriage of a widow to the brother (or sometimes a male relative) of her late husband. This is usually done as a cultural prescription to retain the widow in the same family and ensure social protection. In most cases, the cause of the death of the husband might not be known (which incidentally could be HIV), or the HIV status of the new sexual partner might be unknown. Additionally, sexual cleansing rites for widows are still prevalent in many rural communities in Africa. It is a practice in which a widow (usually) or widower must have sexual relations with a relative of the dead spouse in order to be rid of the spouse's ghost to avert any negative consequence on the future partner (see Kalinda and Tembo 2010).

In addition, the practice of scarification including female genital cutting and other forms of traditional cutting procedures (both curative and aesthetic) in a non-clinical setting has also been implicated in HIV prevalence. Apart from mother-child transmission of HIV, the prevalence of HIV among non-sexually active children in southern Africa is related to a history of prior visits to a traditional healer, especially involving scarification (HRSC 2008). The major reason is that the traditional healers do cuttings with crude equipment, mostly without sterilisation.

12.3.4 Stigmatisation

Stigmatisation in relation to HIV also contributes to the prevalence of HIV in SSA (see Sects. 8.4.1 and 8.4.2 for theories of labelling and stigma). Discrimination against those infected with HIV is responsible for low utilisation of counselling and testing services, forces the people living with HIV/AIDS (PLWHA) to conceal their status, and reduces access to treatment (see Turan et al 2012).

HIV-related stigma is directly detrimental to PLWHA. They often lose community support, individuals may be isolated within their family, or deprived of social goods (housing, employment, and opportunities) required for general well-being (Rankin et al. 2005). For instance, country-level surveys conducted in a number of African countries indicated that PLHWA face barriers to employment, including discrimination in hiring, loss of promotions, and employment termination because of HIV status (Sprague et al. 2011). Discrimination often leads to the development of internal stigma among the PLWHA, thereby causing these people to view themselves as persons doomed to die soon, without hope of life, and a waste to self and society. The major consequences are poor quality of life and accelerated physiological breakdown or death.

12.3.5 Religious Beliefs

A previous section has briefly explained how religion or a spiritual worldview can promote health (see Sect. 3.6.6). This section will focus on how some religious myths could promote risky sexual behaviours. In Africa, a majority of the population is very religious, and expression of sexuality is bound by strict religious values. Such values restrict sexuality education among the underaged in schools and open discourse about sexual matters. The values often promote the culture of silence and shyness about sexual issues as a form of sexual modesty. Despite the religious myths surrounding sexuality, the level of conformity with religious sexual regulation is often low in many communities. This implies that the gap between the religious ideals and social reality is wide, and the reality is sometimes denied because everyone wants to appear modest. For instance, Islam and Christianity often prescribe virginity and abstinence from sex among unmarried persons. In urban Africa, especially among the educated, the age of marriage is increasing and it is often impracticable for a majority of persons to contain their sexual feelings and maintain celibacy until marriage.

It has also been documented that some girls engage in unprotected anal sex to maintain their virginity or have to be married off earlier so that their partners would meet them as virgins. Additionally, some religious myths promote stigmatisation of PLWHA as people who have committed sexual sins, and hence HIV is a penal consequence. Religious beliefs about HIV can also contribute to fatalistic responses and attitudes, which promote a belief in divine cure and hinder participation in treatment, leading to a high rate of HIV-related mortality (Zou et al. 2009).

12.3.6 Cultural Beliefs and Patterns

The first major challenge regarding HIV in Africa was the scepticism about the reality of the disease (Amzat 2010). Many Africans first thought that it was a western conspiracy or that the disease was not real. By the time there was improved knowledge about the reality of HIV, millions of people had already been infected and affected. Then, there were growing misconceptions about the causes and prevention of HIV, especially among those with low level of formal education and little or no access to relevant information on HIV and sexuality. This accounted for a low initial perception of risk factors. The situation is still evident in many rural communities.

More so, the cultural patterns of sexual relations in some African communities also fuel the problem of HIV. Among the rural Maasai and Nuer of East Africa who are mostly semi-nomadic and pastoralists, communal sexual relations, especially within a particular age-grade, is still prevalent. Young girls/men are particularly culturally permitted to gain sexual experience from multiple partners in preparation for adulthood or marriage. Hence STDs (including HIV) are a major cause of morbidity among the Maasai population, with prepubescent girls (starting around eight years of age) frequently presenting with symptoms (of STDs) (Coast 2007). In addition, the Maasai have a widely held belief that semen helps girls to develop physically (especially to help their breasts grow), hence the sexual initiation of prepubescent girls by a number of male members of her age group is condoned (Coast 2007). Such belief also accounts for low utilisation of condoms among the Maasai population.

Girl-child beading in Kenya The practice of "beading" is common among some communities in Samburu and Rendille communities in Kenya. It involves a man (often a relative) buying a beaded necklace, but could include wrist or waist beads for a girl as a sign of sexual engagement. Beading implies a commencement of a community-sanctioned, non-marital sexual relationship between men especially in the "warrior" age group (called the morans) and unmarried girls. Generally, beading is used as adornment but for some communities it also connotes sexual enslavement. The females are often divided into groups: girls, married women, and elderly women. The communities are largely pastoral and semi-nomadic. Most girls perform domestic duties including caring for livestock. Female circumcision (usually performed in a non-clinical setting) is culturally prescribed for girls to prepare them for marriage. The process of beading begins with negotiations between a man and the girl's parents (the girl's choice is violated). Following a mutual agreement between a man and the girl's parents, the girl's mother builds a hut for the girl, where she can be accessed for sex. Girls may be as young as eight years old when they are beaded. Since the sexual relationships often take place within a clan, it is a form of incestuous practice. Therefore, it does not lead to marriage and pregnancy is forbidden despite the nonuse of preventive measures. When pregnancies do result, beaded girls may be forced to have a crude abortion (usually a forced miscarriage performed by older women) or to give up the newborn for infanticide or for adoption by a stranger in another community (one of the options is mandatory according to the culture). In some cases, other members of the man's age grade may also have sexual access to his beaded girl. The sexual risk of HIV is enormous: the girls' age at sexual debut is usually low, the

Table 12.1 Trends in estimates of maternal mortality ratio by five-year periods. (Source: WHO (2012c), p. 26)

Region	MMR					% Change in MMR 1990–2010	Average annual change in MMR 1990–2010
	1990	1995	2000	2005	2010		
World	400	360	320	260	210	−47	−3.1
Developed Region	26	20	17	15	16	−39	−2.5
Developing Region	440	400	350	290	240	−47	−3.1
Africa	760	740	670	570	460	−39	−2.5
North Africa	230	170	120	93	78	−66	−5.3
Sub-Saharan Africa	850	820	740	630	500	−41	−2.6
Eastern Africa	800	770	680	570	450	−45	−2.9
Central Africa	910	900	810	710	600	−34	−2.1
Southern Africa	260	270	350	370	300	19	0.9
Western Africa	970	930	830	700	550	−44	−2.8
Asia	400	320	270	200	150	−61	−4.7

men are usually older with many sexual experiences, and multiple sexual accesses by a number of men could be permitted. Apart from the risk of HIV, the beading practice is a culture of incest, sexual assault, abortion, and infanticide. While the Kenyan constitution does not permit infanticide and sexual assaults or relations with the underage, the extreme culture still persists in several rural communities.

Sources: Samburu Women Trust (2012); McCluskey et al. (2005); Roth et al. (2001).

Progress made in reducing the incidence of HIV/AIDS is partly due to the changing cultural myths and promotion of health education relating to HIV/AIDS. Despite this progress, more efforts still need to be directed to the cultural beliefs and cultural constructions and expressions of sexuality in African communities.

12.4 Maternal and Child Health Problems in Africa

Maternal health refers to the health of women during pregnancy, childbirth, and the postpartum period. There is a growing advocacy to improve reproductive health in order to reduce pregnancy-related morbidity and mortality. Some progress has been made in the control of maternal mortality worldwide, but, unfortunately, the African region still bears the greatest brunt of maternal mortality. WHO (2012b) reported that about 800 women die from pregnancy-related complications every day; 99 % of those deaths occur in developing countries. Globally, an estimated 287,000 maternal deaths occurred in 2010, a decline of 47 % from 1990, but SSA still accounted for 85 % of the global burden (245,000 maternal deaths) (WHO 2012c). Table 12.1 shows estimates of MMR (maternal mortality ratio, expressed as the number of maternal deaths in a given period per 100,000 live births), with SSA bearing the highest burden with 500 maternal deaths per 100,000 live births. Despite the progress made, it is still doubtful whether many of the countries in SSA will meet the Millennium Development Goals (MDGs) target of reducing maternal deaths by 75 % in 2015.

The high burden of maternal mortality in Africa is a result of insufficient progress in control efforts. Many African countries still had a high MMR (defined as MMR ≥ 300 maternal deaths per 100,000 live births) in 2010 (WHO 2012c). The countries with the highest MMR include Chad (1,100), Somalia (1,000), Sierra Leone (890), the Central African Republic (890), Burundi (800), Guinea-Bissau (790), Liberia (770), the Sudan (730), Cameroon (690), and Nigeria (630). The SSA has the largest proportion of maternal deaths attributed to HIV at 10 %; the increasing rate recorded in Southern Africa is partly attributed to HIV-related complications. Central Africa still has the worst MMR in the African region. Malaria-related maternal deaths also account for up to 10 % of maternal mortality (Amzat 2011). While the death rate is very high, it has also been observed that for every woman that dies as a result of pregnancy-related causes, between 20 and 30 more develop short- or long-term disabilities such as vesicovaginal fistula (VVF) and pelvic inflammatory disease (PID). In Africa, up to 10,000/100,000 live births might suffer from such disabilities.

The situation of maternal health is linked to the level of antenatal care (ANC) in Africa. For instance, in Sierra Leone, the 2008 demographic and health survey (DHS) showed that one-quarter of births occurred in health facilities while almost three-quarters of births occurred at home. Home births are more common in rural areas (77 %) than urban areas (57 %); only 42 % of births are delivered by a skilled provider while another 45 % are assisted by a traditional birth attendant and 9 % by untrained relatives or friends (SSL and ICF Macro 2009). In Ghana, about 95 % of pregnant Ghanaian women received some ANC from a skilled provider, but only 59 % of births are delivered by a skilled provider (GSS et al. 2009). In Nigeria, the 2008 DHS showed that up to 58 % of pregnant women received some ANC from skilled providers; however, only 39 % of births were assisted by skilled birth attendants (SBAs) (NPC and ICF Macro 2009). In most African countries, there is a clear disparity between rural and urban areas—while more than half of births take place in the rural areas and at home, only a few (in most cases, less than 30 %) of all births were assisted by SBAs.

The situation of child health is also marked by insufficient progress in control efforts. A UNICEF report indicated that overall, substantial progress has been made towards reducing child mortality, with a 41 % decline between 1990 and 2011. The number of under-five mortalities (or U5MR—expressed as the number of deaths under the age of five per 1,000 live births) worldwide has declined from nearly 12 million in 1990 to about 7 million in 2011. In SSA, as of 2011, the child mortality rate was 109 per 1000 live births (see Table 12.2). Nigeria alone accounts for 11 % of the global child mortality. Countries including DRC, Angola, Somalia, Mali, Sierra Leone, Guinea-Bissau, Chad, and Central African Republic still have U5MR of more than 150/1000 (UNICEF et al. 2012).

At the global level, the leading causes of mortality among under-five children are pneumonia (18 %), preterm birth complications (14 %), diarrhoea (11 %), intrapartum-related complications (9 %), and malaria (7 %) (UNICEF et al. 2012). Globally, more than one-third of under-five deaths are attributable to malnutrition. In SSA, more children die from malnutrition, diarrhoea, and malaria. The factors responsible for insufficient progress in maternal and child health (MCH) include

12.4 Maternal and Child Health Problems in Africa

Table 12.2 Levels and trends in the under-five mortality rate (1990–2011). (Source: UNICEF et al. (2012), p. 9).

Region	Under-five Mortality Rate							Decline (Percent) 1990–2011	Current annual rate of reduction (2011)
	1990	1995	2000	2005	2010	2011	MDG Target		
World	87	82	73	63	53	51	29	41	3.2
Developed Region	15	11	10	8	7	7	5	55	3.5
Developing Region	97	91	80	69	59	57	32	41	3.1
Africa									
North Africa	77	59	45	34	26	25	26	68	5.5
Sub-Saharan Africa	178	170	154	133	112	109	59	39	3.1

limited access to health services (see Sect. 4.9), low socioeconomic status (see Sects. 3.6.2 and 4.3), misconceptions (see Sect. 3.6.1), the ineffective PHC system (see Sect. 10.3.5.1), extremely low coverage of insurance scheme, and a host of other factors (see Sect. 10.3.6).

12.4.1 Some Social Correlates of Maternal and Child Health

Apart from the general challenges of health systems in Africa (see Sect. 10.3.6), there are still a number of social correlates of MCH in Africa. The fertility rate is higher in the developing world than in the developed world. Maternal mortality is correlated with pregnancy that comes too early, too often, and too late. There is still a high value being placed on large family size in most African communities, hence women tend to bear many children. The frequency of birth does not only increase the risk of maternal complications but it could account for a low household carrying capacity which will lead to low levels of care for children.

In many African communities, the age of first marriage is relatively low. Early pregnancy, especially before the age of 18, is associated with pregnancy-related complications. There is still a substantially high level of child marriage due to some cultural and religious reasons. Childbearing at a tender age (as low as age 12) in many societies not only increases the possibility of complications during birth but also questions the preparedness of the child-mother for childcare. In most African countries, there are no effective legal frameworks to prevent child-marriage.

Many underaged girls are withdrawn from school for marriage. This often results in the feminisation of illiteracy, or the relative low level of literacy among women versus men. Invariably, people with a low level of education often have difficulties in understanding health information or are simply denied access to health information. Education is correlated with health condition (see Sects. 3.6.4 and 4.4), hence women's low level of education adversely affects maternal and child health.

In addition, the low level of literacy contributes to inadequate access to formal employment and general low economic security, which all contributes to the feminisation of poverty. While poverty is very high in Africa, the women are poorer. Maternal and child mortalities are generally high among people with low income (see Sects. 3.62 and 4.3 for more discussion on health and SES).

12.5 Towards a Community Approach in Health Care for Africa

From the foregoing examination of health problems in Africa, it is evident that health challenges are entangled in a web of social correlates coupled with limited resources to meet the health needs of the citizens. Community engagement (CE) should constitute a major tool for the PHC workers. Therefore, a community-centered approach in health care intervention could be effective in addressing the health needs of the people, especially in rural areas where the burden of disease is greatly felt. Invariably, strengthening the PHC system requires a community- or people-centered approach. Moreover, PHC efforts to tackle determinants of local ill-health can only be achieved through a community-centered approach. While it should be acknowledged that the CE approach/intervention is not new, this is to stress a need for intensified efforts and to propose a more inclusive approach for health intervention. The approach can capitalise on social solidarity to ensure an appropriate response to community health needs. Principally, the PHC system should utilise the CE approach to deliver better health services to the community. PHC should balance preventive and curative care. This is why the WHO (2008b, p. 41) stressed that primary care should bring health "promotion and prevention, cure and care together in a safe, effective and socially productive way at the interface between the population and the health system." This can only be achieved if there are practical measures to penetrate the communities and mobilise them to achieve set health priorities (WHO 2008b).

The CE approach involves community participatory approach in relations to health maintenance and disease control. Generally, CE involves the application of collective vision for the benefit of the people by building grassroots movement and structures involving community members for actualisation of set goals. CE involves a number of systematic processes of mobilisation emanating from the participatory rapid appraisal approach—social action of the community, by the community (members), and for the community. With regard to population health, it requires sustainable, coordinated activities with the use of manageable and sustainable strategies. Figure 12.2 shows some major components of a CE approach. The following discussion will focus on some major components of a CE approach in health intervention.

12.5.1 Developing and Supporting Local Health Volunteers

Due to limited resources available to organise effective health care, sustainable measures at the community level will help to alleviate the burden of disease. It has

12.5 Towards a Community Approach in Health Care for Africa

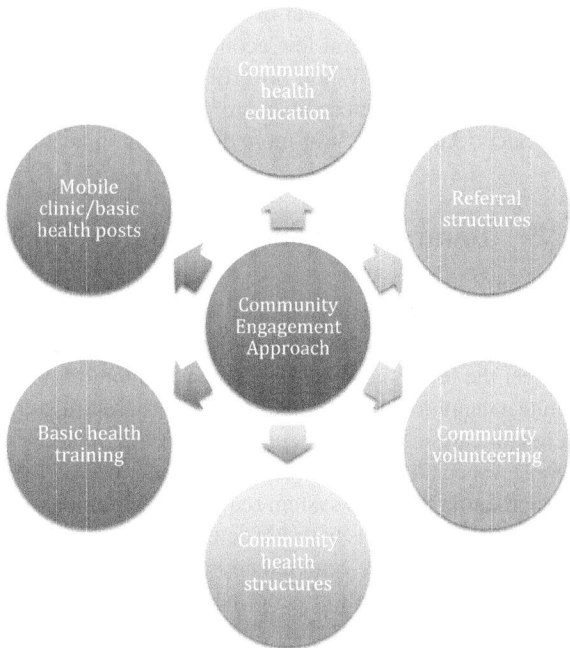

Fig. 12.2 Components of the community engagement approach

previously been observed that in Africa, the number of health workers is extremely insufficient in alleviating the burden of disease (see Sect. 10.3.6). There are many rural communities without any health posts or medical personnel. In such scenarios, it is important to encourage community members to volunteer in addressing their community health needs. This could be done by educating and training a number of people in the community on basic health needs. The most important of such training should involve the dissemination of heath information. This will correct some misconceptions about specific diseases. It will also enhance the knowledge of risk factors and basic preventive and treatment measures. The WHO (2008b, p. 36) observed that "the mobilization of groups and communities to address what they consider to be their most important health problems and health-related inequalities is a necessary complement to the more technocratic and top-down approach to assessing social inequalities and determining priorities for action." One major way this can be done is through local health volunteers.

Volunteering should be undertaken as a humanitarian duty—to serve as a way of contributing to community health and development. In places where there are community development associations, health committees should be developed. This could lead to the development of community "experts" who could play advisory roles on health-related issues or to provide basic medical responses such as giving preventive tips or ensuring appropriate referrals. Generally, community volunteerism is the bedrock of the CE approach, but it can only be achieved when there is an appropriate link to the primary health workers, especially at the primary care centers. Volunteerism ensures that certain individuals take up community roles of passing knowledge to others and provide supportive measures in case of health needs or emergencies.

In a number of communities in Malawi, Tanzania, and Nigeria, the community health volunteers (CHVs) have proven to be effective in addressing basic community health needs with various initiatives in water and sanitation, maternal health, child immunisation, malaria, and HIV prevention (PATH 2010). The CHVs can also provide home-based care. Particularly, encouraging women to help in caring for children and pregnant women might promote access to basic MCH services within the community. The CHVs can serve as a reference group for all health-related matters. The CHVs who are well-trained could serve as links between health facilities and the community. While this will further promote a sense of community, it is also a way of self-defining strategies with the use of minimal resources. Since health problems are internally obvious in the community, a push to make a difference might evolve through the implementation of research focusing on community strategies to addressing their own problems.

12.5.2 Addressing Health Education in the Community

One of the basic problems among the African population is a low literacy rate. The provision of basic health education is a crucial component of the CE approach. It is important for the community members to understand how lifestyle choices, individual health behaviours, and community factors are related to population health. It is also important for community members to understand how some health problems are linked with social, structural, and physical factors in the environment, such as housing arrangement, poor sanitation, exposure to toxic chemicals, occupation, and the lack of supportive interpersonal relationships (Israel et al. 1994). Generally, empowering the community with this basic knowledge can help to improve population health.

While such education cannot be on a one-on-one basis, the volunteers should be the target audience; they should be empowered to be a source of health information in the community. Health education can also be provided through community forums and community-based associations. This is a responsibility of the self-help groups in addressing population health recognised by the WHO. The volunteers can also organise community gatherings during which health issues can be discussed. The various formal health agencies and NGOs can support the volunteers to extend the presence of health systems to local settings and households through health promotion activities, basic home-based care, and community mobilisation to address certain health issues.

12.5.3 Enhancing Community Health Structures

One of the fundamental efforts in primary care is to link the community to the health care posts. This is highly necessary to develop household/community capacities to stay healthy, make healthy decisions and respond to health needs including emergencies (WHO 2008b). Apart from volunteerism and health education, the development of community health structures is also a fundamental aspect of the CE approach. The structure may include the formation of groups of volunteers who will coordinate some health-related services such as community saving/donation, blood donation, emergency transport, and health guest schemes. Community saving could serve as a means of raising money to cater to those in need and in the case of an emergency. It is often difficult for some community members to pay for certain health services because such services are expensive; contributory donations could be a last resort in many circumstances. Community groups could form a blood donor scheme to help in many instances in which a patient requires blood, especially in birth delivery when the mother requires blood. Many communities have to travel more that 5 kilometers to access a health facility. Many community members do not have access to a vehicle. Therefore, organising an emergency transport scheme consisting of individuals who can drive and have access to a vehicle in the community can help to save a lot of lives.

These community health structures have been a vital component of the CE approach implemented by a number of NGOs in SSA (see PATH 2010). It has proven to be effective in enhancing community support in the process of care through some dedicated community structures. Invariably, enhancing the community structures is a major way of strengthening linkages for social support within communities and with the health system.

12.5.4 Basic Health Posts and Mobile Clinics

The PHC system is the first entry into the health care sector and has been a major strategy of providing health care for underserved communities. Unfortunately, many communities in Africa still do not have physical access to health facilities. This is why it is advocated here that basic health posts could be provided as outposts of nearby primary health care centers. The WHO (2008b:53) specifically noted that another strategy in primary care is by "bringing care closer to people, in settings in close proximity and direct relationship with the community, relocating the entry point to the health system from hospitals and specialists to close-to-client generalist primary-care centres." The health posts could serve as a meeting point for health-related matters and house mobile health officials where available. The provision of basic health posts or mobile clinics should also be prioritised to enhance home-based care and appropriate referrals. The idea of mobile health might not necessarily be with the use of specialised or sophisticated ambulance/vehicles but by using motorcycles and bicycles. The use of mobile clinics has also proven effective in a number of communities in Ghana and Kenya. The WHO (2008b) acknowledged that more health benefits accrue when health workers operate more often in the community (i.e., outside the four walls of their consultation room).

In general, the CE approach is based on community efforts but requires mobilisation. Some of the outcomes include the saturation of the community with health information through the use of CHVs to enhance social approval, address misconceptions and increase health care demand. It is in terms of mobilisation that political will is required on the part of the government for some investment in CE to improve population health. The approach is imbued with value for money because of a number of unpaid community volunteering and simple technologies. It has been noted that the CE approach is not new; a number of NGOs and international organisations have implemented the approach to improve community health, and it is sometimes abandoned after the expiration of implementation research. The sustainability of the approach often requires community support in terms of training and basic resources (e.g., drugs). Therefore, there is a need to scale up the CE approach; the approach needs to be adopted by local administrations and incorporated as a tool in the PHC system to address community health needs.

In sum, the challenge of improving population health, especially in developing countries, still remains a challenge yet to be fully resolved. Some progress has been made over the years, but more efforts are constantly needed to avert the huge burden of morbidity and mortality. Medical sociology holds a significant promise to address the social dimension of human health. This dimension is very vital if the goal of considerable reduction of disease burden must be achieved, not only in Africa but also all over the world.

References

Adera, T. D. (2003). Beliefs and traditional treatment of malaria in Kishe settlement area, Southern Ethiopia. *Ethiopian Medical Journal, 41*, 25–33.

African Union (AU). (2006). Universal access to HIV/AIDS, TB and malaria services by a united Africa by 2010. Special Submit of African Union on HIV/AIDS, TB and Malaria (ATM), 2–4 May, 2006.

Agot, K. E., Vander, S. A., Tracy, M., Obare, B. A., Bukusi, E. A., Ndinya-Achola, J. O., Moses, S., & Weiss, N. S. (2010). Widow inheritance and HIV prevalence in Bondo District, Kenya: Baseline results from a prospective cohort study. *PLoS ONE, 5*(11), e14028. doi:10.1371/journal. pone.0014028.

Amzat, J. (2010). Social correlates of HIV among youths in Nigeria. *Hemispheres – Studies on Cultures and Societies, 25*, 1–13.

Amzat, J. (2011). Assessing the progress of malaria control in Nigeria. *World Health and Population, 12*(3), 42–51.

Amzat, J., & Omololu, O. F. (2009). Towards a community model for malaria control in sub-Sahara Africa. *Africana Bulletin, 57*, 166–183.

Bove, R. & Valeggia, C. (2009). Polygyny and women's health in sub-Saharan Africa. *Social Science & Medicine, 68*(1), 21–29. doi:10.1016/j.socscimed.2008.09.045.

Coast, E. (2007). Wasting semen: Context and condom use among the Maasai. *Culture, Health and Sexuality, 9*(4), 387–401. doi:10.1080/13691050701208474.

Comoro, C., Nsimba, S. E. D., Warsame, M., & Tomson, G. (2003). Local understanding, perceptions and reported practices of mothers/guardian and health workers on childhood malaria in a Tanzanian district – implications for malaria control. *Acta Tropical, 87*, 305–313.

De La Cruz, N., Crookston, B., Dearden, K., Gray, B., Ivins, N., Alder, S., & Davis, R. (2006). Who sleeps under bednets in Ghana? A doer/non-doer analysis of malaria prevention behaviours. *Malaria Journal, 5*, 61. doi:10.1186/1475-2875-5-61.

Finger, B. (2004). Non-consensual sex among youth: Lessons learned from research. *Sexual Health Exchange, 3–4*, 12–14.

References

Ghana Statistical Service (GSS), Ghana Health Service (GHS), & ICF Macro. (2009). *Ghana Demographic and Health Survey 2008*. Calverton: GSS, GHS, and ICF Macro.

Gyapong, M., & Garshong, B. (2007). *Lessons learned in home management of malaria implementation research in four African countries*. Geneva: World Health Organization.

Hattori, M. K. & Dodoo, F. N. (2007). Cohabitation, marriage, and 'sexual monogamy' in Nairobi's slums. *Social Science and Medicine, 64*(5), 1067–1078

Heggenhougen, H. K., Hackethal, V., & Vivek, P. (2003). *The behavioral and social aspects of malaria and its control: An introduction and annotated bibliography* (Vol. 03:1). Geneva: TDR/STR/SEB.

HRSC. (2008). HIV infection in children aged 5–14 years: Summary report of an expert group meeting. South Africa: Human Science Research Center (HRSC).

Israel, B. A., Checkoway, B., Schulz, A., & Zimmerman, M. (1994). Health education and community empowerment: Conceptualizing and measuring perceptions of individual, organizational, and community control. *Health Education Quarterly, 21*(2), 149–70.

Jackson, H. (2002). *AIDS Africa: Continent in crisis*. Harare: SAfAIDS.

Jegede, A. S., Amzat, J., Salami, K. K., Adejumo, P. O., & Oyetunde, M. O. (2005). Perceived causes of malaria among market women in Ibadan, Nigeria. *African Journal for the Psychological Study of Social Issues, 8*(2), 335–347.

Kalinda, T., & Tembo, R. (2010). Sexual practices and levirate marriages in Mansa District of Zambia. *Electronic Journal of Human Sexuality, 13*. http://www.ejhs.org/volume13/leverite.htm.

Mabumba, E. D., Mugyenyi, P., Batwala, V., Mulogo, E. M., Mirembe, J., Khan, F. A. & Liljestrand, J. (2007). Widow inheritance and HIV/AIDS in rural Uganda *Tropical Doctor, 37,* 229–231.

MacAuthor, W. (1952). A brief story of English malaria. *Transactions of the Royal Society of Tropical Medicine and Hygiene, 46*(3), 359–366.

Mbonu, N. C., van den Borne, B., & De Vries, N. K. (2009). Stigma of people with HIV/AIDS in sub-Saharan Africa: A literature review. *Journal of Tropical Medicine, 145891,* 14. doi:10.1155/2009/145891.

McCluskey, C. C., Roth, E. & Driessche, P. V. (2005). Implication of Ariaal sexual mixing on gonorrhea. *American Journal of Human Biology, 17,* 293–301.

Mukherjee, J. S., Farmer, P. E., Niyizonkiza, D., McCorkle, L., Vanderwarker, C., Teixeira P., & Kim, J. Y. (2003). Tackling HIV in resource poor countries. *British Medical Journal, 327,* 1104–1106.

National Population Commission (NPC) [Nigeria], & ICF Macro. (2009). *Nigeria Demographic and Health Survey 2008*. Abuja. Nigeria: National Population Commission and ICF Macro.

Onwujekwe, O., Uzochukwu, B., Ezumah N. & Shu, E. (2005). Increasing coverage of insecticide-treated nets in rural Nigeria: Implications of consumer knowledge, preferences and expenditures for malaria prevention. *Malaria Journal, 4,* 29. doi:10.1186/1475-2875-4-29.

Opiyo, P., Mukabana W. R., Kiche, I., Mathenge, E., Killeen G. F., & Fillinger U. (2007). An exploratory study of community factors relevant for participatory malaria control on Rusinga Island, western Kenya. *Malaria Journal, 6*(48). doi:10.1186/1475-2875-6-48.

PATHS (Partnership for Transforming Health Systems). (2010). Increasing access to safe motherhood services. Technical Brief, UK Department for International Development (DFID).

Population Reports (PR). (2001). Youth and HIV/AIDS: Can we avoid the catastrophe? *Population Reports, xxix*(3), 1–39.

Rankin, W. W., Brennan, S., Schell, E., Laviwa, J., & Rankin, S. H. (2005). The stigma of being HIV-positive in Africa. *PloS Medicine, 2*(8), e247. doi:10.1371/journal.pmed.0020247.

Reniers, G., & Tfaily, R. (2012). Polygyny, partnership concurrency, and HIV transmission in sub-Saharan Africa. *Demography, 49*(3), 1075–1101. doi:10.1007/s13524-012-0114-z.

Roth, E., Fratkin, E., Ngugi. E., & Glickman B. (2001). Female education, adolescent sexuality and the risk of sexually transmitted infection in Ariaal Rendille culture. *Culture, Health & Sex, 3,* 35–48.

Samburu Women Trust (2012). Silent Sacrifice: Girl-child beading in the Samburu Community of Kenya. A report prepared by Samburu Women Trust, Nairobi, Kenya.

Sharp, P. M. & Hahn, B. H. (2011). Origin of HIV and the AIDS pandemic. *Cold Spring Harbor Perspectives in Medicine, 1,* a006841.

Sprague, L., Simon S., & Sprague, C. (2011). Employment discrimination and HIV stigma: Survey results from civil society organisations and people living with HIV in Africa. *African Journal of AIDS Research, 10*(supplement), 311–324.

Statistics Sierra Leone, & ICF Macro. (2009). *Sierra Leone Demographic and Health Survey 2008.* Calverton: SSL and ICF Macro.

Turan, J. M., Hatcher, A. H., Medema-Wijnveen, J., Onono, M., Miller, S., Bukusi, E. A., Turan, B., & Cohen, C. R. (2012). The role of HIV-related stigma in utilization of skilled childbirth services in rural Kenya: A prospective mixed-methods study. *PLoS Med, 9*(8), e1001295. doi:10.1371/journal.pmed.1001295.

UNAIDS (2012a). Global report: UNAIDS report on the global AIDS epidemic 2012. UNAIDS: Geneva.

UNAIDS (2012b). UNAIDS World AIDS Day Report: 2012. UNAIDS: Geneva.

UNICEF, WHO, World Bank, & UNDESA (2012). *Levels and trends in child mortality: Report 2012.* New York: UNICEF.

Wellcome News (2002). Research directions in malaria (Supplement 6). London.

WHO. (2002). *Community involvement in rolling back malaria.* Geneva: WHO.

WHO. (2008a). *World malaria report 2008.* Geneva: WHO.

WHO. (2008b). *The world health report 2008: primary health care now more than ever.* Geneva: WHO.

WHO. (2009). Integrating gender into HIV/AIDS programmes in the health sector: tool to improve responsiveness to women's needs. WHO: Geneva.

WHO. (2011). *World malaria report 2011.* Geneva: WHO.

WHO. (2012a). *World malaria report 2012.* Geneva: WHO.

WHO. (2012b). Maternal Mortality: Fact Sheet N°348. http://www.who.int/mediacentre/factsheets/fs348/en/index.html. Accessed 25 Sep 2012.

WHO. (2012c). *Trends in maternal mortality: 1990 to 2010 -WHO, UNICEF, UNFPA and The World Bank estimates.* Geneva: WHO.

Zou, J., Yamanaka, Y., John, M., Watt, M., Ostermann, J., & Thielman, N. (2009). Religion and HIV in Tanzania: Influence of religious beliefs on HIV stigma, disclosure, and treatment attitudes. *BMC Public Health, 9,* 75 doi:10.1186/1471-2458-9-75.

Index

A
Abdel-Hameed, A.A., 222
Abdullahi, A.A., 216, 218
Abraham, F., 133, 134
Abraham, J., 188, 189, 191
Acceptability
 of health care, 79
Accessibility
 of health care, 6
Accidents, 27, 30, 32, 34, 36, 40, 41, 47, 52, 62, 74, 151, 201
Acharya, S.N., 231
Acquired immunodeficiency syndrome (AIDS), 8, 11, 31, 45, 119, 131, 265, 269, 270, 273, 275
Actual social identity, 165
Acupuncture, 207
Acute diseases/illness, 30, 31
Acute phase, 160
Ademiluyi, I.A., 221
Adeokun, L., 11
Adequacy
 of health care, 78
Adera, T.D., 268
Adesina, S.K., 211, 215
Adherence, 50, 52
Adlam, J., 172
Adudans, M.K., 45
Adultery gene, 192
Adulthood, 54, 185, 274
Aetiology *see* Social aetiology, 9
Affective action, 135
Affective neutrality, 138
Affordability
 of health care, 78
Afolabi, B.M., 50
Africa, 3, 8, 11, 27, 32, 36, 41, 43–47, 49–54, 64, 65, 67, 74, 77, 99, 119, 178, 180, 188, 194, 198, 199, 210, 215, 219, 220, 222, 224, 231, 235, 236
African traditional medicine, 208
Age, 5, 54, 64, 95, 116, 149, 217, 226, 230, 270, 276
Agot, K.E., 272
Agriculture, 3, 74, 270
Ajzen, I., 143–146
Akighir, A., 217
Alaba, O., 101
Albinism, 36, 168, 169
Albouy, V., 67
Alcohol use, 44
Alcoholism, 112, 166, 188
Alexander, K., 119
Algeria, 221
Allan, K., 137
Allhoff, F., 195, 249
Allied health professionals (AHPs), 226, 234
Allwood, C.W., 46
Alonzo, A.A., 39, 40, 47, 49, 50, 140
Alrawi, S., 216
Altruistic suicide, 94
Alubo, O., 11, 216
Alubo, S.O., 216
Aluko-Arowolo, S., 221
Alves, R.R.N., 208, 209
American Sociological Association (ASA), 1
Amzat, J., 40, 51, 53, 65, 85, 108, 131, 233, 254, 268, 270, 271, 274, 276
Ancestors, 35, 209–212
Andersen's model, 129, 139
Andersen, R.M., 150, 151
Anderson, J.W., 72
Andersson, N., 45
Angola, 64, 276
Animal byproducts, 209
Animal parts, 209, 211, 219

Annandale, E., 122, 123
Anomic suicide, 94
Anopheles mosquitoes, 266
Anorexia, 46, 188, 193
Antenatal care (ANC), 276
Anti-malarial drugs, 40, 221
Anti-psychiatry movement, 186
Apartheid, 222
Aphrodisiac drugs, 188
Appleton, S., 67
Armitage, C.J., 146
Artemisinin-based combination therapy, 236
Artificial insemination, 196, 252, 253
Artificial ventilation, 198, 256
Ashforth, A., 219
Assisted death, 198
Assisted reproductive technology, 14, 253
Asthmatic patients, 158
Asylums, 8, 172
Attention-deficit/hyperactivity disorder (ADHD), 195
Attitudes, 16, 28, 100, 144, 145, 151, 168, 209, 273
Audo, M.O., 232
Autonomy, 122, 124, 149, 157, 174, 175, 200, 255, 257, 259, 260
Auvert, B., 194
Availability
   of health care, 77, 151
Awofeso, N., 23
Ayurveda, 208

B
Băban, A., 46
Bad death, 17
Baer, H.A., 109–111, 113, 114
Baker, M., 70
Baller, R.D., 95
Bandura, A., 139
Bantu, 34
Barbie, E., 131
Barbour, R.S., 8
Barker, K.K., 155, 158, 161
Bati, J., 119
Baumann, A., 256
Baylis, F., 249
Beauchamp, T.M., 245, 256–258
Becker, H., 162
Becker, H.S., 155, 162
Becker, M.H., 139, 141
Beiersmann, C., 47
Belgium, 198, 220
Bell, S.E., 185

Belmont report, 248
Beneficence, 258
Benin, 74, 168
Bhasin, V., 34
Bhootra, B.L., 219
Bice, T., 23
Bilton, T., 91
Bio-statistical theory (BST), 26
Bioethics
   biotech, 248, 249
   clinical/health care, 246, 247
   cultural, 251, 252
   history and notions of, 243, 244
   policy and regulatory, 251
   principlism, understanding, 256, 257
   public health, 249–251
   research, 247, 248
   sociology of, 14, 15
   theoretical, 245, 246
   varieties of, 245
Biographic disruption model, 159, 164
Biographical work, 161
Biological discontinuity, 27
Biomedical reductionism, 2
Biomedicalism, 189
Biotech bioethics, 248, 249
Bircher, J., 24
Bird, C.E., 124
Birth control, 121
Bisexuality, 193, 194
Bjerk, P.K., 231
Black, N., 172
Blackburn, J., 119
Blame-the-victim, 112
Blaxter, M., 25
Bloland, P.B., 51
Bloom, G., 232
Bloom, S.W., 7
Body modification, 26, 179
Body-without-organ (BwO), 179
Bone-setters, 214
Boorse, C., 26, 28, 29
Botswana, 45
Bourdieu, P., 96, 97, 179
Bourgeoisie, 108, 111, 113
Bove, R., 272
Bradby, H., 88
Branaman, A., 174, 175
Breast augmentation, 197
Breyer, F., 228
Britain, 194, 220
Brodish, A.B., 77
Brown, J.B., 158

Brown, P., 155–158
Brown, S., 95
Brown, T.N., 143
Bruegel, I., 103
Brunello, G., 67
Bryant, C.D., 17
Buiting, H.M., 198
Bunton, R., 179, 180
Bureaucracy, 12, 136–138, 231
Bureaucratic rationality, 7, 129, 138
Burke-Gaffney, H.J.O'D., 220–222
Burkina-Faso, 269
Burns, A.C., 139
Burrell, G., 133
Burrows, S., 95
Burton, C.R., 159
Burundi, 64, 276
Bury, M., 157, 161
Busfield, J., 189, 191
Buttock enhancement, 197

C

Callahan, D., 23, 241, 243, 245, 250, 251
Cameroon, 276
Campbell, C., 101, 166
Canada, 117, 230
Cancer, 31, 36, 39, 77, 225
Capes, T., 119
Capitalism, 5, 108, 109, 115
Capitalist health care, 151
Capitalist heath care system, 13, 229, 230
Career status, 162
Carpenter, L.M., 194
Carpiano, R.M., 101
Carver, A., 56
Castellani, B., 5, 7, 8
Castro, A.L., 196
Casuistry, 260, 261
Catholics, 94, 95
Cause-effect *see* Determinism, 85
Celibacy, 273
Central Africa, 276
Central African Republic, 64, 74, 276
Chafet, J.S., 121
Charles, C., 200–202
Charmaz, K., 158
Chattopadhyay, S., 245
Child health, 232, 276
Child labour, 2, 70
Child mortality, 276
Childbirth, 26, 64, 124, 188, 195, 196, 225, 253
Childhood, 40, 41, 45, 46, 50, 54, 185, 253
Childress, J.F., 257, 258

Chloroquine, 191, 269
Chola, L., 101
Chrisman's stages of illness behaviour, 84
Chrisman, N.J., 48, 49
Christian healers, 216
Christianity, 34, 54, 215, 273
Chronic diseases, 31
Chronic obstructive pulmonary disease (COPD), 53
Clark, E.G., 41
Clarke, J.N., 123
Class division, 111, 113, 114, 179
Class relations, 109, 112
Classen, T.J., 95
Clausen, R., 8
Client-practitioner relationship, 199, 200
Clinical bioethics, 242, 246
Clinical gaze *see* Medical gaze, 180
Clinical trials, 15, 114, 200, 248, 261
Coast, E., 274
Cobb, S., 49
Cockerham, W.C., 6, 71, 177, 179, 180
Coerced sex *see* Forced sex, 45
Cohen, P.S., 135
Cole, D., 74
Coleman, J.S., 96, 98, 99
Coleman, J.W., 3
Collective consciousness, 87
Colonialism, 113, 220, 221, 223
Commercial sex work, 112, 120
Commercial sex workers (CSWs), 45
Commercialisation of sex, 45
Commodification of health, 112
Communicable disease, 2, 53
Communitarianism, 246
Community engagement (CE), 5, 233, 278
Community health volunteers (CHVs), 280
Community health workers (CHWs), 47, 52, 227
Community psychiatry, 12, 13
Comoro, C., 11, 268
Complementary and alternative medicine (CAM), 14, 207
Comte, A., 6, 84, 85
Conco, W.Z., 34
Concoction, 209, 211, 214, 215
Condoms, 45, 145, 274
Confidentiality, 246, 248, 254, 261
Conflict, 12, 84, 91, 108, 114, 149, 227, 259
Congo (DR), 64, 213
Conley, S.B., 72
Conner, M., 146

Conrad, P., 7, 155, 158, 161, 185, 186, 188, 193, 194, 199
Consumerism, 189, 199, 201
Control beliefs, 143–146
Cooley, C.H., 162
Cooley, M.E., 159
Coovadia, H., 222
Copeland-Linder, N., 77
Corbin, J., 159, 161
Corbin, J.M., 161
Corbin-Strauss trajectory model, 159
Coser, L.A., 4, 96, 135
Cosmetic surgery, 195, 197, 225, 229, 242
Cote d'ivoire, 35
Council for the Development of Social Science Research in Africa (CODESRIA), 9
Course of illness, 11, 49, 155, 157, 159
Crăciun, C., 46
Cramm, J.M., 52
Crane, C., 54
Crespo-fierro, M., 51
Crime, 2, 3, 70, 92, 93, 122
Crisis phase, 160
Criticisms against traditional medicine, 218
Cruz-Inigo, A.E., 168
Cuba, 114, 230
Cues for action, 139
Cultural bioethics, 251, 252
Cultural differentialism, 178, 179
Culture of silence, 273
Cutler, D.M., 54, 67, 68

D
Dada, A.A., 215
Dake, J.A., 43
Daniels, N., 195, 228, 230
Darulis, Z., 5
Davidhizar, R., 143
Dawson, A., 257
Day, A., 95
Day, L.H., 95
de Beauvoir, S., 120, 121, 123
De La Cruz, N., 268
De Silva, M.J., 101, 102
De Vries, R., 14, 245
Deacon, H., 166
Deafness, 74, 169, 173
Deconstruction, 178, 180
Dehumanisation, 168, 244
Deinstitutionalisation, 172
Deities, 34, 212, 219
Delamater, P.L., 78
Delamonica, E., 68

Deleuze, G., 179
Deliberative model, 202, 203
Delinquent homes, 172
Delisle, H.F., 72
Demedicalisation, 188, 193, 194, 199
Dementia, 33
Demographic and health survey (DHS), 276
Denial of illness, 148
Dentistry, 225
Denzin, N.K., 181
Deoxyribonucleic acid (DNA), 191
Depersonalisation, 168, 172
Deprofessionalisation, 136
Deprofessionalism, 232
Deregulation, 189, 229
Deressa, W., 47
Derman, E.W., 44
Desocialisation
 definition, 186
Determinism, 107, 130, 191
Devolder, K., 247
Diabetes, 31, 46, 68, 71, 73, 169
Diagnostic categories, 135
Diagnostic imperialism, 187
Dialectic materialism, 120
Dietary behaviours, 45, 46, 54, 71, 72, 91
Dietary fibre, 71
Dignity, 195, 248, 249, 259
Discontinuity, 27, 147, 177
Disenchantment, 137
Distributive justice, 228, 258
Diviners, 212, 214
Divorce, 93, 95, 272
Do-not-resuscitate (DNR), 251
Dodoo, F.N., 272
Domestic violence, 64
Domestication of women, 121
Downward phase, 160
Doyal, L., 114, 123
Drug resistance, 51, 191, 269
Drug use, 44, 55, 71
Dunn, R.A., 95
Durkheim, E., 6, 84, 85, 93, 94, 96
Duxbury, J., 176
Dying phase, 161
Dysfunctionality, 27, 87

E
Early marriage, 265
Ecological bioethics, 244
Education, 53, 67–69, 280
 low level of, 235
 medical, 17
Efficacy of expectation *see* Self-efficacy, 139

Egalitarian, 114, 228, 230, 231
Egoistic suicide, 93–95
Egwuatu, V.E., 213
Egypt, 45, 65, 95, 220
Elder, J.P., 140
Emanuel, E., 200–202
Emanuel, L.L., 200–202
Embryos, 247, 252
Emile Durkheim, 92, 130
Emke, I., 88
Empiricism, 85, 178, 220
Enabling factors, 145, 151, 152
Enchantment, 137, 209, 212
End-of-life care
 ethics in, 255, 256
Engels, F., 110
Epidemiology, 109, 110, 220
 social, 16
Erinosho, O., 11
Ethical
 legal and social implications, 191, 249, 252
Ethics of care, 246
Ethiopia, 45, 46, 268
Ethno-medicine, 14
Ethnomethodology, 130
Eugenics, 193, 195, 254
Euthanasia, 198, 246, 247, 252, 255, 258
Evenson, K.R., 55
Everyday life work, 161
Ex-patient phase, 176
Exploitation, 91, 112, 113, 115, 138, 191, 200, 220–222, 253, 255

F
Fabrega, H., Jr., 27, 29, 30, 49, 156
Faith-based healers (FBHs), 35, 50, 54, 211, 215–217
Faith-Based Organisation (FBO), 234
Falciparum, 266
Falk, G., 165, 166
Family planning, 26, 213, 233
Famine, 45
Farr, J., 96, 99
Fatalistic suicide, 94
Fathalla, M.F., 61, 67
Female body, 121, 122, 196, 253
Female circumcision, 214
Feminine, 122, 123
Feminisation, 124, 253, 277
Feminism, 107, 120, 122, 125, 176, 246, 270
Feminist analysis of health, 120, 122, 123, 125, 130
Fertility rate, 277

Feyisetan, B.J., 11
Figert, A.E., 185
Filc, D., 185
Finger, B., 270
Firestone, S., 120, 121
Fishbein, M., 143
Flight to health, 148
Folk medicine, 208
Fonseca, R., 68, 69
Forced sex, 45, 122, 271
Formal rationality, 137
Formalisation, 137
Foster, G.M., 34, 35
Foucault, M., 130, 131, 155, 177, 179, 180, 186, 187
Fox, J.N., 179, 180
Fragmentation of care, 147
France, 67, 114, 220, 222, 230
Frankenberg, R., 156
Free market health care see Capitalist health care, 228
Freese, J., 192
Freidson, E., 7, 157, 187
Functionalism, 7, 84–87, 108, 112, 114, 115, 130, 132, 176
Fundamental causes, 3, 107, 109, 114, 116–119, 250

G
Gabe, J., 108, 114, 199, 207
Garfinkel, H., 168
Garrard, E., 257
Garro, L.C., 29, 35
Garshong, B., 269
Gates, T., 167, 168
Geissler, P.W., 114, 261
Gender, 2, 5, 10, 11, 17, 53, 61–64, 76, 107, 120–123, 125, 140, 145
Gender division of labour, 63, 121
Gender dysphoria, 193
Gender inequality, 10, 53, 63, 64, 121, 122, 253, 271
Gender roles, 121, 123
Gender stratification, 120
Generalisation, 85
Genetic causes, 35, 36
Genetic determinism, 192
Genetic engineering, 195, 243
Genetic testing, 15, 191, 192, 196, 248, 253, 254
Geneticisation, 191–193, 199
Genetics, 3, 35, 191–193
Georgianna, S., 95
Germ theory, 33, 220

Germany, 220
Ghana, 221, 269, 276, 281
Gilbert, L., 8
Gillon, R., 257–259
Gjerberg, E., 227
Glanz, K., 143
Glaser, B.G., 8, 131
Glenn, L.M., 249
Global bioethics, 244
Globalisation, 120, 178, 191, 199
God of thunder, 210
Godlee, F., 23
Goffman, E., 8, 13, 165, 166, 172–174, 176
Good death, 199, 256
Gordijn, B., 249, 260
Gorman, B.K., 123–125
Gove, W., 164
Govender, T., 70
Gracia, J.R., 192
Grandi, G., 53, 254
Grant, U., 65
Greif, M.J., 44
Guattari, F., 179
Guinea-Bissau, 64, 276
Gulliford, M., 77, 79
Guten, S., 40, 41
Gyapong, M., 269

H
Haas, S., 158
Hafferty, F.W., 5, 7, 8
Hahn, B.H., 269
Halfmann, D., 194
Han, G., 208
Hanifan, L.J., 96, 97
Harkness, S.K., 164
Harpham, T., 55
Harris, D.M., 40, 41
Harris, S.R., 3
Hart, N., 115
Haslanger, S., 120
Hattori, M.K., 272
Hausas, 169
Hausmann, L.R.M., 77
Haviland, W.A., 99
Health
  definition, 21, 23–26
Health behaviour (HB)
  definition, 39–41
Health Belief Model (HBM), 84, 112, 129, 139–143
Health education, 41, 233, 275, 280, 281
Health financing, 224

Health inequalities, 6, 67, 107, 112, 113, 116, 117, 222
Health information, 54, 65, 68, 101, 224, 235, 250, 277, 280
Health insurance, 113, 151, 161, 229, 230, 236, 258
Health maintenance, 42, 142, 278
Health needs, 9, 124, 189, 217, 234, 236, 249, 278–281
Health policy, 6, 16, 165
Health politics, 15, 16, 108
Health workforce, 223, 224
Healthcare ethics *see* Clinical bioethics, 246
Hean, S., 95
Hedgecoe, A.M., 191
Heggenhougen, H.K., 136, 267
Heinemann, L., 42, 43
Helmut, T., 95
Helsinki Declaration, 248
Hendel, T., 227
Henly, S.J., 159
Herbalists, 211, 212, 216
Hereditary causation *see* Genetic causes, 35
Herek, G.M., 171
Herzlinger, R.E., 229
Heterosexual, 194
Hierarchisation, 137, 138
High risk behaviour, 42
High risk group (HRG), 42
Hippocrates, 61, 265
Hippocratic Oath, 243, 246, 256
Hirst, M., 212
Hochbaum, G.M., 139
Hollender, M.H., 200
Holtz, T.H., 3, 7, 111
Homans, H., 7
Home management of malaria (HMM), 269
Home treatment, 50
Home-based care, 280, 281
Homeostasis, 27
Homosexuality, 28, 156, 166, 193, 194, 252
Hooyman, N., 95
Hospitalisation, 49, 149, 172, 176
House, J.S., 116
Housing, 10, 69–71, 74, 76, 110, 117, 120, 168, 173, 273
Huber, M., 22–24
Hulka, B.S., 44
Human enhancement *see* Medical enhancement, 195
Human Genome Projects (HGP), 13, 191, 192

Human immunodeficiency virus (HIV) *see*
    Acquired immunodeficiency syndrome
    (AIDS), 2
Humphreys, S.J., 15
Hunchback *see* Kyphosis, 168
Hunt, K., 122, 123
Hypertension, 27, 31, 68, 69, 71

I
Iatrogenesis, 113
Ideal type, 133, 136
Idealism, 130
Identity kit, 174
Idiographic approach, 130, 155, 178
Igun, U.A., 48, 51
Ijaiya, M.A., 119
Illich, I., 113, 187, 188, 198
Illness behaviour
    definition, 46, 47
Illness perception, 10, 49, 52
Illness work, 161
Immunisation, 40, 41, 250, 280
In vitro fertilisation (IVF), 196, 247, 253
In-patient phase, 176
Incantation, 209, 210, 212, 217, 218
Individualism, 100
Industrial revolution, 2
Industrialisation, 2
Industrialism, 115
Infanticide, 10, 63, 64
Infertility, 27, 188, 210, 213, 253
Informal care
    definition, 50
Informal sector, 232, 236
Information and Communication Technology, 13
Informative model, 201
Informed consent, 201, 248, 254, 257, 261
Injuries, 27, 32, 34, 36, 49, 52, 64, 65, 74, 112, 214, 233, 247
Insecticide-treated bed nets (ITNs), 267–269
Institutional review boards (IRBs), 247, 248, 260, 261
Instrumental-rational action, 134, 135
Integrity, 255, 259
Intentions, 144, 146
Intermittent preventive treatment (IPT), 269
Interpretive model, 202
Irving, Z.K., 186
Irwin, A., 65
Islam, 34, 54, 215, 273
Islam, M.K., 97–101
Islam, S.M.S., 45
Islamic healers, 216
Israel, B.A., 280
Italy, 67, 220
Ityavyar, D.A., 220, 221
Izugbara, C.O., 213

J
Jackson, H., 3, 270
Jackson, J.S., 77
Jadad, A.R., 23, 24
Jahr, F., 243
Jameson, F., 177
Janssens, L., 254
Janz, N.K., 139, 141
Janzen, J.M., 108
Jayapoorani, N., 171
Jegede, A.S., 11, 16, 35, 40, 114, 261, 268
Jennings, B., 250
Johanson, R., 196
Johnson, C.A., 45
Jones, E., 165, 169
Jonsen, A.R., 260
Justice, 15, 61, 228, 242, 244, 251, 256, 258, 259

K
Kahabuka, C., 232
Kalekin-Fishman, D., 76
Kaler, A., 248
Kalinda, T., 272
Kaminskas, R., 5
Kantianism, 243, 246
Karanja, J., 40
Kasl, S.U., 39, 49
Kass, N.E., 249, 250
Katzung, B.G., 51
Kawachi, I., 70, 95, 101, 103
Keith, B., 177
Kenya, 41, 45, 69, 221, 252, 268, 269, 281
Kerbo, H.R., 3
Khan, M., 45
Kickbusch, I.S., 68
Kidney dialysis, 243
King, M., 235
Kingma, E., 26
Kirigia, D.G., 237
Kirigia, J.M., 237
Kirscht, J.P., 139
Kiyak, H., 95
Kjølsrød, L., 227
Kleinman, A., 138, 156–158
Kofi-Tsekpo, M., 218
Kor, K., 146

Kottack, C.P., 99
Kozloff, M.A., 91
Kranz, S., 72
Krieger, N., 16, 107, 112
Krogstad, U., 227
Kronemer, A., 231
Kroska, A., 164
Kruk, M.E., 232
Kushner, H.I., 94
Kwashiorkor, 43
Kyphosis, 168

L
Labellers, 163
Labelling, 25, 156, 187
Labelling theory, 155, 162–164, 186
Labels, 131, 135, 162–164, 167, 168, 187, 208, 215
Labinjo, J., 134, 135
Laflamme, L., 95
Lairon, D., 72
Lamont, J.A., 91
Lancaster, K.J., 72
Larson, J.S., 21, 22, 24
Latimer, E.J., 255
Lay consultation, 48, 49
Leavell, H.R., 41
Lemert, E.M., 162
Lengermann, P.M., 120
Leprosy, 166, 169
Lequien, L., 67
Lesbian, gay, bisexual, transgender (LGBT), 194
Lesotho, 45, 67
Levels of health care delivery, 232
Levine, S., 91
Levitt, N., 46
Li, Y.C., 74
Liberia, 52, 276
Libertarianism, 246
Lichtenstein, R., 227
Life expectancy, 10, 17, 45, 67, 71, 110, 125, 179, 270
Life extension, 195, 249
Lifestyle, 10, 54, 71, 72
    sedentary, 44
Light, D.W., 17
Lin, N., 96, 97, 101
Lin, P., 195, 249
Link, B.G., 99, 107, 116–118, 120, 164, 165, 167–169
Lippman, A., 191, 192
Literacy, 67, 235, 277

Lleras-Muney, A., 54, 67, 68
Lochner, K., 99, 100
Lochner, L., 68
Lofholm, P.W., 51
Looping, 175
Lumpen-proletariat, 113
Lundberg, P., 44
Lupton, D., 87, 113
Lurie, P., 248
Lyman, S.M., 2
Lynch, J., 95, 101, 103

M
Maasai, 274
Mabumba, E.D., 272
MacAuthor, W., 265
Mackenbach, J.P., 67
Macroanalysis, 109
Macroscopic, 86
Madagascar, 45
Maiman, L.A., 139
Maimon, D., 95
Malaria, 3–5, 28, 40, 265, 267
Malawi, 45, 46, 67, 269, 280
Male circumcision, 194, 213, 214
Male hegemony, 10
Mali, 64, 67, 74, 276
Malingering, 89
Malnutrition, 34, 46, 110, 113, 276
Malton, M., 255
Manstead, A.S.R., 144, 145
Marital infidelity, 192
Marmorstein, N.R., 44
Marmot, M., 67
Marson, S.M., 95
Martin, M., 54
Martinez, P., 44
Marx, K., 111
Marxism, 108, 246
Marxist analysis of health, 110, 112
    criticisms, 114, 115
Masculine, 122, 123
Mashita, R.J., 45
Masturbation, 193
Material condition, 110
Material life, 108, 121
Maternal and child health (MCH), 233, 265, 276, 277
Maternal health, 64, 123, 212, 276, 280
    definition, 275
Maternal mortality, 119, 213, 275–277
Maternal mortality ratio (MMR), 275
Mauritania, 74
Mbanya, J.C.N., 46

Mbonu, N.C., 271
McCombie, S.C., 50
McCorkle, R., 159
McLean, M.R., 249
Mead, G.H., 162
Mechanic, D., 7, 9, 18, 46, 49, 50
Media
  role in medicalization, 199
Medical education, 17, 18
Medical enhancement, 15, 188, 195
Medical expansionism, 187
Medical experimentation, 114
Medical gaze, 187
Medical hegemony, 185
Medical pluralism, 207, 208, 216, 265
Medical sociology
  definition, 5, 6
  history of, 6–9
Medicalisation, 7, 26, 91, 124, 162, 185–189
  of beauty, 196–198
  of death and dying, 198, 199
Medicinal ingredient sellers, 211
Medicine murder, 219
Menopause, 121, 188
Menstruation, 26, 121
Mental diseases, 12
Mental health hospitals, 172, 176
Metaphysical belief, 209
Methodological triangulation, 181
Microanalysis, 130, 139, 150, 155
Middle-range theories, 84, 246
Midwives, 79, 212, 234
Migration, 2, 3, 236
Miles, S.H., 213
Military, 94, 172
Millennium Development Goals (MGDs), 233, 275
Millett, K., 121, 122
Mini-narrative, 130, 178
Missionaries, 220, 221, 223
Mobile clinics, 281
Modern health care, 14, 55, 212, 216, 219–221, 224, 226, 235
Modern health professionals, 219
Modern social theory, 176
Modernisation, 2, 207, 220
Modifying factors, 132, 139, 140, 142
Mohammed, S.A., 77
Mokhtar, N., 72
Molyneux, C., 114, 261
Monger, M., 171
Moomal, H., 77
Moorman, P.G., 44

Moral ethics, 243, 245
Moral perplexities, 14, 246, 247
Morality, 87, 242, 244, 245, 251, 252
Morgan, G., 133
Morgan, J.H., 133, 134
Morgan, L.M., 109
Morland, K.B., 55
Morocco, 221
Mortification of self, 174–176
Mozambique, 45, 67
Mpofu, E., 44
Mukanga, D., 47
Mukherjee, J.S., 270
Mullan, B.A., 146
Multiple causality, 34, 85
Muntaner, C., 95
Murdock, G.P., 35
Muscular dystrophy, 161, 247
Muzur, A., 243, 244
Mwenesi, H., 49
Mystical causation, 35, 215, 217
Mystification, 209

N
Namibia, 41, 45, 248, 269
Natality inequality, 124
Nathanson, C.A., 123, 125
Natural causation, 30, 34
Navarro, V., 112, 113, 116, 123
Nazi, 248
Need factors, 151
Neighbourhood, 43, 55, 65, 71, 99, 118
Netherlands, 198
Nettleton, S., 123
Neuhauser, D., 172
Neumam, W.L., 83
Neurosis, 33
Ngwena, C., 222
Niebrugge, G., 120
Niger, 45, 64, 67
Nigeria, 31, 34, 35, 40, 50, 67, 74, 168, 210, 215, 220, 221, 234
Nijmegen Method, 260
Nominalism, 130
Nomothetic assumption, 86
Non-adherence, 51, 141, 142
Non-communicable diseases (NCDs), 31, 53, 235
Non-governmental organisations (NGOs), 9, 234
Non-maleficence, 199, 251, 255, 257
Non-probability sampling, 131, 132
Nordenfeldt, L., 28, 29
Normative stigma, 166

North Africa, 45, 79, 221, 252
Novignon, J., 119
Nsimba, S.E.D., 50
Nuer, 274
Nuremberg Code, 248
Nutbeam, D., 68
Nuwaha, F., 40

O
O'Grady, L., 23, 24
O'Neil, D., 34
Oakley, A., 121, 196
Obesity, 28, 31, 46, 55, 68, 71, 77, 117, 132, 156, 166, 169, 194
Objectivity, 86
Obrist, B., 77
Obsiye, M., 102
Occupation, 2, 10, 17, 61, 64, 67, 73, 74, 116, 140, 151, 270, 280
Officialdom, 137, 138
Ololo, H., 213
Oman, D., 55
Omololu, F., 85, 108, 131
Omololu, O.F., 268
Omonzejele, P.F., 34, 35
Onoge, O.F., 114, 116
Onwujekwe, O., 268
Opiyo, P., 268
Oral infection, 225
Organ transplantation, 243, 252
Organismic analogy, 6, 84, 86
Orphanages, 172
Over-the-counter (OTC), 44, 47, 147, 189
Overmedicalisation, 253
Owumi, B.E., 215

P
Palliative care, 26, 198, 255
Pannenborg, C., 23
Paradies, Y.A., 77
Paradigm
  definition, 83
Parameswari, S.J., 171
Parsons, T., 7, 24, 88–91, 96, 138, 187, 200
Pasacreta, J.V., 159
Pascoe, E.A., 77
Pasman, J., 164
Passage rite, 17
Pastoralists, 74, 274
Patel, V., 215
Paternalism, 199–201, 257
Paternalistic model, 200, 201
Pathologisation, 186

Pathophysiology, 157
Patient-practitioner relations see Client-practitioner relationship, 90
Patienthood, 149, 155, 172, 176
Patriarchy, 121, 123, 125, 196
Pattern variables, 90
Pauperisation, 108, 112, 270
Pavone, V., 192
Pearce, N., 101
Peden, M., 32
Peltzer, K., 41, 214
Penile enlargement, 197
Pennell, I., 114
People living with HIV/AIDS (PLWHA), 52, 168, 171, 273
Perceived barriers, 139, 141
Perceived behavioural control, 143–146
Perceived benefits, 139, 141
Perceived severity, 139, 141
Perceived susceptibility, 139–141
Perceived threats see Perceived severity, 141
Peril, 169
Personalism, 246
Personalistic cause, 35
Personality, 22, 145, 192
Personhood, 254, 255
Persons, 9, 50, 70, 88, 90, 95, 98, 156, 163, 165, 167, 168, 173, 175, 194, 243, 254, 255, 257, 270, 273
Pescosolido, B.A., 95, 170
Peters, E., 68
Petersen, A., 14, 15, 179, 180
Petrie, K.J., 52
Pharmaceutical expansionism, 188
Pharmaceuticalisation, 188, 189, 191
Pharmacy, 226
Phelan, J., 99, 107, 116–120
Phelan, J.C., 107, 116, 165, 167–169, 193
Phenomenology, 130
Philips, S.D., 167, 168
Physician assisted suicide (PAS), 198
Picker, L., 68
Pilgrim, D., 12
Place, 5, 14, 15, 42, 61, 88, 151, 167, 172, 186, 193, 216, 221, 229, 236, 258, 276
Plateau, 161
Policy and regulatory bioethics, 251
Political economy of health (PEH), 108, 114, 265
Political economy of health care, 109
Political economy of illness/disease, 109
Political inequality, 109

Political organisation of health systems
  utilitarianism, 219
Pollution, 65, 70, 110, 113, 244
Polygyny, 271
Portes, A., 96, 99
Portugal, 220
Positivism, 85, 107
Postmodernism, 178
  in medical sociology, 179, 180
  note on, 176, 177
Postmodernity, 178, 180
Poststructuralism, 177, 179
Potter, L., 244
Potter, V.R., 243, 244
Povar, G.J., 228
Poverty, 2, 3, 43, 52, 53, 55, 64, 67, 73, 95,
  119, 120, 235, 267, 271, 278
Powell, R.M., 95
Power relations, 7, 12, 53, 61, 112, 114, 136,
  138, 163, 169, 200
Pre-patient phase, 176
Pre-trajectory
  phase, 159
Pregnancy, 27, 28, 43, 53, 64, 124, 162, 195,
  196, 225, 253, 277
Prenatal diagnosis, 243
Preventive health behaviour (PHB), 39, 40
Primary care, 189, 216, 218, 223, 225, 227,
  232–234, 278, 280, 281
Primary health care (PHC), 213, 218, 231, 232
Primary prevention, 41
Prince, M., 33
Principlism, 15, 256
Prisoners, 95
Probability sampling, 86
Procrastination, 147, 148, 157, 267
Professionalisation, 7, 136
Professionalism, 7, 136, 161
Proletariat, 108, 111
Protective health behaviour (PHB), 40
Protestants, 94, 95
Psychological reductionism, 132
Psychosis, 33
Public health, 8, 43, 136, 191, 200, 220, 250
  bioethics, 250, 251
Purdy, L.M., 253
Putnam, R., 96, 98

Q

Qualitative approach, 131
Quaternary care, 235

R

Racism, 117, 120, 121

Ramlagan, S., 101
Rankin, W.W., 273
Rationalisation, 136, 185, 252
Rawls, J., 228
Read, J.G., 123–125
Realism, 85, 107
Realist tradition *see* Realism, 85
Reeve, J., 158
Referral system, 232
Refractory symptoms, 160, 255, 256
Regimentation, 175
Rehabilitee, 149
Rehmann-Sutter, C., 252
Reich, W.T., 241
Reidy, A., 115
Relativism, 130, 178, 180, 242, 260
Religion, 5, 17, 54, 55, 86, 93, 95, 166, 179,
  217, 220, 223, 241, 252, 273
Remedicalisation, 188, 193, 194
Rendtorff, J.D., 259
Reniers, G., 272
Rensburg, H.C.J., 222
Reproductive autonomy, 53
Reproductive restrictiveness, 193
Research bioethics, 247, 248
Ricci, F., 119
Richman, L.S., 77
Ricoeur, P., 257
Rieker, P.P., 124
Rinčić, I., 243, 244
Risk behaviour, 41, 43, 44, 54, 103, 109, 120,
  139, 229
Rituals, 50, 168, 212, 214
Ritzer, G., 83, 87, 92, 93, 130, 131, 133, 137,
  138, 176–178
Robert, J.S., 249
Roberts, L., 219
Rogers, A., 12
Roll Back Malaria (RBM), 267
Rosa, I.L., 208, 209
Rose, D., 168
Rosenstock, I.M., 139, 140
Rutta, A.S.M., 47
Rwanda, 46, 67

S

Sánchez-Barriga, J.J., 68
Safe sex, 272
Salisbury, S., 219
Saracci, R., 23
Sarkar, C., 56
Sartorius, N., 33
Scambler, G., 178

Scarification, 213, 272
Scheff, T.J., 164
Schnall, P., 110
Secondary health care (SHC), 234
Secondary prevention, 42
Segall, A., 49, 90
Selective reproduction, 193, 196, 253
Self-diagnosis, 52
Self-efficacy, 139, 141, 144, 145, 165, 170
Self-fulfilling prophecy, 164
Self-medication, 47, 52, 67, 147, 202
Sen, A., 63, 124
Senegal, 65, 74, 269
Severe acute respiratory syndrome (SARS), 2, 30
Sex differences, 122, 123
Sex selection, 213, 248, 253
Sexting, 43
Sexual behaviour, 8, 43, 45, 54, 77, 117, 194, 270, 273
Sexual enhancement, 188
Sexual freedom, 122
Sexual network, 10, 271, 272
Sexualisation, 197
Sexuality, 120, 121, 123, 188, 271, 273, 275
Sexually transmitted diseases (STDs), 40, 45, 64, 213, 214, 272, 274
Sharp, P.M., 269
Shopping, 147, 149
Shostak, S., 192
Shuper, P.A., 44
Sick role, 7, 29, 49, 84, 89, 91, 92, 148, 200
  Parsons, 88
Sierra Leone, 64, 67, 74, 276
Significant others, 12, 47, 49, 89, 96, 136, 145, 148, 149, 159, 161, 171, 175, 202, 217
Simmel, G., 4, 96
Simmons, S.J., 23
Singer, M., 112, 116, 155
Slums, 55, 65, 69
Smelser, N., 1
Smelser, N.J., 3
Smith, G.D., 101
Smoking behaviour, 44
Snadden, D., 158
Social action
  definition, 130, 133
Social action theory
  Weberian, 132–134
Social aetiology, 10, 61
Social alienation, 76, 77, 93, 113

Social capital, 76, 77, 89, 95–100, 116, 117, 136
  horizontal, 100
  vertical, 100
Social cognitive theory, 141, 145
Social construction of illness, 131, 155, 162, 187, 265
Social constructionism, 129, 132
Social death, 17, 256
Social determinants of health (SDH), 9, 10, 16, 61, 63, 67, 92, 110, 112, 114, 117, 259
Social epidemiology, 16
Social factors, 5, 6, 9, 17, 61, 62, 93, 124, 132, 193, 230
Social facts, 3, 92, 93, 131, 180, 242
Social forces, 2, 155, 163
Social influence, 102, 143
Social integration, 94
Social interdependence, 99, 136
Social model
  of health, 24, 186
Social order, 84, 88, 92, 96
Social organism, 87
Social parenthood, 253
Social pathology, 4, 22
Social problem
  definition, 2
Social production of health (SPH), 107, 109, 132
Social psychiatry, 12
Social referrals, 50
Social regulation, 7, 94
Social sciences, 7, 12, 21, 84, 96, 177, 191, 241
Social support, 55, 95, 97, 99–101, 170, 281
Social system, 1–4, 7, 12, 16, 30, 51, 87–90, 93, 107
Socialised health care, 13, 73, 114, 230
Socialist heath care system, 219, 228, 230
Societal disruption, 195, 243, 249, 252
Socioeconomic inequality, 110
Socioeconomic status (SES), 53, 62, 64, 65, 67, 94, 99, 101, 116, 117, 230, 277
Sociological theory
  definition, 83
Sociology
  definition, 1
Sociology in medicine, 7, 9
Sociology of bioethics, 14, 242
Sociology of medicine, 9
Solidarity, 101, 136, 230, 278
Somalia, 46, 64, 67, 276
Song, L., 96, 97
Sontag, S., 158

Index

Sorsdahl, K., 217
Sosa-Estani, S., 42
South Africa, 8, 34, 44, 45, 52, 67, 70, 77, 101, 168, 267
Southern Africa, 270, 272, 276
Spain, 67, 220
Specialisation, 6, 8, 90, 137, 138, 224, 225
Spencer, H., 6, 84, 85
Spiritual power, 35, 55, 209, 215
Spiritual worldview, 273
Sprague, L., 273
Stable phase, 160
Stacey, J., 123
Stacey, M., 7
Stages of illness behaviour, 48
  Chrisman's, 84
  Suchman's, 129
Standing, H., 232
Statistical normality, 27
Status loss, 167, 168
Steinkamp, N., 260
Stem cell research (SCR), 14, 15, 247
Stempsey, W.E., 26, 28
Steptoe, A., 43
Stereotyping, 167
Stigma, 8, 13, 33, 52, 71, 91, 117, 131
Stigmatisation, 13, 30, 71, 76, 95, 164, 165, 168–170, 271, 273
Stoler, J., 56
Straus, R., 9
Strauss, A.L., 8, 131, 159, 161
Strecher, V.J., 139, 140
Street children, 65, 168
Sub-Saharan Africa (SSA), 10, 46, 213, 215, 236, 266
Subjective norms, 145, 151
Subjectivity, 155
Substantive theories, 8, 84, 86–88, 129, 138, 181
Suchman's stages of illness behaviour, 129
Suchman, E., 147–149
Suchman, E.A., 49
Sudan, 221, 222, 276
Sui generis, 92, 130
Suibhne, S.M., 172
Suicide, 6, 92, 93, 198
Supernatural causation, 34, 35, 212
Surrogate motherhood, 253
Swaziland, 45, 67
Sylvia, O., 33
Symbolic interactionism, 130, 162
Symptom definition, 48, 49
Symptom experience, 49, 148

Szabo, C.P., 46
Szasz, T., 186
Szasz, T.S., 200

T
Tönnies, F., 100
Tannenbaum, F., 162
Tanner-Smith, E.E., 143
Tanzania, 45, 168, 221, 231, 268, 280
Tarlov, A., 61
Taye, O.R., 210
Technologies, 44, 177, 192, 195, 224, 241, 248, 256, 282
Tella, A., 210
Temple, J.R., 43
Temple, L.K.F., 28
Ten Have, H.A.M.J., 191, 244
Tengland, P., 28
Terminal sedation, 26, 161, 198, 255
Tertiary Health Care (THC), 234
Tertiary prevention, 41, 42
Tfaily, R., 272
The Gambia, 74
Theoretical bioethics, 245, 246
Theoretical triangulation, 181
Theory of planned behaviour (TPB), 139, 143–146
Theory of social stigma, 155, 162, 165
Therapeutic abortion, 193
Therapeutic cloning, 247, 252
Thomas theorem, 164
Thomas, D.S., 164
Thomas, W.I., 164
Thoral, M., 220, 222
Thoresen, C.E., 55
Thorne, B., 123
Timmermans, S., 158
Tlili, A., 102
Togo, 74, 269
Tooth decay, 225
Total institution, 8, 11, 13, 131, 171–174, 176
Total institution theory, 155, 172–174, 176
Toulmin, S.E., 260
Traditional action, 135, 136
Traditional birth attendants (TBAs), 211–213
Traditional birth homes (TBHs), 213
Traditional medicine (TM), 14, 55, 135, 207, 208
  African, 208–210
  determinants of utilisation, 216–218
  shortcomings of, 218, 219
Traditional psychiatrists, 211, 215
Trajectory of chronic illness, 155, 159–161
Transactional sex see Commercial sex work, 45

Transexualism, 193
Transhumanism, 179, 195, 249
Transplantation, 14, 15, 247, 249
Treatment failure, 51
Triage, 251
Triangulation, 181
Tribal stigma, 166
Truog, R.D., 199
Tuberculosis (TB), 2, 70, 110, 117, 119, 139
Tunisia, 221, 252
Turan, J.M., 273
Turner, L., 242
Turrell, G., 56
Tuskegee Syphilis Study, 248
Twaddle, A.C., 49
Two-tier heath care system, 219
Twumasi, P.A., 221, 223

U
Udosen, A.M., 215
Uganda, 40, 41, 47, 69, 221, 269
Ukwaja, K.N., 119
Ukwayi, J.K., 213
Umeora, O.U.J., 213
UNAIDS, 194, 270
Under-Five Mortality Rate, 276
United Kingdom, 8, 198, 230
United Nations Children's Fund (UNICEF), 276
United Nations Population Fund (UNFPA), 64
United States, 3, 8, 95, 119, 139, 166, 194, 198, 229, 269
Universal coverage, 231
Unprotected sex, 45, 115
Unstable phase, 160
Urbanisation, 2, 46
Use of health services, 151, 229
Use of tobacco, 31, 64
Utilisation of traditional medicine, 216, 218

V
Vaccination *see* Immunisation, 41
Valeggia, C., 272
Value-rational action, 135
Van Poppel, F., 95
Vandemoortele, J., 68
Vearey, J., 55
Veatch, R.M., 258
Verbrugge, L.M., 123, 124
Verstehen, 131, 133
Vesicovaginal fistula (VVF), 10, 64, 276
Vicious cycle, 110, 112, 120
Vincent, L., 219

Violence, 2, 10, 13, 32, 64, 271
Virchow, R., 111
Virginity, 273
Virtual social identity, 165
Virtue ethics, 246
Vlassoff, C., 123
Volitional control, 144
Volkers, A.C., 73
Voluntarism, 130, 155
Vulnerability, 2, 10, 13, 43, 53, 61, 62, 65, 67, 68, 124, 140, 259, 267, 271, 272

W
Waitzkin, H., 110, 111, 113
Wamala, S., 70
Wardle, J., 43
Washington, H.A., 114, 248, 261
Water-borne diseases, 71
Waters, A., 70, 71
Weaver, J.H., 231
Weber, L.R., 2
Weber, M., 131, 133, 134, 136–138
Weinstein, R.M., 172
Weisheit, A., 218
Weiss, E., 219
Weiss, H.A., 194
Whelton, S.P., 72
Widowhood rites, 272
Widows, 94, 166, 272
Wilcken, A., 213, 214
William, S.J., 89
Williams, D.R., 77
Williams, S., 188
Wilson, A., 212
Winter, M.F., 163
Wirtz, V., 201
Witchcraft, 35, 223
Withholding and withdrawal of treatment, 251
Wolfe, S.M., 248
Women's health, 63, 124
Wood, P.H.N., 23
Woodward, C., 91
Working class, 100, 110, 111, 113
Working conditions, 110
World Health Organization (WHO), 269, 278, 280, 281
World system, 114
Wright, K., 176

Y
Yoruba, 34–36, 168, 210
Young, J.T., 89, 129
Yusuf, O.B., 65

Z

Zaidi, S.A., 123
Zambia, 45, 65, 269
Zheng, Y., 68, 69
Zimbabwe, 41, 45, 67, 213, 248, 252

Zola, I.K., 91, 187
Zoonoses, 74
Zoosexuality, 156
Zou, J., 273

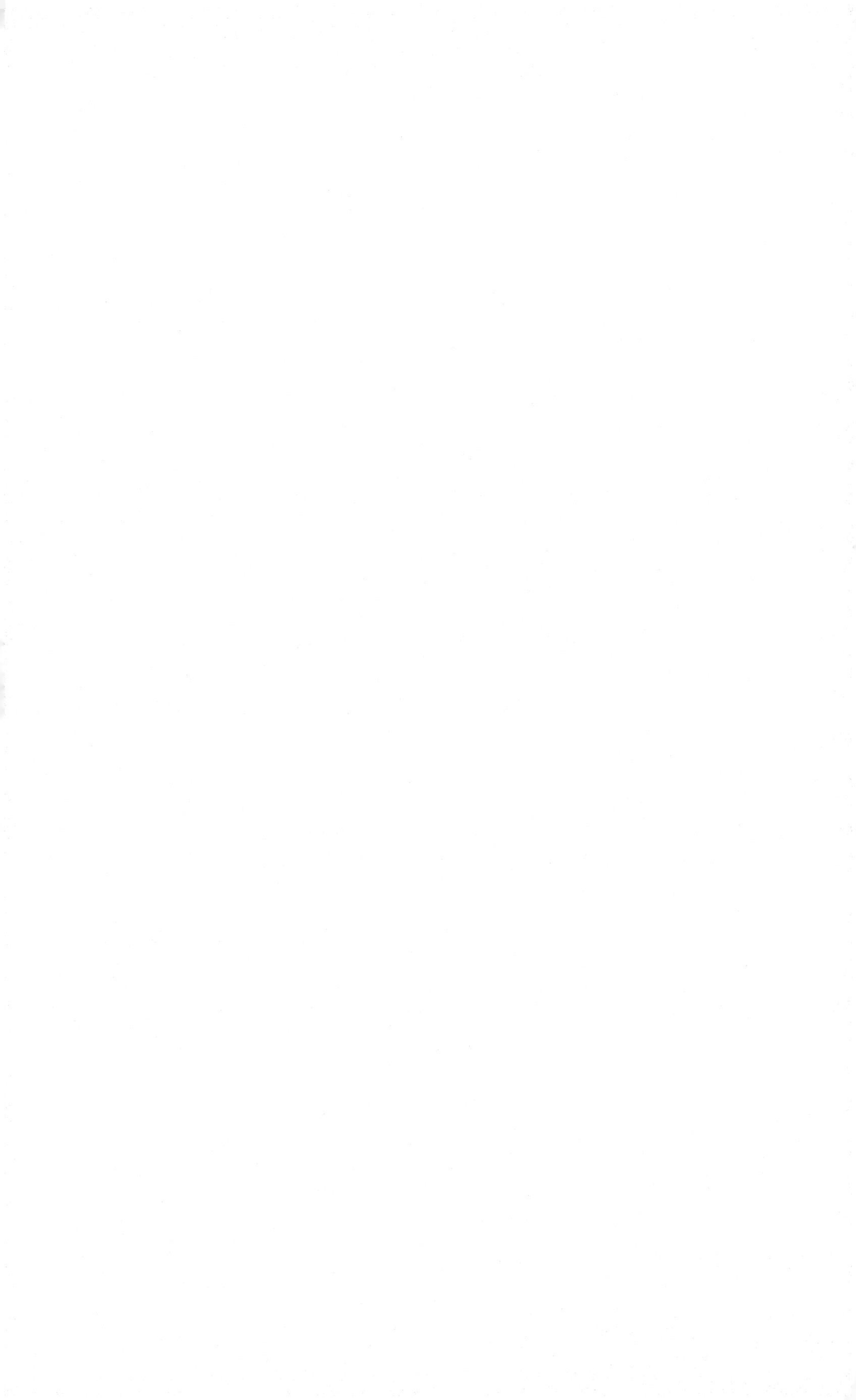

The manufacturer's authorised representative in the EU is Springer Nature Customer Service Centre GmbH, Europaplatz 3, 69115 Heidelberg, Germany. If you have any concerns regarding our products, please contact ProductSafety@springernature.com

Printed and bound by CPI Group (UK) Ltd, Croydon, CR0 4YY
23/03/2026
02076671-0002

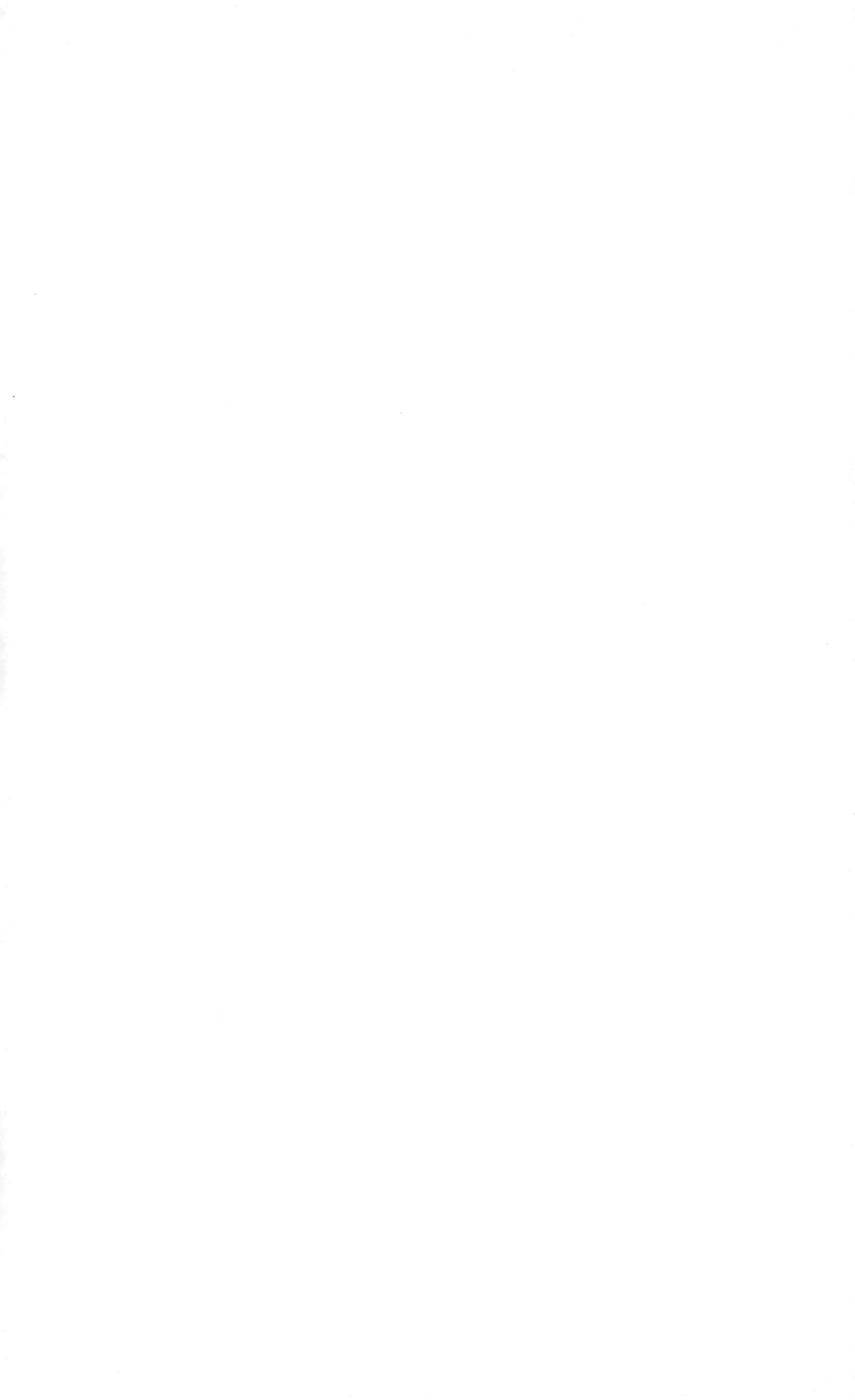

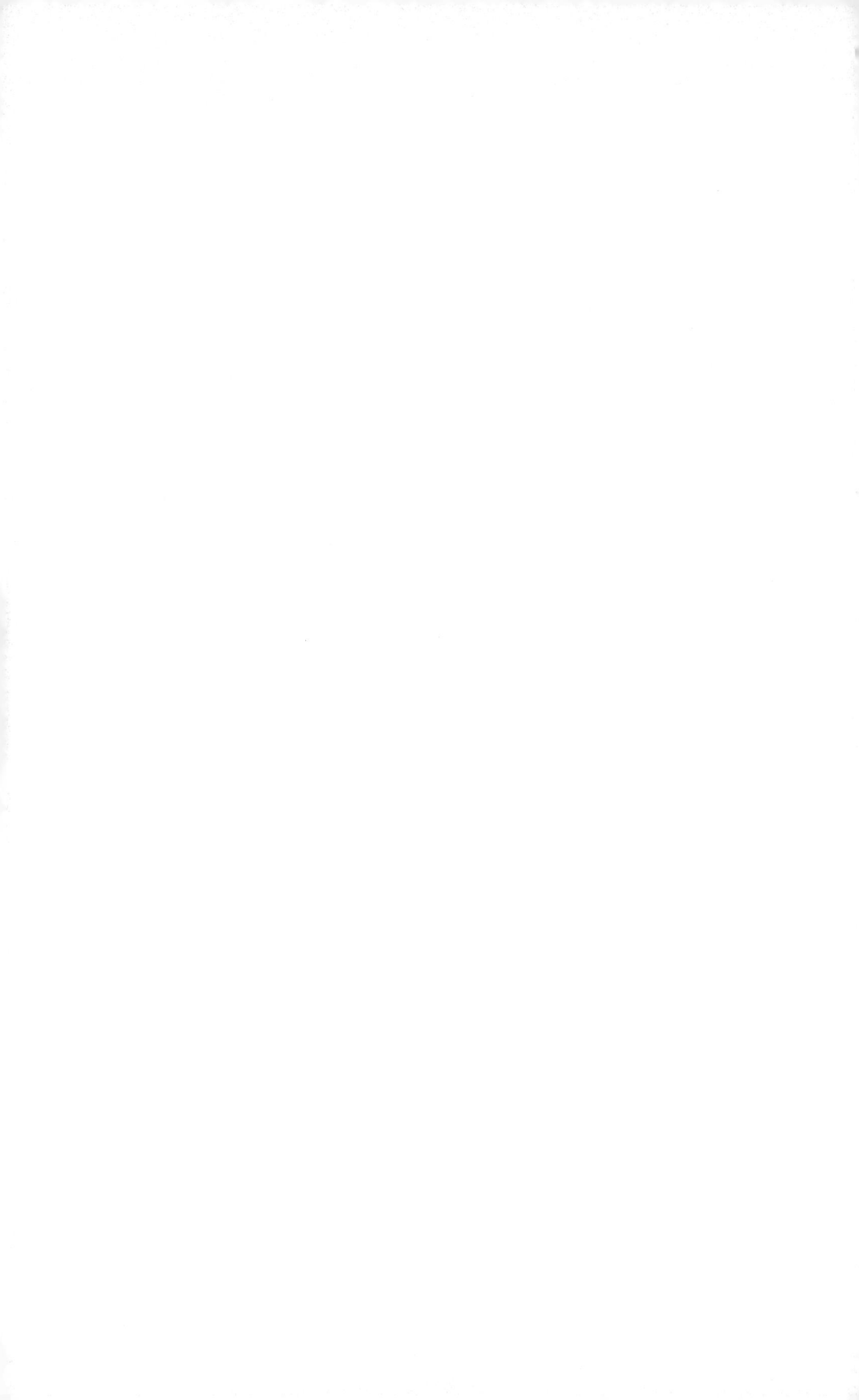